CLINICAL HAEMATOLOGY ILLUSTRATED

CLINICAL HAEMATOLOGY ILLUSTRATED

AN INTEGRATED TEXT AND COLOUR ATLAS

A. Victor Hoffbrand MA, DM, FRCP, FRCPath, FRCP(Edin)
Professor of Haematology
Royal Free Hospital and School of Medicine
London, UK

John E. Pettit MD Otago, FRCPA, MRCPath
Associate Professor of Haematology
University of Otago Medical School
Dunedin, New Zealand

Now at
Pearson Laboratory
Christchurch
New Zealand

Churchill Livingstone Edinburgh · London · New York

Distributed in all countries except USA, Canada and Japan by:
Churchill Livingstone
Robert Stevenson House
1-3 Baxter's Place
Leith Walk
Edinburgh EH1 3AF

Distributed in the USA and Canada by:
W. B. Saunders Company
West Washington Square
Philadelphia, PA 19105
USA

Distributed in Japan by:
Nankodo Co. Ltd.,
Tokyo International P.O. Box 5272,
42-6, Hongo 3-chome,
Bunkyo-ku, Tokyo 113, Japan.

ISBN: 0-443-03905-4

British Library Cataloguing in Publication Data:
Hoffbrand, A.V.
  Clinical haematology illustrated: an integrated text and colour atlas.
  1. Hematology
  i. Title   ii. Pettit, J.E.
  616.1'5   RB145

Project Editor: Sharyn Wong
Design & Illustration: Marie McNestry
Line Artist: Marion Tasker

Type set in Bembo 11/12pt.

Printed in Hong Kong by Imago Publishing Limited.

PREFACE

There are excellent atlases of haematology which illustrate peripheral blood and bone marrow appearances in the various diseases of the blood. Haematology, however, is an increasingly complex clinical discipline. There are a vast number of clinical signs that may occur in blood diseases. Moreover, the haematologist must call on many specialized invasive or non-invasive techniques to reach a diagnosis and decide on patient management. The purpose of our book is to bring together in a visual form the clinical features, peripheral blood and bone marrow morphology, special laboratory tests, radiographic, computerized tomographic and isotope scan appearances in diseases of the blood. The newer technique of surface membrane marker analysis using monoclonal antibodies and DNA probes for haemo-globinopathies and immunoglobulin gene rearrangements are also included. A small selection of electronmicroscopic appearances of some leukaemic cells is included in Appendix II. Treatment of blood diseases is not covered.

This book is aimed primarily at the haematologist in training and haematologists practising both laboratory and clinical haematology, and also teachers of the subject. It should also be of value to medical students and physicians generally. The text provides a brief summary of the clinical features, pathological processes and differential diagnosis of each disease. The anaemias, and benign and malignant white cell disorders as well as the lymphomas, coagulation and platelet disorders, and tropical diseases of the blood are included, and one chapter is devoted to the bone marrow appearances in systemic diseases. The first chapter deals not only with normal appearances of the blood and bone marrow but also with some of the more fundamental biological and biochemical aspects of normal haemopoiesis and the function of normal blood cells which form a basis for the subsequent chapters dealing with the various diseases.

The illustrations are largely from our collections made over many years from our own cases and laboratories. Our colleagues at the Royal Free and Dunedin Hospitals, however, have been most generous in helping with slides of particular interest and importance, and we are indebted to them as well as to the many other experts around the world who have contributed material and advice.

We are particularly grateful to Mr. Cedric Gilson of the Department of Medical Illustration at the Royal Free Hospital and Mr. Derek Birchan of the Department of Medical Illustration, Otago Medical School, for their help and skill in preparing many of the clinical illustrations, to Mrs. Jackie Wilkinson and Miss R. Neilson for typing the manuscript and for their expert and cheerful secretarial assistance. Finally, we wish to thank Miss Sharyn Wong and all the staff of Gower Medical Publishing for their skilful cooperation and unstinting efforts in preparing this book.

A.V.H. & J.E.P.
London, 1987

ACKNOWLEDGEMENTS

We gratefully acknowledge the contribution of the following who have provided slides, radiographs or other illustrative material from their personal collections and given us valuable advice:

Royal Free Hospital and School of Medicine

Dr. L. Berger
Dr. M.K. Brenner
Dr. D. Campana
Dr. R. Dick
Dr. G.E. Francis
Mr. J. Griffiths
Dr. A. Hilson
Mr. P.J. Humphries
Dr. R.A. Hutton
Mrs. B.F.A. Jackson
Prof. G. Janossy
Dr. P.B.A. Kernoff
Dr. S.M. Knowles
Dr. J.E. McLaughlin
Dr. D. Nag
Dr. J.D. Norton
Dr. U. O'Callaghan
Mr. A.B. Parsonson
Dr. R.E. Pounder
Dr. H.G. Prentice
Dr. I. Sarkany
Prof. P.J. Scheuer
Dr. L.M. Secker-Walker
Dr. M.R. Taheri
Dr. E.G.D. Tuddenham
Dr. B. Wonke

Otago Medical School

Dr. L. Beale
Dr. B.B. Berkeley
Prof. J.B. Blennerhassett
Prof. V. Chadwick
Dr. N.W. Fitzgerald
Dr. M.D. Holdaway
Mr. J.E. Lucas
Prof. J.C. Parr

Other Hospitals and Medical Schools

Dr. M. Arrabel
Dr. A.S. Awidi
Dr. M. Bilter
Dr. K.F. Bradstock
Dr. P.G. Bullough
Dr. D. Catovsky
Dr. J.M. Chessells
Dr. M. Chilosi
Dr. J.W. Clark
Dr. C.R. Dowding
Dr. Y.S. Erosan
Dr. L. Fry
Dr. H. Furze
Dr. M.Y. Gordon
Dr. I.M. Hann
Mr. J.W. Keeling
Prof. R.J. Levinsky
Prof. G. Luccarelli
Dr. S.J. Machin
Prof. I. Magnus
Dr. E. Matutes
Dr. J. Melo
Dr. M.R. Moore
Dr. J. Old
Dr. G. Pizzolo
Dr. A. Price
Mrs. D. Robinson
Prof. C.H. Rodeck
Prof. J. Rowley
Dr. G. Serjeant
Prof. H. Stein
Dr. P.V. Srivastava
Dr. J.S. Stewart
Dr. S.L. Thein
Prof. D. Todd

CONTENTS

I

NORMAL HAEMOPOIESIS
AND BLOOD CELLS

HAEMOPOIETIC STEM AND PROGENITOR CELLS

Haemopoietic stem cells have the property of self-renewal and also, through cell division and differentiation, form populations of progenitor cells which are committed to the main marrow cell lines: erythroid; granulocytic and monocytic; megakaryocytic; and lymphocytic (Fig. 1.1). The earlier progenitor cells are multipotent but, as division and differentiation proceed, later progenitors are formed which are committed to only one or two cell lines. Most evidence suggests that the haemopoietic stem and progenitor cells morphologically resemble small and intermediate-sized lymphocytes.

The marrow contains a stromal matrix which provides the correct microenvironment for stem cell growth (Figs. 1.2 & 1.3). A stromal layer can be grown *in vitro* in long-term cultures on which haemopoietic cells grow. In the embryo, the yolk sac and subsequently, in the fetus, the spleen and

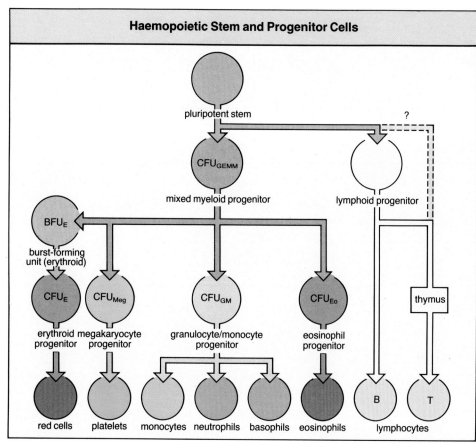

Fig. 1.1 Haemopoietic stem and progenitor cells: bone marrow pluripotent stem cell and the cell lines arising from it. The various progenitor cells can be identified by culture in semisolid media by the type of colony they form. CFU = colony-forming unit; GEMM = mixed granulocyte/erythroid/monocyte/megakaryocyte; E = erythroid; Meg = megakaryocyte; GM = granulocyte/monocyte; Eo = eosinophil; BFU_E = burst-forming unit, erythroid.

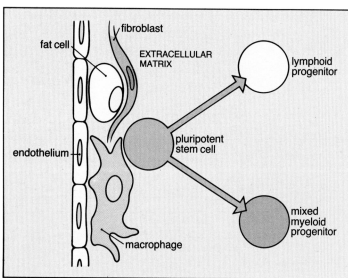

Fig. 1.2 Haemopoiesis in a suitable microenvironment provided by a stromal matrix on which stem cells grow and divide.

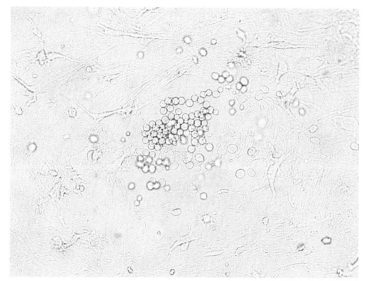

Fig. 1.3 Blast colony: produced by adding normal human bone marrow cells to preformed cultured marrow stromal cells. The blast colony-forming cells adhere to the stromal cultures and are stimulated to proliferate and form colonies. The elongated cells in the background are fibroblastoid cells and macrophages of the stromal layer. Courtesy of Drs. M.Y. Gordon and C.R. Dowding.

liver provide the correct environment for stem cells to grow and replicate. Although not distinguishable from other lymphocyte-like cells morphologically, the presence of progenitor cells can be shown by marrow culture techniques. The human pluripotential stem cell itself cannot be cultured *in vitro* but, in the mouse, stem cells form colonies in the spleen of an irradiated recipient. A number of culture systems have been developed which permit proliferation of the committed progenitor cell for the major marrow cell lines (Figs. 1.3–1.8).

In culture media, the progenitor cells are defined as 'colony-forming units' (CFU). Thus, the earliest detectable haemopoietic progenitor cell which gives rise to granulocytes, erythroblasts, monocytes and megakaryocytes is termed CFU_{GEMM} or CFU_{mix}. More mature and specialized precursor cells are termed CFU_{GM} (granulocytes and monocytes), CFU_{Eo} (eosinophils), CFU_E (erythroid) and CFU_{Meg} (megakaryocytes). BFU_E (burst-forming unit, erythroid) refers to an earlier erythroid progenitor than the CFU_E (Fig. 1.8).

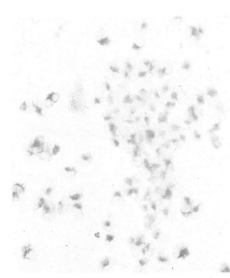

Fig. 1.4 Bone marrow culture: granulocyte/macrophage (GM) colony in semisolid agar culture after 7 days' growth. The cell giving rise to this colony is termed CFU_{GM}. Staining: see Fig. 1.5. Courtesy of Dr. G.E. Francis.

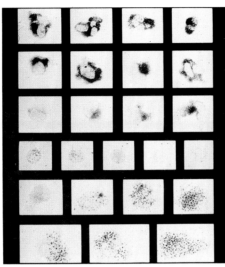

Fig. 1.5 Bone marrow culture: cells in diffuse granulocyte/macrophage colonies can be identified using a dual esterase method. Chloracetate esterase (CAE) activity present in cells of the granulocytic series is demonstrated by a blue-staining reaction; non-specific esterase (NSE), present in cells of macrophage lineage, is demonstrated by an amber-staining reaction. Courtesy of Dr. G.E. Francis.

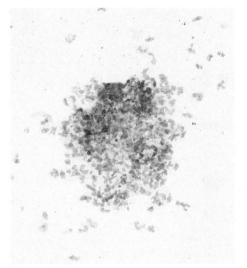

Fig. 1.6 Bone marrow culture: mixed granulocyte/erythrocyte colony (CFU_{mix}). The haemoglobin-containing cells are stained with o-dianisidine (reddish-brown). The neutrophils stain only with the haematoxylin counterstain. Colonies containing granulocytes (G), erythrocytes (E), monocytes (M), and megakaryocytes (Meg) are termed CFU_{GEMM}. Courtesy of Dr. G.E. Francis.

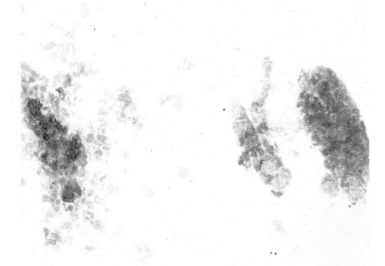

Fig. 1.7 Bone marrow culture: mixed granulocyte/erythrocyte colony adjacent to an eosinophil colony. Luxol-fast blue stain. Courtesy of Dr. G.E. Francis.

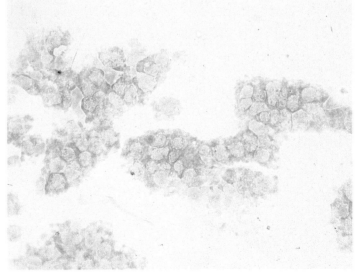

Fig. 1.8 Bone marrow culture: an erythroid 'burst'. This type of multicentric colony develops from a single cell termed 'burst-forming unit, erythroid' (BFU_E). The cultures are stimulated by both erythropoietin and burst-promoting activity (BPA) derived from phytohaemagglutinin (PHA)-stimulated lymphocytes or other sources. Courtesy of Dr. G.E. Francis.

Proliferation of the stem and progenitor cells is under the control of the hormone-like inducers of growth and differentiation, produced by stromal cells of the micro-environment and by the haemopoietic cells themselves, for example, the colony-stimulating factors, interleukins and erythropoietin (Fig. 1.9).

MEMBRANE–GROWTH FACTOR INTERACTIONS

The mechanisms by which the signal to proliferate or differentiate, carried by an extracellular factor, is transmitted from the cell membrane to its nucleus is only now becoming apparent (Fig. 1.10). Binding of the growth factor to a specific receptor on the cell surface causes a transmembrane signal to alter the cell membrane. The enzyme phosphatidyl-inositol biphosphate phosphodiesterase (PPDE) is then activated to break down membrane lipid, thus releasing two secondary messengers, diacylglycerol (DG) and inositol triphosphate (IP_3). A GTP binding (G) protein may act as an intermediary between the membrane receptor and the enzyme PPDE. This G protein is activated by binding GTP which it then hydrolyzes to GDP via its GTPase activity in order to return to its inactive form. DG activates an enzyme, protein kinase C which, in turn, phosphorylates proteins mainly on threonine and serine residues. IP_3 causes release of intracellular calcium ions. The exact way in which these two biochemical changes subsequently cause signal transduction to the nucleus is unclear. The intracytoplasmic filaments, intermediate, actin and tubulin, may act as solid-state transducing elements.

Stromal Cells	Extracellular Matrix	Growth Factors	Monokines and Lymphokines	
macrophages	fibronectin	Multipotent IL-3 (BPA)	IL-1	IL=interleukin
fibroblasts	laminin		IL-2	BPA=burst-promoting activity
reticulum ('blanket') cells	collagen	Committed GM-CSF G-CSF	interferons, α & γ	CSF=colony-forming factor
fat cells	proteoglycans (acid mucopolysaccharides)	M-CSF Eo-CSF erythropoietin	tumour necrosis factor (TNF)	G=granulocyte
endothelial cells		? thrombopoietin	BCGF	M=monocyte
			BCDF	Eo=eosinophil
				BCGF=B-cell growth factor
				BCDF=B-cell differentiation factor

Fig.1.9 The stromal cells, extracellular matrix, growth factors, and monokines and lymphokines on which haemopoiesis depends.

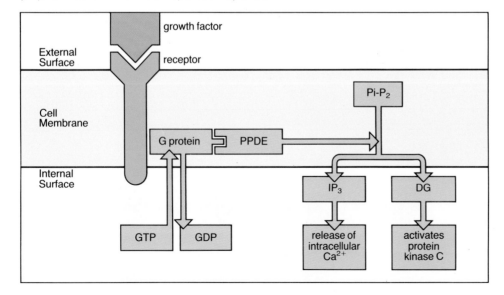

Fig.1.10 Suggested pathway for transduction of a growth factor signal from the cell membrane to the cell interior. Binding of a growth factor to its receptor causes a conformation change in a GTP-binding (G) protein, which activates PPDE to release DG and IP_3 from the lipid membrane substrate. The mechanism by which the signals transmit the message to the nucleus is unclear; cytoskeletal proteins may be involved. Hydrolysis of GTP by a GTPase activity intrinsic to the G-protein attenuates the signal.

Pi-P_2=phosphatidylinositol biphosphate

Binding of a growth factor to its membrane receptor may also activate adenylate cyclase in the cell membrane and so increase the intracellular cyclic AMP levels; this may lead to a cellular response. It remains to be seen how far these general biochemical pathways vary with different cell types, growth factors and receptors. It is clear that, in some systems, tyrosine kinase enzymes, which phosphorylate proteins on tyrosine residues and may be coded by cellular oncogenes, are involved in the pathways.

ONCOGENES

Studies of animal RNA tumour viruses have revealed that many possess genes termed viral oncogenes (v–oncs) capable of transforming cells in culture from a benign to a malignant phenotype. Human and other eukaryotic cells contain genes, cellular proto-oncogenes (c-oncs) which are closely homologous to viral oncogenes. Proto-oncogenes are highly conserved in vertebrate evolution and, in general, code for proteins involved in cell proliferation or differentiation (Fig. 1.11). One class of oncogenes codes for growth factor or receptor-like molecules, for example, v–sis for the β chain of platelet-derived growth factor, erb-B for the epidermal growth factor receptor, and fms for the receptor for CSF-1 which autophosphorylates on tyrosine. Others code for protein tyrosine kinases, such as abl, fes, ros, src and yes, or for protein serine-threonine kinases, for example, mos and raf, or for GTP-binding proteins such as H–ras, K–ras and N–ras. The specific function of some oncogenes, for instance, those whose products are located in the nucleus as myc, ets or fos, remains unknown.

Name	Viral Strain	Probable Animal Origin	Chromosome Locality	Function of Protein Product
abl	Abelson murine	Mouse	9q34	Tyrosine kinase
src-1	Rous sarcoma	Chicken	20q12-13	
src-2			1p34-36	
fes	Synden-Theilen feline sarcoma	Cat	15q26	
fps	Fujinami sarcoma		15q24-25	
ros	Avian sarcoma	Chicken	6q16-22	
yes	Y73 sarcoma		18q21	
mos	Moloney sarcoma		8q22	Serine/threonine kinase
fms	McDonough sarcoma	Cat	5q32	Receptor for CSF-I
rel	Reticuloendotheliosis	Turkey	2p	Unknown
raf-1	Murine sarcoma	Mouse	3p25	Serine/threonine kinase
K-ras-1	Kirsten murine leukaemia	Rat	6p11/12	GTP binding & hydrolysis
K-ras-2			12p12	
H-ras-1	Harvey sarcoma		11p14-15	
N-ras	Nasheed rat sarcoma		1p11-13	
myc	Avian myelocytomatosis	Chicken	8q24	Unknown; all active in nucleus
Lmyc			1p32	
myb	Avian myeloblastosis		6q22-24	
fos	FBJ osteosarcoma	Mouse	14q21-31	
ets-1	Avian oncogenic	Avian	11q23-24	
ets-2			21q22	
sis	Simian sarcoma	Woolly monkey	22q13	Platelet-derived growth factor
erb-A	Avian erythroblastosis	Chicken	17q21-22	Thyroid hormone receptor
erb-B			7p11-13	Epidermal growth factor receptor*

N.B. Other oncogenes less well characterized include Blym-1, fgr, lsk, ski, trk, bcl-1, bcl-2, N-cam and akt-1.
 * tyrosine kinase & intramembrane portion only

Fig.1.11 Oncogenes, their viral strain, probable animal origin, chromosomal location and, where known, the function of the protein product.

Activation of a cellular oncogene by point mutation, gene amplification, translocation or insertion of a new promoter by a retrovirus ('promoter insertion') may lead to enhanced and uncontrolled expression of that oncogene and may play a role in the malignant transformation of the cell.

The location of many of the oncogenes in the human genome has now been elucidated (Fig. 1.12). It is also becoming apparent that the cytogenetic abnormalities found in many cases of acute or chronic leukaemia or in myelodysplasia (see Appendix) may involve movement of oncogenes to new sites in the genome where they become abnormally expressed. In some lymphoid tumours, these translocations may juxtapose immunoglobulin or T-cell receptor genes and oncogenes.

CYTOGENETICS (see also Appendix)

The human somatic cell contains forty-six pairs of chromosomes. These are numbered 1 to 22 with one pair, the sex chromosomes, being XX in females and XY in males. The appearance of these chromosomes in a preparation from

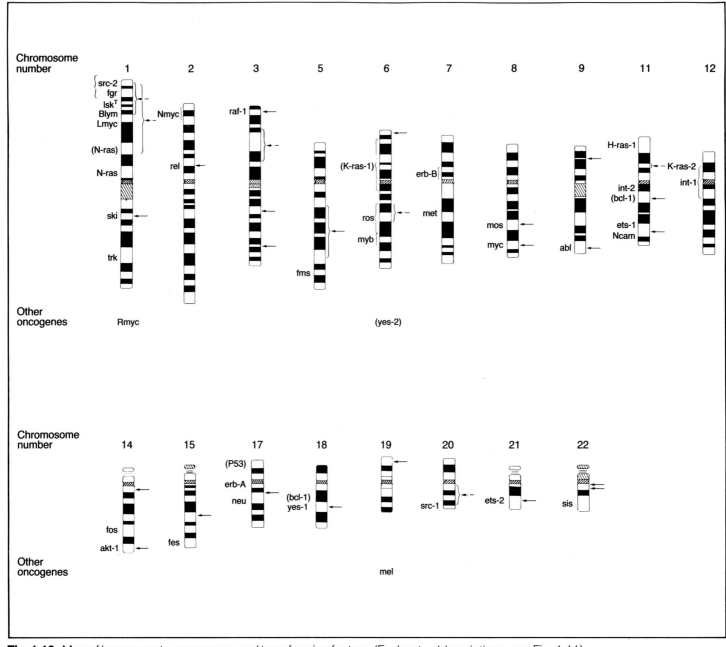

Fig. 1.12 Map of human proto-oncogenes and transforming factors. (For key to abbreviations, see Fig. 1.11) Courtesy of Prof. J. Rowley.

dividing cells is termed the karyotype (Fig.1.12). The letters 'p' and 'q' refer to the short and long arms of the chromosomes respectively; translocations are indicated by 't' followed by the chromosomes involved in the first set of brackets and the chromosome bands involved in a second set of brackets. The dark or lighter staining bands are detected by the Giemsa (G) or quinacrine (Q) techniques and are numbered from the centromere outwards. 'Inv' indicates an inversion, 'ins' an insertion and 'del' a deletion; + or − in front of a number indicates gain or loss of the whole chromosome while + or − after a number means a gain or loss of part of the chromosome.

BONE MARROW EXAMINATION

Bone marrow aspirates provide films on which the cytological details of developing cells can be examined (Figs.1.13 & 1.14). The proportional numbers of the different cell lines is assessed (Fig.1.15), appearances of the individual cells noted and a search made for the presence of cells foreign to the normal marrow, such as metastatic deposits from carcinoma. Iron stores may also be assessed (see Fig.1.36).

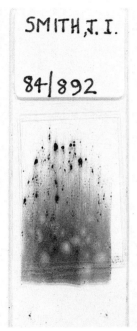

Fig.1.13 Bone marrow aspirate: this normal aspirate has been spread, allowed to dry and stained by the May-Grünwald/Giemsa technique. Bone marrow fragments are clearly visible at the tail end of the smear.

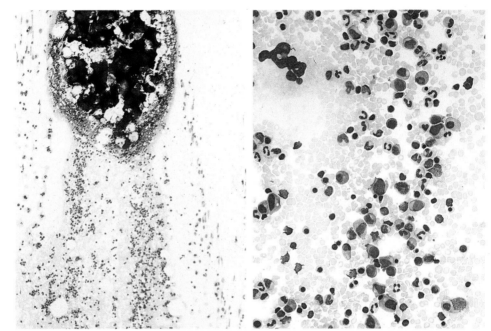

Fig.1.14 Normal marrow fragment and cell trails: the marrow fragment (left) contains haemopoietic cells, supporting reticuloendothelial cells and some fat spaces. During the spreading procedure, representative cells of each haemopoietic cell line spill out into 'trails' behind the marrow fragments; (right) higher magnification.

Fig.1.15 Normal myelogram: the normal myeloid:erythroid ratio is 2.5 – 15:1. The different colours indicate broad postulated developmental groups.

Normal Myelogram			
Cells	Percent	Cells	Percent
Pronormoblasts	0.5-5.0	Myeloblasts	0.1-3.5
Normoblasts		Promyelocytes	0.5-5.0
basophilic	1-3		
polychromatic	2-20	Myelocytes	
pyknotic	2-10	neutrophil	5-20
		eosinophil	0.1-3.0
Megakaryocytes	0.1-0.5	basophil	0-0.5
Lymphocytes	5-20	Metamyelocytes	
		& band forms	10-30
Plasma cells	0-3.5	Segmented forms	
		neutrophils	7-25
Monocytes	0-0.2	eosinophils	0.2-3.0
Macrophages	0-2	basophils	0-0.5

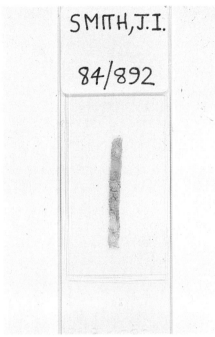

Fig.1.16 Normal trephine biopsy: gross appearance of a section prepared from a trephine biopsy of the posterior iliac crest. Haematoxylin and eosin stain.

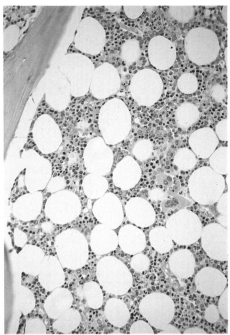

Fig.1.17 Normal trephine biopsy: representative histology taken from the posterior iliac crest. Approximately half of the inter-trabecular space is occupied by haemopoietic tissue and half by fat. Haematoxylin and eosin stain.

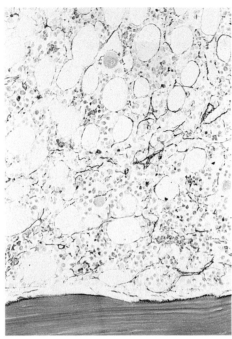

Fig.1.18 Normal trephine biopsy: the reticulin fibres are thin and delicate, and form a network around the haemopoietic cells. Silver impregnation stain.

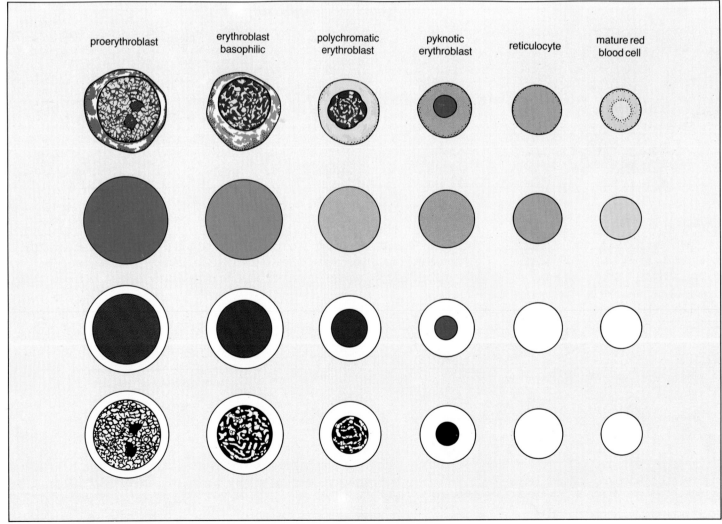

Fig.1.19 Red cell differentiation and maturation: the second, third and fourth rows show cytoplasmic colour maturation, nuclear size and staining, and nuclear chromatin patterns respectively. The first row shows the composite appearance.

Bone marrow trephine biopsies produce cores of bone and marrow which are decalcified and processed for histological assessment (Figs.1.16–1.18). The trephine provides an excellent sample for examination of marrow architecture and cellularity. It is the most reliable method of detecting marrow infiltrates.

Erythropoiesis

A diagrammatic representation of the nuclear and cytoplasmic changes during erythropoiesis is shown in Fig.1.19. The earliest recognizable erythroid cell in the marrow is the pronormoblast, a large cell with dark blue cytoplasm and a primitive nuclear chromatin pattern (Fig.1.20). Kinetic studies have identified four cell cycles between the pronormoblast and the late non-dividing erythroblast (normoblast).

The more differentiated normoblasts are progressively smaller and contain increasing amounts of haemoglobin, giving an acidophilic cytoplasm; the nuclear chromatin becomes progressively more condensed. Basophilic (early), polychromatic (intermediate) and pyknotic (late) stages of normoblast development are recognized (Figs.1.21 & 1.22).

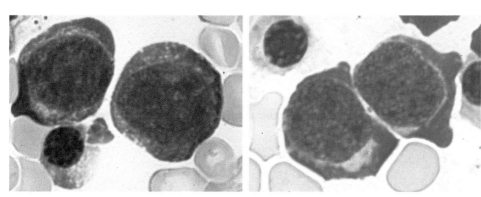

Fig.1.20 Erythropoiesis: proerythroblasts and smaller polychromatic normoblasts.

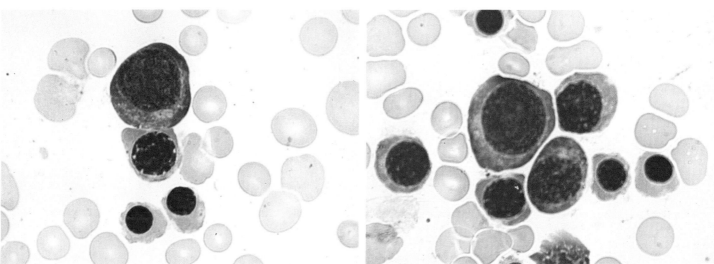

Fig.1.21 Erythropoiesis (left) from top to bottom, basophilic, polychromatic and two pyknotic normoblasts; (right) further examples of basophilic, polychromatic and pyknotic normoblasts.

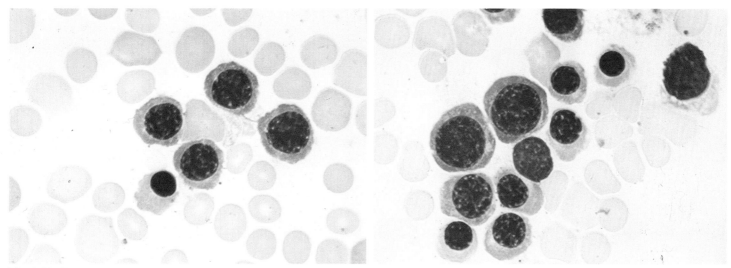

Fig.1.22 Erythropoiesis: polychromatic and pyknotic erythroblasts.

The nucleus is finally extruded from the late normoblast within the marrow, producing a reticulocyte which still contains some ribosomal RNA (Fig.1.23) and is capable of synthesizing haemoglobin. This cell spends one to two days in the marrow and then a further one to two days in the peripheral blood and spleen, where the RNA is completely lost and an orthochromatic or pink-staining erythrocyte (red cell) results. In the marrow, erythroblasts are associated closely with their supportive macrophages (Figs.1.24 & 1.25).

Granulopoiesis and monocyte production
In granulopoiesis (Fig.1.26), the first recognizable cell of the granulocytic series is the myeloblast. Following division and differentiation, the following sequence of cells may be seen: promyelocyte (which contains primary granules); myelocyte; metamyelocyte; band cell; and segmented or mature granulocyte (Figs.1.27-1.30). Specific (secondary) granules (neutrophil, eosinophil or basophil) appear from the promyelocyte stage onwards.

In line with the dominance of neutrophils among the granulocytes of the peripheral blood, neutrophil precursors form the majority of granulocyte precursors in the marrow, with a few eosinophil precursors and rare basophil precursors present. Only small numbers of monocytes and their precursors, the monoblasts and promonocytes, are seen in normal marrow.

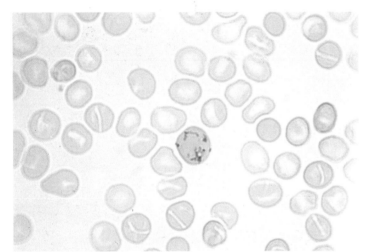

Fig.1.23 Reticulocyte: reticular material (precipitated RNA and protein) is clearly visible in the central reticulocyte. Supravital new methylene blue stain.

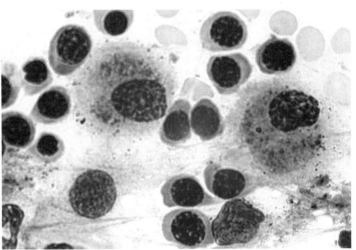

Fig.1.24 Bone marrow macrophages: close association of polychromatic normoblasts with two pigmented macrophages

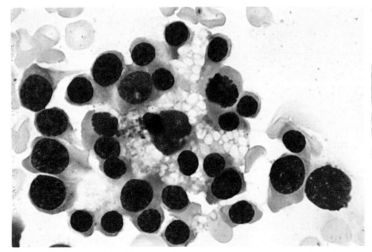

Fig.1.25 Erythroblast/macrophage nests: normoblasts in tight clusters around central macrophages with lipid-laden cytoplasm.

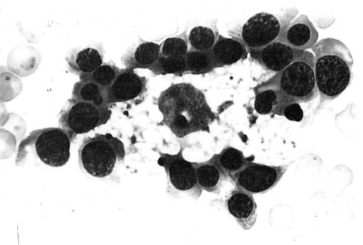

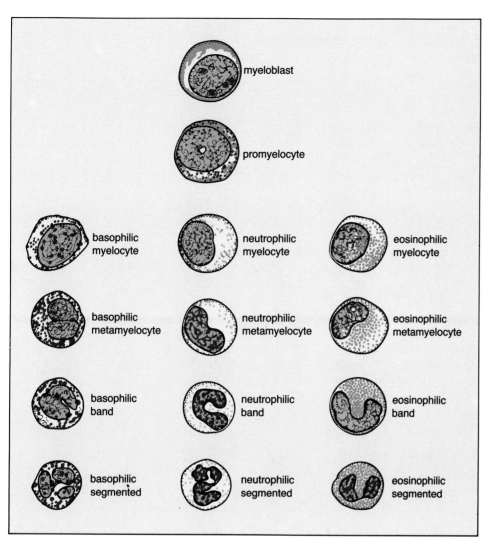

myeloblast

promyelocyte

basophilic myelocyte | neutrophilic myelocyte | eosinophilic myelocyte

basophilic metamyelocyte | neutrophilic metamyelocyte | eosinophilic metamyelocyte

basophilic band | neutrophilic band | eosinophilic band

basophilic segmented | neutrophilic segmented | eosinophilic segmented

Fig.1.26 Granulocyte differentiation and maturation: the myeloblast and promyelocyte give rise to three different cell lines according to the type of secondary granules and nuclear morphology.

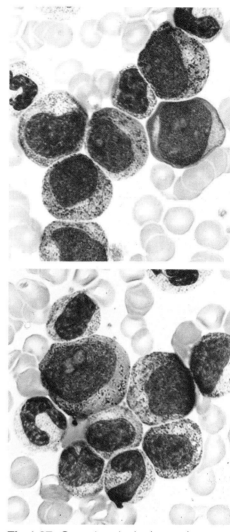

Fig.1.27 Granulopoiesis: (upper) a myeloblast, late promyelocytes and myelocytes; (lower) a promyelocyte, myelocytes and metamyelocytes.

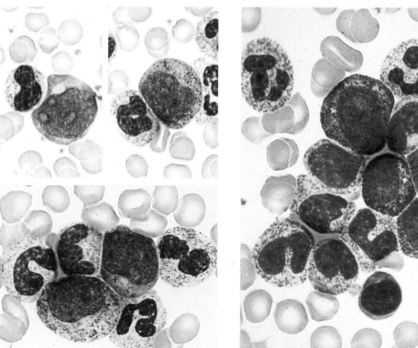

Fig.1.28 Granulopoiesis: (upper left) myeloblast and (upper right) promyelocyte; (lower) early promyelocyte, myelocyte, metamyelocyte and band neutrophils.

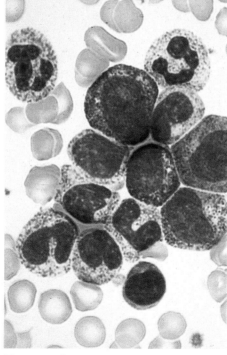

Fig.1.29 Granulopoiesis: sequence of cells from myelocytes through metamyelocytes and band forms, and a single segmented neutrophil.

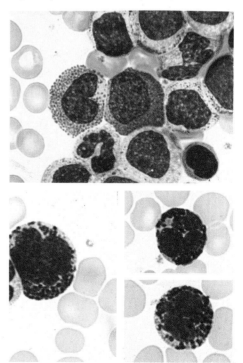

Fig.1.30 Granulopoiesis: (upper) eosinophil myelocyte and metamyelocyte; (lower left) basophil myelocyte; (lower right) more mature basophils.

1.11

Megakaryocyte and platelet production

The earliest small progenitor cells of the megakaryocytic line are not easily differentiated from myeloblasts. They may be identified by electronmicroscopic immunological techniques. The megakaryocyte matures by a process of endomitotic synchronous nuclear replications, enlarging the cytoplasmic volume as the number of nuclei increases in multiples of two. These polypoid cells contain the equivalent of four, eight, sixteen, or thirty-two sets of chromosomes. At a variable stage of development, usually at the four-, eight- or sixteen-nucleus stage, further nuclear replication and cell growth ceases; the cytoplasm becomes granular and platelets are produced (Figs.1.31–1.33)

Lymphocytes and plasma cells

Although the marrow remains the principal site of 'virgin' lymphocyte formation, the majority of circulating lymphoid cells (mature T and B cells) are produced in peripheral lymphoid tissue: lymph nodes, spleen, thymus and lymphoid tissue of the gastrointestinal and respiratory tracts. Lymphocytes usually comprise less than ten percent of the normal myelogram and the progenitor lymphoblasts are difficult to differentiate from other blast cells. Isolated plasma cells (Fig.1.34) are generally not difficult to find in marrow cell trails. They comprise up to four percent of the normal marrow cell population.

Assessment of iron status

In the assessment of iron status, marrow films are stained by the Perls' reaction. Tissue (macrophage) stores are observed in the marrow fragments, and one or two siderotic granules are normally present in about a third of developing erythroblasts (Fig.1.36).

Osteoblasts and osteoclasts

Osteoblasts and osteoclasts are occasionally seen during bone marrow examination (Figs.1.37 & 1.38). When present in significant numbers, it is important not to confuse them with metastatic malignant cells.

Cells in mitosis

Although bone marrow is one of the most rapidly dividing tissues in the body, only small numbers of dividing cells are seen in normal marrow aspirate cell trails (Fig.1.39).

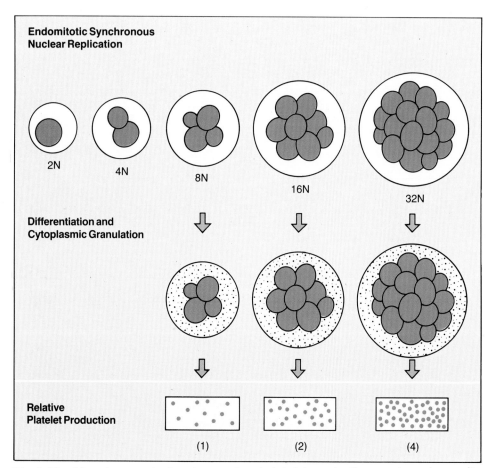

Fig.1.31 Megakaryocyte development and platelet production: each nuclear unit has two sets of chromosomes. N = number of sets of chromosomes or 'ploidy'.

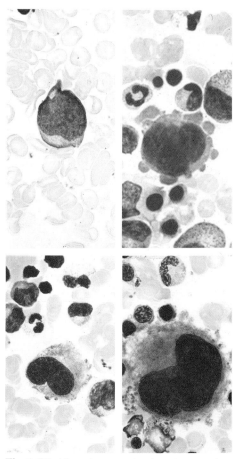

Fig.1.32 Megakaryocyte development: (upper) megakaryoblasts with nucleoli; (lower left) early bilobed megakaryocyte without obvious cytoplasmic granulation; (lower right) larger megakaryocyte with obvious early granulation of cytoplasm.

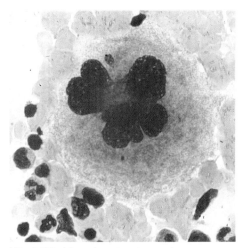

Fig.1.33 Megakaryocyte: mature megakaryocyte with many nuclear lobes and pronounced granulation of its cytoplasm.

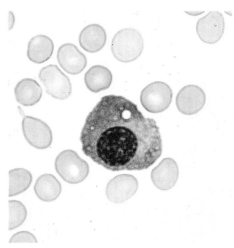

Fig.1.34 Plasma cell: typical appearance of an eccentric nucleus with basophilic cytoplasm, prominent perinuclear clearing and a single vacuole.

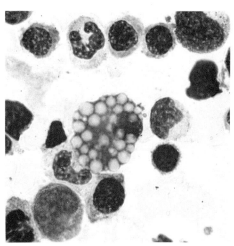

Fig.1.35 Plasma cell: this type contains many spherical cytoplasmic inclusions and is sometimes referred to as a 'Mott' cell.

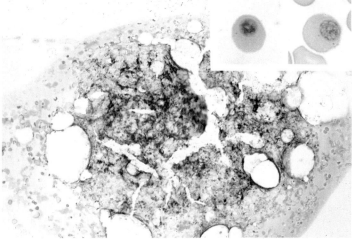

Fig.1.36 Bone marrow iron assessment: bone marrow fragment stained for iron by the Perls' reaction. Abundant Prussian blue positivity indicates iron as haemosiderin in reticuloendothelial cell macrophages; (inset) in the cell trails, some of the normoblasts contain one, two or three Prussian blue-positive 'siderotic' granules.

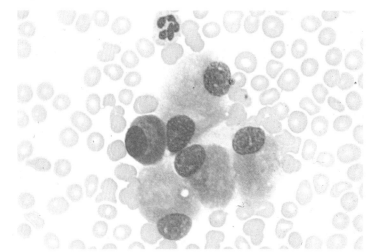

Fig.1.37 Osteoblasts: a group of five osteoblasts and a plasma cell (on the left) with a neutrophil (uppermost) for comparison. The osteoblasts are large cells resembling plasma cells, but their chromatin pattern is more open, their cytoplasm less basophilic and they tend to occur in clumps.

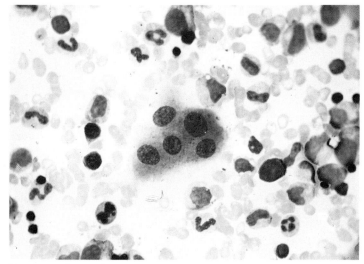

Fig.1.38 Osteoclasts: these multinucleated cells are occasionally seen in normal marrow aspirates. In contrast to megakaryocytes, the nuclei of osteoclasts are usually discrete, round or oval, and often contain nucleoli.

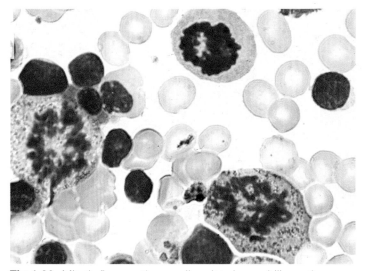

Fig.1.39 Mitotic figures: three cells, a late basophilic erythroblast (upper field) and two myelocytes, in metaphase. Only a small fraction of the cells seen in normal marrow are in mitosis.

PERIPHERAL BLOOD CELLS

The usual initial diagnostic approach to blood disorders is blood counting and blood film examination. Various parameters make up the normal blood count (Fig. 1.40). Blood films on glass slides (Fig. 1.41) are usually stained with one of the Romanowsky stains (for example, May-Grünwald/Giemsa or Wright's).

Red cells in normal peripheral blood are circular and fairly uniform in size with a mean cell diameter of 8μm. Only mild variation in size (anisocytosis) and shape (poikilocytosis) is seen (Fig. 1.42). In the ideal part of the blood film for examination, which is where the red cells are just beginning to touch and overlap, their biconcave shape produces a central pallor.

Platelets appear as granular basophilic forms with a mean diameter of 1-2μm (Figs. 1.42 & 1.43). Small numbers of large platelets with diameters up to 7μm may also be found (Fig. 1.44). The volume of platelets diminishes as they mature and age in the circulation.

During blood film examination, the white cell numbers and morphology are assessed and a differential count is performed, if this has not been provided by an electronic laboratory blood counter. Representative examples of white cells found in normal blood are shown in Figs. 1.45 to 1.50.

Normal Blood Count		
Haemoglobin	♂ 13.5-17.5g/dl ♀ 11.5-15.5g/dl	
Red cells (erythrocytes)	♂ 4.5-6.5 × 10^{12}/l ♀ 3.9-5.6 × 10^{12}/l	
PCV (haematocrit)	♂ 40-52% ♀ 36-48%	
MCV	80-95fl	
MCH	27-34pg	
MCHC	30-35g/dl	
White cells (leucocytes): total neutrophils lymphocytes monocytes eosinophils basophils	4.0-11.0 × 10^9/l 2.5-7.5 × 10^9/l 1.5-3.5 × 10^9/l 0.2-0.8 × 10^9/l 0.04-0.44 × 10^9/l 0.01-0.1 × 10^9/l	
Platelets	150-400 × 10^9/l	

Fig.1.40 Blood count: normal adult values.

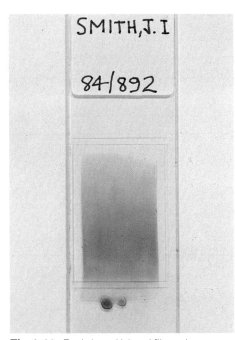

Fig.1.41 Peripheral blood film: glass slide of a well spread blood film stained by the May-Grünwald/Giemsa technique

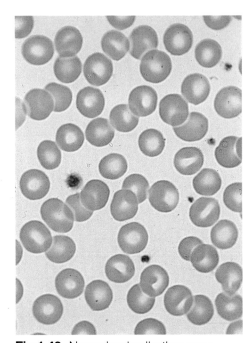

Fig.1.42 Normal red cells: these are 7-8μm in diameter with minor variations in size (anisocytosis) and shape (poikilocytosis). Their outside portions have a good depth of staining reaction, but the majority show a central pale area of diminished staining. Platelets, varying in size between 1-3μm, are also evident.

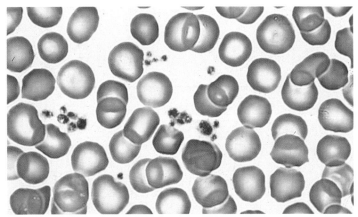

Fig.1.43 Normal platelets: in this blood film, made from a finger-prick sample, the platelets have agglutinated into small clumps. This is a regular feature of blood films prepared from blood which has not been collected into an anticoagulant.

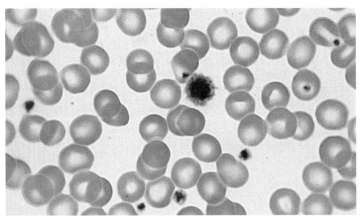

Fig.1.44 Normal platelets: these platelets show more variation in size than those in Fig. 1.43, the largest measuring approximately 6μm in diameter. Platelets of this size are seen only rarely in normal blood films.

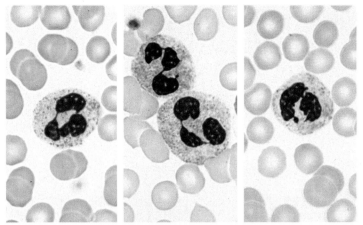

Fig.1.45 Normal neutrophils: mature forms showing typical nuclear lobe separation by fine filaments. Normal segmented neutrophils may show up to five lobes; (right) a 'Barr body' is attached to a lobe of the nucleus. This is typical of a female neutrophil and due to the possession of two X chromosomes.

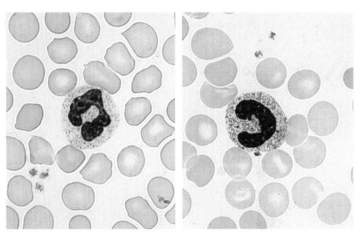

Fig.1.46 Normal neutrophils: stab or band forms. The nuclear segmentation of these less mature cells is incomplete.

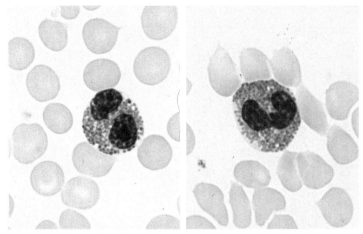

Fig.1.47 Normal eosinophils: each of these cells shows two nuclear segments and the typical coarse eosinophilic granulation of the cytoplasm.

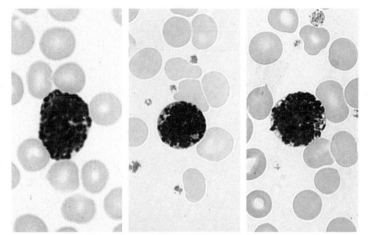

Fig.1.48 Basophils: the coarse basophilic granules of these cells often overlie the nucleus, thus obscuring the detail of its segmented structure. Only small numbers of basophils are found in the normal blood film.

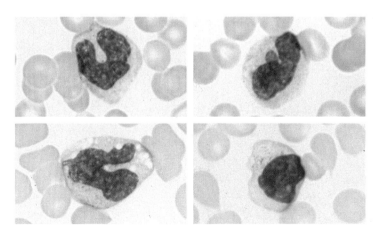

Fig.1.49 Monocytes: these cells are usually the largest white cells found in normal blood. The nucleus is usually folded or convoluted with a moderately fine chromatin pattern. The cytoplasm typically has a grey (ground-glass) appearance with fine azurophilic granules. Some (lower left) have rather prominent cytoplasmic vacuoles.

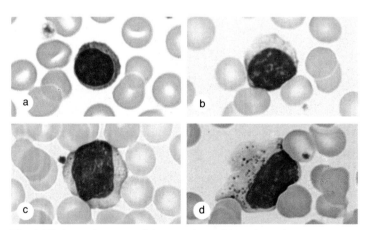

Fig.1.50 Lymphocytes: (a) normal small lymphocytes are 7-12μm in diameter. The light blue cytoplasm is scanty and the central round nucleus has a condensed amorphous chromatin pattern; (b & c) some lymphocytes have diameters up to 20μm, and even larger forms are found during lymphocytic reactions in other diseases (see Fig.7.36). Cells with azurophilic granules (d) are called 'large granular lymphocytes' and usually show natural killer (NK) cell function.

1.15

Very occasionally, either epithelial (Fig.1.51) or endothelial (Fig.1.52) cells are seen during blood film examination. It is likely that these have been aspirated from the skin or the blood vessel wall during venesection. Other rare appearances include neutrophil–platelet rosetting (Fig.1.53) and neutrophil aggregation (Fig.1.54), neither of which are usually of clinical significance.

RED CELLS

The main function of red cells is to carry oxygen to the tissues and return carbon dioxide from the tissues to the lungs. The protein haemoglobin is responsible for most of this gaseous exchange. The principal adult haemoglobin molecule (Hb A) has a molecular weight of 68,000 and comprises two alpha and two beta polypeptide chains (α_2,β_2), each with its own haem group. There are small

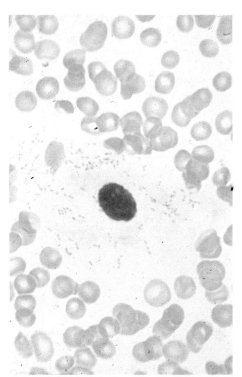

Fig.1.51 Epithelial cell: occasional isolated squamous cells are found in normal blood films. These very large cells are an artifact collected from the epidermis during venepuncture.

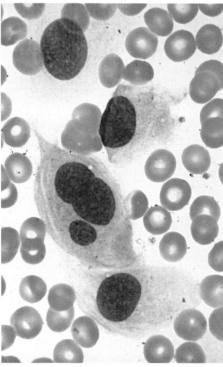

Fig.1.52 Endothelial cells: isolated clusters of vascular endothelial cells are a rare finding in normal blood films. These cells are dislodged from the intima of the vein during venepuncture.

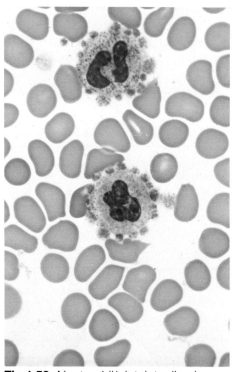

Fig.1.53 Neutrophil/platelet adhesion: rosetting of platelets around neutrophils is an interesting but unexplained finding in occasional blood films. This aggregation only occurs in the presence of the anticoagulant ethylenediaminetetraacetic acid (EDTA).

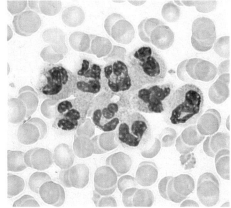

Fig.1.54 Neutrophil agglutination: clusters of aggregated neutrophils are also an occasional and unexplained finding during blood film examination. The phenomenon is sometimes seen in patients with viral infections.

	Globin Chain Synthesized	
Embryo	$\zeta_2\varepsilon_2$	Gower 1
	$\zeta_2\gamma_2$	Portland
	$\alpha_2\varepsilon_2$	Gower 2
Fetus	$\alpha_2\gamma_2$	Hb F
Adult	$\alpha_2\delta_2$	Hb A$_2$
	$\alpha_2\beta_2$	Hb A

Fig.1.55 Haemoglobins in the embryo, fetus and adult: there are two genes each on chromosome 16 for the ζ and α chains, and genes on chromosome 11 for Aγ and Gγ chains as well as one each for ε, δ and β chains.

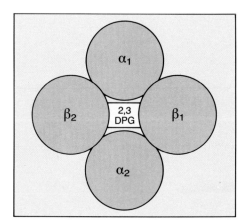

Fig.1.56 Normal adult haemoglobin A: there are two α and two β chains. 2,3 DPG fits into a pocket between the β chains and displaces oxygen.

quantities of Hb F (α_2, γ_2) and Hb A$_2$ (α_2, δ_2) (Fig.1.55). In the embryo, haemoglobin Gower 1 (ζ_2,ϵ_2), Portland ($\zeta_2\gamma_2$) and Gower 2 ($\alpha_2\epsilon_2$) are formed and, in the fetus, Hb F predominates. Two types of γ chain exist (Aγ and Gγ) according to whether alanine or glycine respectively are present at position 136.

Haem synthesis occurs mainly in the mitochondria by a series of biochemical reactions, commencing with the substrates glycine and succinyl–CoA, and globin chains are assembled on polyribosomes (see Fig.2.1). Two-thirds of the total cell content of haemoglobin is synthesized in erythroblasts, the remainder at the reticulocyte stage.

As the haemoglobin molecule takes up and releases oxygen, the individual globin chains move on each other. When oxygen is released, the ß chains are pulled apart, permitting the entry of the glycolytic metabolite 2,3 diphosphoglycerate (2,3 DPG ; Fig.1.56). This results in a lower affinity of the molecule for oxygen and improved delivery of oxygen to the tissues. It is also responsible for the sigmoid form of the oxygen dissociation curve (Fig.1.57).

For successful gaseous exchange, the flexible biconcave red cell, 8µm in diameter, has to pass through the micro-circulation, whose minimum diameter is only 3.5µm; it has to maintain haemoglobin in a reduced state and maintain osmotic equilibrium, despite having an inherently leaky membrane and an osmotic pressure approximately five times that of plasma. Devoid of mitochondria and the enzymes required for oxidative phosphorylation, the mature red cell is dependent on the glycolytic pathway (see Fig.4.24) to provide ATP for its energy requirements to maintain its volume, shape and flexibility. It is also able to generate reducing power as NADH by this pathway and as NADPH by the pentose-phosphate shunt pathway (see Fig.4.24). The iron atoms in normal haemoglobin are in the ferrous form. The enzymes methaemoglobin reductase use NADH or NADPH to reduce methaemoglobin (which contains ferric iron) formed normally during the lifespan of the red cell. Deficiency of NADH-methaemoglobin reductase leads to cyanosis with up to thirty percent methaemoglobin present and consequent deoxygenation of the haemoglobin (Fig. 1.57, right).

The Luebering-Rapoport shunt (see Fig.4.25) regulates the concentration of 2,3 DPG vital to the release of oxygen from the haemoglobin tetramer. As enzymes cannot be replaced in the mature red cell, there is a gradual deterioration in red cell metabolism and the cells become less viable with age. After a mean lifespan in the circulation of one hundred and twenty days and an estimated vascular journey of about three hundred miles, ageing red cells are destroyed extravascularly by macrophages of the reticuloendothelial system (see Fig.4.1).

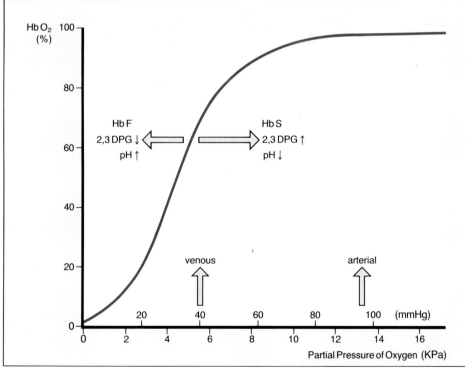
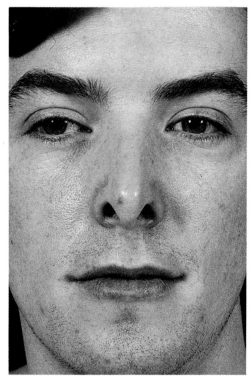

Fig. 1.57 Haemoglobin oxygen dissociation: (left) normal sigmoid curve relating Hb saturation to the partial pressure of oxygen to which it is exposed. The curve is shifted to the left (less oxygen is released at any given PO$_2$) by a fall in 2, 3 DPG, rise in pH (Bohr effect), if Hb A is replaced by Hb F or by a high affinity Hb. The curve is shifted to the right by a rise in 2, 3 DPG attached to the Hb, a fall in pH, if Hb A is replaced by Hb S or an Hb M (in which the haem iron is stabilized in the ferric form) or if haemoglobin is oxidized to methaemoglobin; (right) cyanosis due to NADH-methaemoglobin reductase deficiency in a man of 22 showing a typical slate-grey appearance. The blood count was normal.

1.17

GRANULOCYTES

All cells of this group (neutrophils, eosinophils and basophils) play an essential role in inflammation. They are primarily phagocytes and, with antibodies and complement, are responsible for the defence against microorganisms.

Neutrophils (polymorphs)

Neutrophil production and differentiation in the bone marrow takes from six to ten days. Large numbers of band and segmented neutrophils are held in the marrow as a 'reserve pool' which, in the normal state, contains ten to fifteen times the number of neutrophils in the peripheral blood. Following their release from the marrow, they spend six to twelve hours in the circulation before migrating into tissue where they perform their phagocytic function. They survive two to four days in the tissues before being destroyed during defensive action or as a result of senescence.

Following chemotactic attraction to sites of inflammation, offending microorganisms are ingested and contained within phagosomes (Fig.1.58). The neutrophil granule enzyme contents are released into these spaces. The primary azurophilic granules contain lysozyme and other enzymes. These enzymes are partly responsible for bacterial destruction; a second killing mechanism consists of oxidant damage by hydrogen peroxide and superoxide generated by glucose metabolism through NADH and NADHP. Lactoferrin, secreted by granulocytes, leads to bacteriostasis by depriving infected cells of iron.

Eosinophils

Although less is known about the kinetics of eosinophil production, differentiation, circulation and migration, it is likely that the mechanism is similar to that of neutrophils. Eosinophils are also capable of phagocytosis. The granules are membrane-bound organelles with a 'crystalloid' core. These cells are particularly important in allergic and parasitic diseases. Following appropriate stimulation, the granule contents may be released outside the cell at large targets, such as helminthic parasites. Eosinophils release histaminase and aryl-sulphatase, which inactivate histamine and a slow-reacting substance of anaphylaxis (SRS–A) released from mast cells.

Basophils

Although both basophils and tissue mast cells are of bone marrow origin, their relationship is not entirely clear. The granules of both cells contain heparin and pharmacological mediators such as SRS–A and histamine. Release of these substances follows an allergen–IgE complex binding to the cell surface via Fc receptors for IgE (see Fig.1.67). Mast cells may be important in the defence against parasites; they are also responsible for many of the adverse symptoms in allergic disorders.

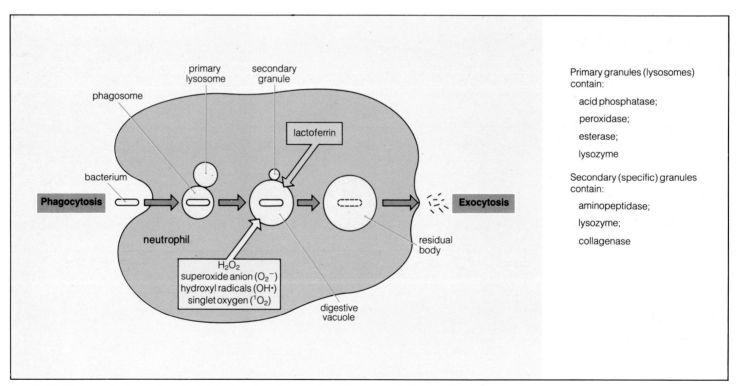

Fig.1.58 Phagocytosis and bacterial destruction: the neutrophil surrounds the bacterium with an invaginated surface membrane to form a phagosome by fusion with a primary lysosome. The lysosomal enzymes attack the bacterium. Secondary granules also fuse with the phagosomes, and new enzymes and lactoferrin attack the organism. Various types of activated oxygen generated by glucose metabolism also help to kill bacteria. Undigested residual bacterial products are excreted by exocytosis.

MONONUCLEAR PHAGOCYTIC SYSTEM
Monocytes

Monocytes spend only a short time in the marrow. Their precursors (monoblasts and promonocytes) are difficult to distinguish from myeloblasts and monocytes.

Monocytes are active phagocytes. Ingestion and adherence to microorganisms are facilitated by special surface receptors for the Fc position of IgG and for complement (for example, C3b) with which the microorganisms may be coated. Monocytes carry other surface markers including HLA-DR and those for lymphokines, such as γ-interferon and migration inhibition factor. Monocytic lysosomes contain acid hydrolases and peroxidase, which are important in the intracellular destruction of microorganisms. They also produce complement components, prostaglandins, interferons, tumour necrosis factor (TNF) and monokines, such as interleukin 1.

After circulating for twenty to forty hours, monocytes leave the blood to enter the tissues where they mature and carry out their principal functions. Their extravascular lifespan may be as long as several months or sometimes years. These cells are divided into the phagocytic macrophages, whose role is to remove particulate antigens, and the antigen-presenting cells, whose main function is to present antigens to lymphocytes (Figs. 1.59 & 1.60).

Reticuloendothelial system: phagocytes and antigen-presenting cells

In addition to the wandering or free tissue macrophages, the monocyte-derived phagocytic cells form a network known as the reticuloendothelial system (RES) and are found in many organs (Fig. 1.59). This system includes the Küpffer cells in the liver, alveolar macrophages in the lung, macrophages of various serosal surfaces, mesangial cells of the kidney, brain microglia and macrophages of the bone marrow, splenic sinuses and lymph nodes.

Antigen-presenting cells (APCs) are found primarily in the skin, lymph nodes, spleen and thymus. Following stimulation, the Langerhans cells of the skin migrate via the afferent lymphatics into the paracortical areas of draining lymph nodes where they 'interdigitate' with T cells, presenting them with antigens carried from the skin (Fig. 1.60). Other specialized APCs include the follicular dendritic cells found in the germinal centres of lymph nodes and other lymphoid tissues, and the interdigitating follicular cells found in the thymus.

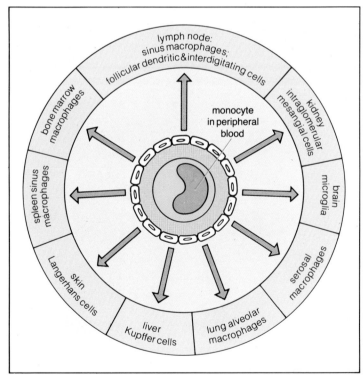

Fig.1.59 Reticuloendothelial system: distribution of macrophages.

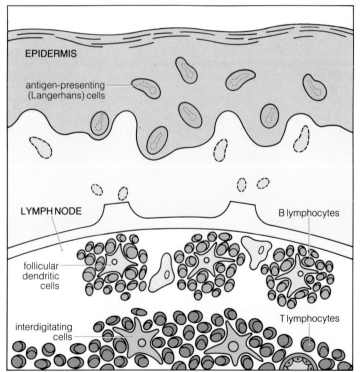

Fig.1.60 Antigen-presenting cells in the skin and lymph nodes: Langerhans cells in the epidermis are characterized by the presence of Birbeck bodies (tennis racquet-shaped collections of granules). These antigen-carrying cells migrate via afferent lymphatics to the neighbouring lymph nodes and become interdigitating cells in the T-cell paracortical zone. Follicular dendritic cells, bone marrow-derived as are Langerhans cells, are found in the B-cell germinal centres.

LYMPHOCYTES

Lymphocytes assist the phagocytes in the defence of the body against infection and other foreign invasion, and add specificity to the attack. There are two main groups of lymphocytes with different functions, T cells and B cells, which are indistinguishable by traditional Romanowsky staining. T cells are processed initially in the thymus and B cells are produced in the bone marrow. In birds, B cells differentiate in an organ known as the bursa of Fabricius.

T cells

Mature T cells carry a marker (antigen CD5) which binds

sheep erythrocytes (Fig.1.61) and comprise sixty-five to eighty percent of the circulating lymphocyte population. Other surface markers may be defined by indirect immunofluorescence or by immunoperoxidase-linked specific antibodies (Fig.1.62), some of which are able to define subpopulations of T cells, such as the CD4 (T4) marker on T-helper cells and CD8 (T8) marker on T-suppressor/cytotoxic cells (see Fig.7.33). CD4 cells predominate in the peripheral blood and CD8 cells form the major subpopulation in the bone marrow. T cells also contain a number of lysosomal acid hydrolases, such as ß–glucuronidase, and acid phosphatase, which may be detected cytologically as discrete

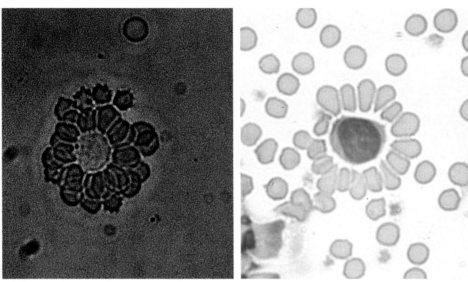

Fig.1.61 T lymphocytes: following centrifugation together, human T lymphocytes and sheep red cells bind to each other in rosettes. Phase-contrast microscopy (left), May-Grünwald/Giemsa stain (right)

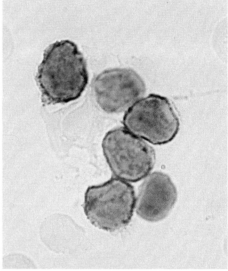

Fig.1.62 T lymphocytes: human T cells identified by (brown) staining of surface antigen (four of the six central cells are T cells). Immunoperoxidase technique using OKT11 (CD5) monoclonal antibody.

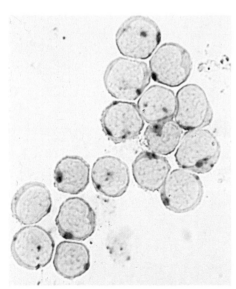

Fig.1.63 T lymphocytes: using acid phosphatase, the cells show polar positive (red) staining in the Golgi zone.

Gene	Chromosome (band)	
Immunoglobulin		
heavy	14	(q32)
light		
ϰ	2	(p12)
λ	22	(q11)
T-cell receptor		
α	14	(q11)
β	7	(q35)
γ	7	(p14-15)

Fig.1.64 Chromosomal locations of the genes for immunoglobulins and the T-cell receptor.

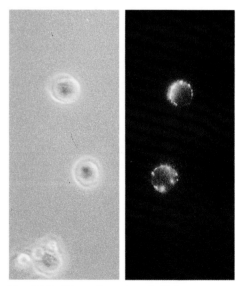

Fig.1.65 B lymphocytes: (left) three peripheral blood lymphocytes seen by phase-contrast microscopy; (right) patchy fluorescence under UV light using fluoresceinated anti-human Ig shows that only two of the cells carry surface Ig.

masses in the Golgi zone in the cytoplasm (Fig.1.63).

The T-cell surface contains an antigen receptor consisting of α and β chains, each with variable and constant portions (see Chapter 7). A γ chain is also present but its function is as yet unclear. The genes for these polypeptide chains, on chromosomes 14 and 7 (Fig.1.64), are rearranged in T cells in a manner similar to the rearrangement of immunoglobulin genes in B cells, resulting in a wide diversity among T lymphocytes (see Chapter 7). Close by the T-cell receptor is a complex of proteins termed the CD3 complex, which consists of γ, δ and ε chains. This complex is probably responsible for transducing signals derived from interaction of antigen with the T-cell receptor to the cell interior. The sequence of gene rearrangements and antigen expression during T-cell development in the cortex and medulla of the thymus is illustrated in Fig.7.33.

B cells

This subpopulation of lymphocytes comprises five to fifteen percent of the circulating lymphocyte population. Mature B cells are defined by the presence of endogenously produced immunoglobulin (Ig) molecules inserted into the surface membrane where they act as receptors for specific antigens. Fluorescein-labelled specific antibodies may be used to demonstrate these surface-bound Ig molecules (Fig.1.65) and B cells can be identified by monoclonal antibodies to certain surface cell antigens, for example, CD19, detected by B4 antibody (Fig.1.66).

The surface immunoglobulins are individual to each clone of B cells and are identical to those secreted as antibodies by the B lymphocyte or plasma cell. The Ig may be one of five classes: IgM, IgD, IgG (divided into four subtypes), IgE or IgA (divided into two subtypes). Each immunoglobulin molecule consists of light chains (κ or λ) and heavy chains (μ, δ, γ, ε or α respectively) which determine the class of immunoglobulin (Fig.1.67). The heavy-chain genes are arranged in the order given above on chromosome 14 and the light-chain genes on chromosomes 2 (κ) and 22 (λ) (see Fig.1.64).

The sequence of antigen expression and gene rearrangements in early B-cell development, which occurs in the bone marrow, is illustrated in Fig.7.29. The immunoglobulins are expressed in the cytoplasm (in pre-B cells; Fig.1.68) before they can be detected on the surface while the nuclear enzyme, terminal deoxynucleotide transferase (TdT), is expressed early in B-cell ontogeny. Diversity is produced by differences in the rearrangement of the genes for the variable (V), diversity (D), joining (J) and constant (C) regions of the immunoglobulins they secrete. The majority of B cells carry HLA-DR antigens, which are important in the regulation of the immune response. Complement receptors for C3b and C3d are also found on more mature B cells.

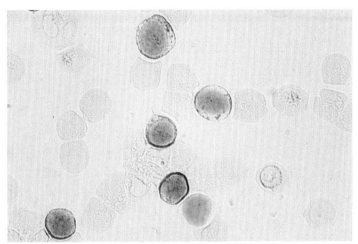

Fig.1.66 B lymphocytes: identification by (brown) staining of antibody fixed to a surface antigen using the immunoperoxidase technique and B4 (CD19) monoclonal antibody.

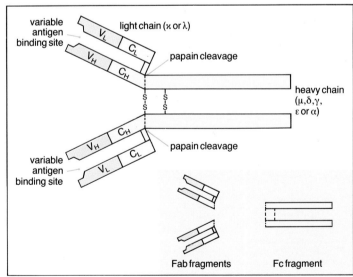

Fig.1.67 Basic structure of an immunoglobulin molecule: each molecule is made up of two light (κ or λ) and two heavy chains, and each chain is made up of variable (V) and constant (C) portions, the V portions including the antigen binding site. The heavy chain (γ, μ, δ, ε or α) varies according to the immunoglobulin class. IgA molecules form dimers while IgM forms a ring of 5 molecules. Papain cleaves the molecules into an Fc fragment and two Fab fragments.

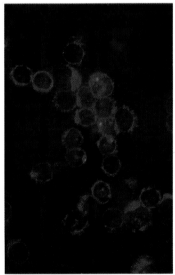
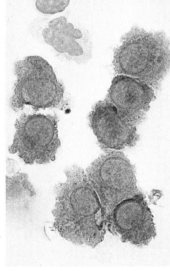

Fig.1.68 Pre-B lymphoid cells: peripheral blood cells expressing intracytoplasmic IgM as (left) a crystalline appearance using indirect immunofluorescence, from a patient with chronic lymphocytic leukaemia, and (right) using the indirect immunoperoxidase method, from a case of hairy cell leukaemia. Courtesy of Dr. J.V. Melo.

'Null' cells

There is a minor population of 'lymphocytic' cells which do not carry markers of either T or B cells and are known as 'non-T, non-B' cells or 'third population' cells. The sequence of differentiation of these cells is not known. The majority of 'null' cells appear as large granular lymphocytes (see Fig.1.50) in the peripheral blood. It appears likely that this population of cells contains the majority of natural-killer (NK) cells and antibody-dependent cellular cytotoxic (ADCC) cells which are able to kill tumour and virus-infected cells. Small numbers of circulating 'null' cells are immature T or B cells and myeloid or erythroid progenitor cells.

Lymphocyte proliferation and differentiation

T and B cells proliferate and develop in reactive lymphoid tissue, for example, lymph nodes, and lymphoid tissues of the alimentary and respiratory tracts and spleen. Both T and B cells acquire receptors for antigens, which commit them to a single antigenic specificity, and are activated when they bind their specific antigen in the presence of accessory cells. Antigen-presenting cells (APCs) interact with T cells bearing the appropriate receptor for that particular antigen providing there is major histocompatibility complex (MHC; see below) recognition (class I for CD8 and class II for CD4 cells). B cells with the appropriate surface receptor (immuno-globulin) for the antigen are also stimulated (Fig.1.69). Subsequently, these stimulated T and B cells proliferate and differentiate under the stimulus of factors released from antigen-presenting cells (interleukin 1) and activated helper T cells (interleukin 2; Fig.1.70). The helper T lymphocytes also secrete B-cell growth factor (BCGF), which causes B cells to multiply, and B cell differentiation factor (BCDF), which stimulates the B cells to produce antibodies and to stop replication. Clones of both effector and memory B cells are produced. When the memory cells are stimulated at a later date by their specific antigen, they are able to proliferate again in an accelerated fashion (secondary response).

Activated T cells become responsible for cell-mediated immunity and secrete a number of lymphokines, including interleukins 2 and 3, interferons α and γ, migration inhibition factor, lymphotoxins, tumour necrosis factor and others which activate killer T cells, enabling them to attack an

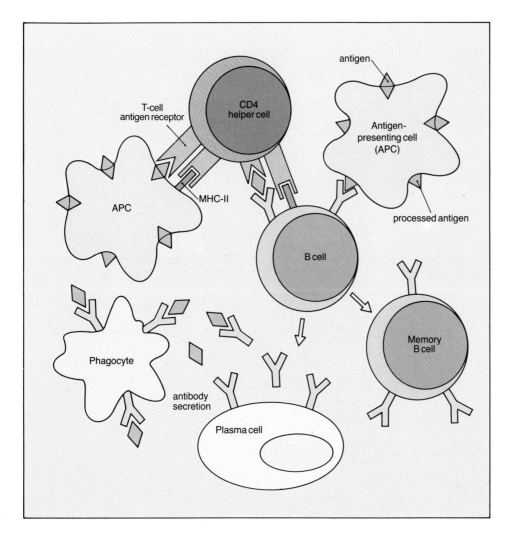

Fig.1.69 The immune response: there is interaction between an APC and a CD4$^+$ (helper) T cell, with MHC-II and antigen–T-cell receptor recognition, and both cells interact with a B cell with recognition between its surface immunoglobulin and the antigen. As a result, clones of T cells and B cells are stimulated to proliferate (see Fig.1.70), the B cells becoming either plasma cells secreting antibody to the antigen or memory B cells. A phago-cyte takes up the antigen–antibody complex.

invading organism or cell and induce macrophages to stay at the site of infection and help to digest the cells they have phagocytosed. T–helper cells are important in the initiation of a B-cell response to antigens; T-suppressor cells reduce the B-lymphocytic response, and T-cytotoxic cells are capable of directly damaging cells recognized as foreign or virus–

infected (Fig. 1.71).

Activated B cells are responsible for humoral immunity. Many B-cell blasts mature into plasma cells which produce and secrete antibodies of one specificity and immunoglobulin class (Fig. 1.72). B lymphocytes at different stages of differentiation and activation are shown in Fig. 1.73.

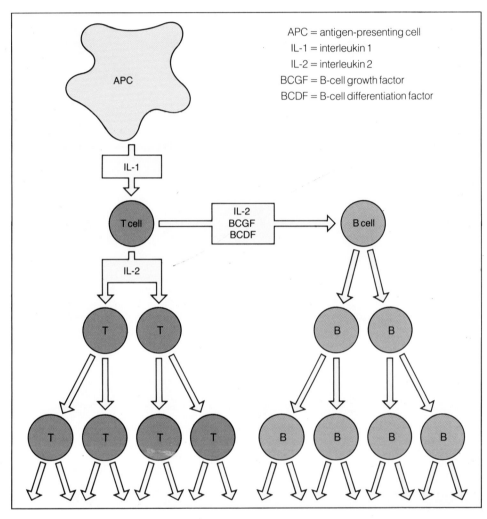

APC = antigen-presenting cell
IL-1 = interleukin 1
IL-2 = interleukin 2
BCGF = B-cell growth factor
BCDF = B-cell differentiation factor

Fig.1.70 Roles of interleukins 1 and 2 (IL-1 & -2), and B-cell growth and differentiation factors (BCGF & BCDF) in the immune response: reaction between an APC and a T cell leads to secretion of IL-1 by the APC, which stimulates the T cell to secrete IL-2, thus stimulating T cells to undergo cell division. The T cell also secretes BCGF which, with IL-2, stimulates interacting B cells to proliferate, and BCDF, which switches off the proliferative response and stimulates the B cells to terminal differentiation and antibody secretion. A proportion of the B cells become memory cells which react with an accelerated response if re-challenged with the same antigen.

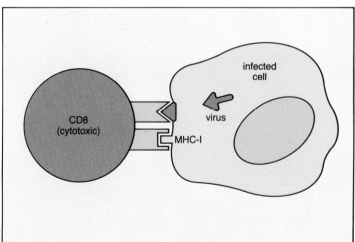

Fig.1.71 Interaction between a CD8⁺ (cytotoxic) T cell and a virus-infected cell: when there is MHC-I recognition between the two cells as well as correspondence between the antigens of the virus expressed on the cell surface and the T cell antigen receptor on the surface of the CD8⁺ cell, the CD8⁺ cell kills the virus-infected cell.

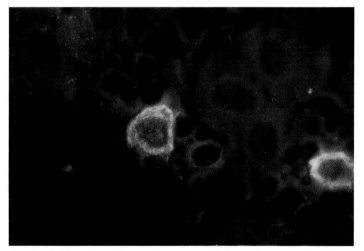

Fig.1.72 Plasma cells: two plasma cells from a bone marrow aspirate show intense intracytoplasmic fluorescence. Fluoresceinated anti-IgG, Evans blue counterstain.

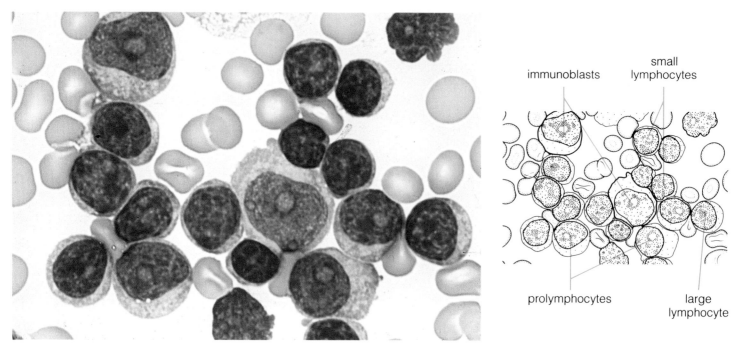

Fig.1.73 B lymphocytes: peripheral blood film of a patient with chronic lymphocytic leukaemia with prolymphocytoid transformation shows B lymphocytes at various stages of development. Courtesy of Dr. J.V. Melo.

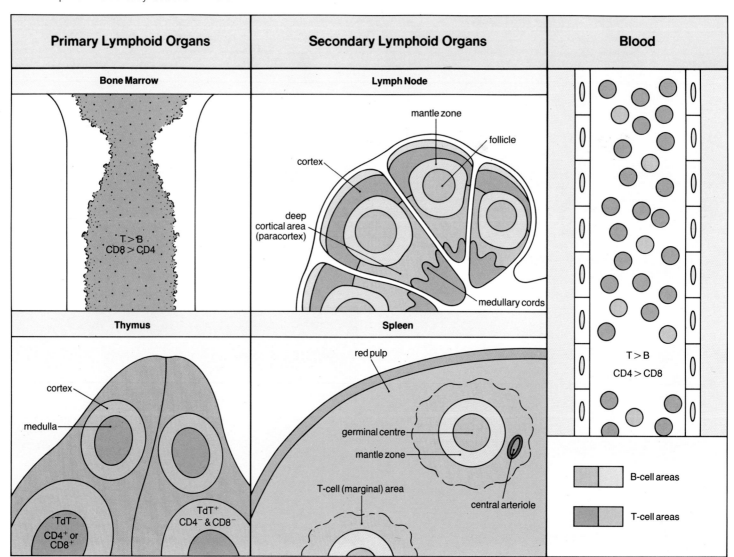

Fig.1.74 Lymphocyte distribution: primary and secondary lymphoid organs and blood. Aggregates of secondary lymphoid tissue are found elsewhere in the body, e.g. Peyer's patches of the small intestine. The mantle zones of the lymph nodes and spleen also contain macrophages and APCs, and the paracortex also contains many interdigitating reticulum cells (IDC).

Lymphocyte circulation

Lymphocytes from the primary lymphoid organs of the marrow and thymus migrate via the blood through post-capillary venules into the substance of lymph nodes, into unencapsulated lymphoid collections of the body and into the spleen. T cells home to the paracortical areas of the nodes and to the periarteriolar sheaths of the spleen. B cells accumulate selectively in germinal follicles of lymphoid tissue, in the subcapsular periphery of the cortex and in the medullary cords of the lymph nodes (Figs. 1.74 & 1.75). Lymphocytes return to the peripheral blood by the efferent lymphatic system and the thoracic duct. The median duration of a complete circulation is about ten hours. The majority of recirculating cells are T cells. B cells are mainly sessile cells and spend long periods in lymphoid tissue and the spleen. Many more lymphocytes have long lifespans and may survive as memory cells for several years.

HUMAN LEUCOCYTE ANTIGEN (HLA) SYSTEM

The short arm of chromosome 6 contains a cluster of genes known as the major histocompatibility complex (MHC) or the human leucocyte antigen (HLA) region (Fig. 1.76).

Among the genes in this region are those that code for the proteins of the HLA antigens which are present on the cell membranes of many nucleated cells. As well as playing a major role in transplant rejection, these antigens are involved in many aspects of immunological recognition and reaction.

MHC proteins are classified into three types. Class I proteins comprise two polypeptides, the larger of which is encoded by the MHC. The small component, a β–micro-globulin, is encoded outside the MHC. Class II proteins comprise an α and a β chain, both of which are encoded by the MHC. Class III proteins are the complement components encoded by the MHC region.

In man, the main regions of the MHC gene complex are A, B, C, and D. The class I proteins encoded by the A, B and C regions act as surface recognition antigens which can be identified by cytotoxic (CD8–positive) T lymphocytes. The D region genes encode class II proteins which are involved in cooperation and interaction between helper (CD4–positive) lymphocytes and antigen-presenting cells. HLA-A, –B and –C antigens are present on all nucleated cells and platelets, and those encoded by the D region are present on B lympho-cytes, monocytes, macrophages and some activated T cells.

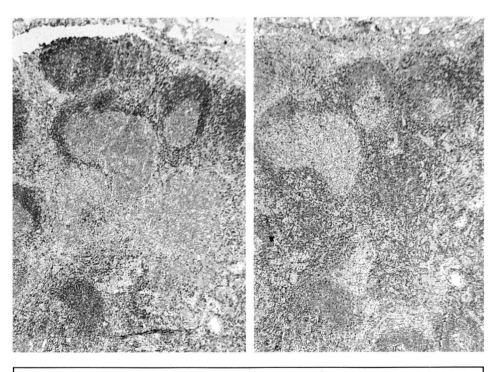

Fig. 1.75 B- and T-lymphocyte distribu-tion: lymph node section showing (left) B cells in the germinal centres, their coro-nas (heavy staining) in the subcapsular cortex and medullary cords; (right) T-cells are most numerous in perifollicular areas of the deeper cortical region. Immuno-peroxidase technique using (left) pan-B monoclonal antibody B4 (CD19) and (right) OKT11 (CD2) monoclonal anti-body.

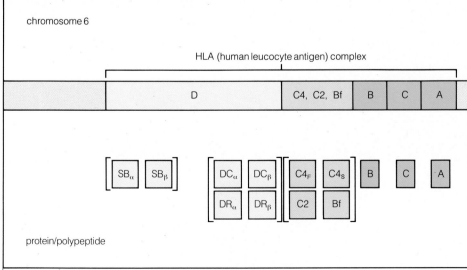

Fig. 1.76 HLA gene complex on chromo-some 6: regions B,C, and A encode MHC-I molecules; D encodes α and ß chains of MHC-II proteins SB, DC and DR (carrying specificities DP, DQ and DR respectively). The region between D and B encodes class 3 (complement; C3) proteins, including tandem alleles of C4 and genes for C2 and factor B (Bf). The polypeptides are bracketed because the precise gene order is uncertain.

HLA-A, -B and -C typing is usually carried out on peripheral blood lymphocytes. Originally, antigens of the D system were identified by non-reactivity in a mixed lymphocyte culture (MLC) reaction (a lymphocyte reaction proliferation assay) against rare homozygous D-locus cells.

More recently, it has been possible to detect HLA-D region antigens serologically and these are referred to as HLA-DR and are subdivided into three groups: DR, DP and DQ. A current list of HLA antigens is presented in Fig. 1.77.

A	B		C	D	DR	DQ	DP
A1	B5	Bw50(21)	Cw1	Dw1	DR1	DQw1	DPw1
A2	B7	B51 (5)	Cw2	Dw2	DR2	DQw2	DPw2
A3	B8	Bw52(5)	Cw3	Dw3	DR3	DQw3	DPw3
A9	B12	Bw53	Cw4	Dw4	DR4		DPw4
A10	B13	Bw54(w22)	Cw5	Dw5	DR5		DPw5
A11	B14	Bw55(w22)	Cw6	Dw6	DRw6		DPw6
Aw19	B15	Bw56(w22)	Cw7	Dw7	DR7		
A23 (9)	B16	Bw57(17)	Cw8	Dw8	DRw8		
A24 (9)	B17	Bw58(17)		Dw9	DRw9		
A25(10)	B18	Bw59		Dw10	DRw10		
A26(10)	B21	Bw60(40)		Dw11(w7)	DRw11(5)		
A28	Bw22	Bw61(40)		Dw12	DRw12(5)		
A29(w19)	B27	Bw62(15)		Dw13	DRw13(w6)		
A30(w19)	B35	Bw63(15)		Dw14	DRw14(w6)		
A31(w19)	B37	Bw64(14)		Dw15	DRw52		
A32(w19)	B38(16)	Bw65(14)		Dw16	DRw53		
Aw33(w19)	B39(16)	Bw67		Dw17(w7)			
Aw34(10)	B40	Bw70		Dw18(w6)			
Aw36	Bw41	Bw71(w70)		Dw19(w6)			
Aw43	Bw42	Bw72(w70)					
Aw66(10)	B44(12)	Bw73					
Aw68(28)	B45(12)						
Aw69(28)	Bw46						
	Bw47	Bw4					
	Bw48	Bw6					
	B49(21)						

Fig.1.77 Recognized HLA specificities: established specificities are denoted by a number, and those not fully confirmed are prefixed by a 'w' (workshop). More restricted specificities are included in a broader group ('splits') shown in brackets following the firmer specificity. Antigens Bw4 and Bw6 are very broad ('public') and include splits which have been further subdivided

2

HYPOCHROMIC ANAEMIAS

The hypochromic anaemias are characterized by hypochromic cells in the peripheral blood with a reduced mean cell haemoglobin (MCH) of less than 27pg. The cells are also usually microcytic with a mean cell volume (MCV) of less than 80fl. With manual methods of haemoglobin and haematocrit (packed cell volume, PCV) estimation, the mean corpuscular haemoglobin concentration (MCHC) is also reduced (to less than 32g/dl); but this estimation is not of value when using modern electronic counters.

The hypochromasia is due to failure of haemoglobin synthesis (Fig.2.1), most commonly as a result of iron deficiency; but it may also arise from a block in iron metabolism as in the anaemia of chronic disorders, failure of protoporphyrin and haem synthesis as in the sideroblastic anaemias, or failure of globin synthesis as in the thalassaemias (see Chapter 5) or crystallization of haemoglobin in some of the other haemoglobin disorders, for example, haemoglobin C (see Chapter 5). Lead inhibits both haem and globin synthesis and may cause a hypochromic anaemia, but also causes haemolysis probably because of failure of RNA breakdown.

IRON DEFICIENCY ANAEMIA

The symptoms of iron deficiency are caused by anaemia (if sufficiently severe) as well as, in some cases, by damage to epithelial tissues. Also, there may be symptoms of the underlying disease which is causing the deficiency. On rare occasions, the patient has a craving for bizarre food (pica), such as ice, chalk or paper.

The patient with iron deficiency anaemia may show pallor of the mucous membranes, which is usually recognized clinically only if the haemoglobin is less than about 9.0g/dl. There is pallor of the lips, conjunctivae, creases of the palms and nail beds (Figs.2.2-2.4). Skin colour, however, is not a reliable sign of anaemia since it depends on the state of the skin circulation as well as on the haemoglobin content of the blood. The patient's nails frequently are ridged and brittle (Fig.2.5) or may show koilonychia (spoon nails; Fig.2.6). There may be angular cheilosis (stomatitis; cracking at the corners of the mouth), especially in those with badly fitting false teeth (Fig.2.7).

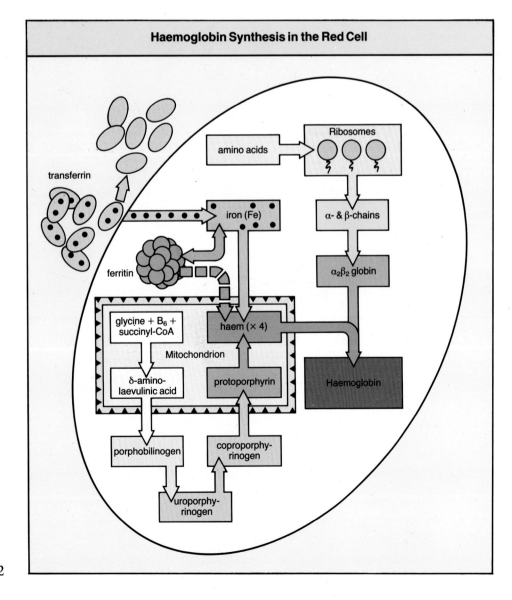

Haemoglobin Synthesis in the Red Cell

Fig.2.1 Haemoglobin synthesis in developing red cell: iron enters the cell from transferrin and is combined with protoporphyrin which is synthesized largely from glycine and succinyl-CoA in mitochondria to form haem. One molecule of haem attaches to one of the globin polypeptide chains and one haemoglobin molecule is made up of four haem/globin units. Hypochromic anaemias arise due to lack of iron (iron deficiency or anaemia of chronic disorders), failure of haem synthesis (sideroblastic anaemia or lead poisoning), failure of α- or β-globin chain synthesis (α- or β-thalassaemias) or the presence of an abnormal haemoglobin (such as haemoglobin C).

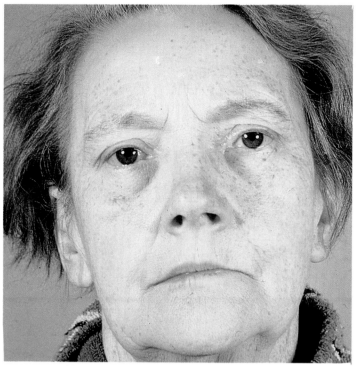

Fig.2.2 Iron deficiency anaemia: pallor of mucous membranes (lips) and skin in a 69-year-old female. *Hb:8.1g/dl; RBC:4.13x10^{12}/l; PCV:26.8%; MCV:65fl; MCH:19.6pg.*

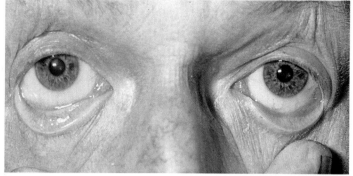

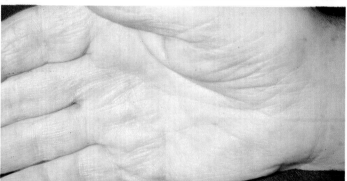

Fig.2.3 Iron deficiency anaemia: (upper) pallor of conjunctival mucosa. Mucous membrane pallor becomes clinically apparent when the haemoglobin concentration is below 9.0g/dl; (lower) pallor of palmar skin creases.

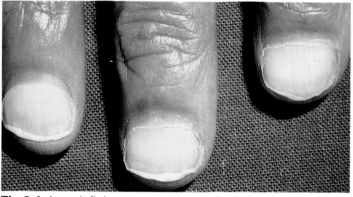

Fig.2.4 Iron deficiency anaemia: marked pallor of the nail beds in a dark-skinned patient. The nails are flattened.

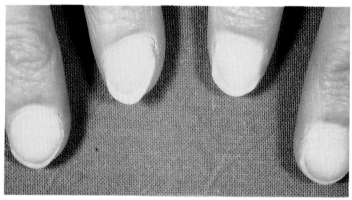

Fig.2.5 Iron deficiency anaemia: although there is no obvious concavity, these nails are flattened and brittle with marked pallor of the nail beds.

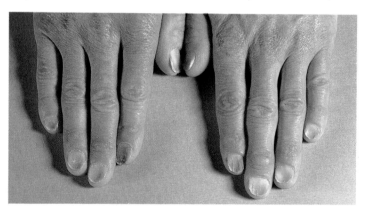

Fig.2.6 Iron deficiency anaemia: koilonychia. The nails are concave, ridged and brittle. This patient's anaemia had been rapidly corrected by blood transfusion prior to an operation for caecal carcinoma. The cause of the nail changes in iron deficiency is uncertain, but may be related to the iron requirement of many enzymes present in epithelial and other cells. Courtesy of Dr. S.M. Knowles.

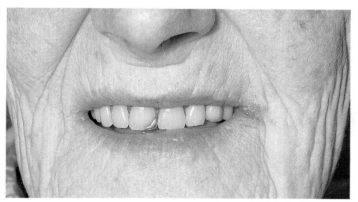

Fig.2.7 Iron deficiency anaemia: angular cheilosis. There is fissuring and ulceration at the corners of the mouth. The biochemical mechanism is uncertain but may be similar to that for nail, mucosal and pharyngeal changes (see Figs. 2.4-2.6, 2.8 & 2.9).

In severe cases especially in older patients, an atrophic glossitis with loss of filiform papillae (Fig.2.8) may be present.

There may also be dysphagia due to postcricoid webs (Plummer-Vinson or Paterson-Kelly syndrome), especially in middle-aged women (Fig.2.9).

The biochemical explanation for these epithelial cell abnormalities is unclear; it may be related to a reduction in haem–containing enzymes, for example, cytochromes, cytochrome c oxidase, succinic dehydrogenase, catalase, peroxidase, ribonucleotide reductase, xanthine oxidase and aconitase. When the anaemia is very severe and of rapid onset, there may be retinal haemorrhages (Fig.2.10).

Blood and bone marrow appearances

The blood film shows the presence of hypochromic microcytic red cells (Figs.2.11-2.13) with abnormally shaped cells ('pencil' or cigar-shaped poikilocytes) and occasional target cells. The severity of the blood film changes and of the fall in the MCH and MCV are related to the degree of anaemia. The platelet count is often raised, particularly if haemorrhage is occurring.

The bone marrow is of normal cellularity, sometimes with normoblastic hyperplasia, and the developing erythroblasts show a ragged vacuolated cytoplasm (Fig.2.14). Perls' staining shows a complete absence of iron stores (Fig.2.15) and of siderotic granules from developing erythroblasts (Fig.2.16).

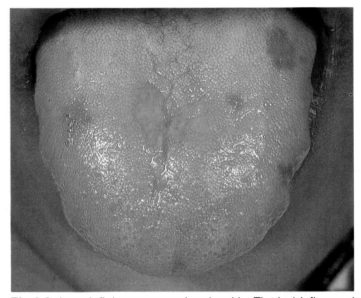

Fig.2.8 Iron deficiency anaemia: glossitis. The bald, fissured appearance of the tongue is due to flattening and loss of papillae.

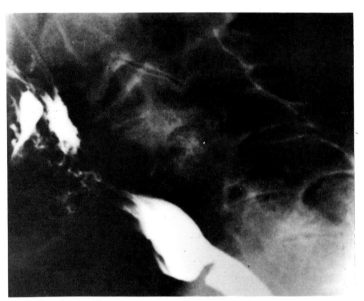

Fig.2.9 Iron deficiency anaemia: barium swallow radiograph showing a postcricoid web causing a filling defect, in a 50-year-old female with the Plummer-Vinson (Paterson-Kelly) syndrome who complained of dysphagia.

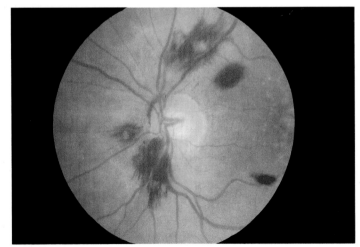

Fig.2.10 Iron deficiency anaemia: multiple retinal haemorrhages in a 25-year-old female with chronic iron deficiency due to severe haemorrhage (menorrhagia). *Hb:2.5g/dl.*

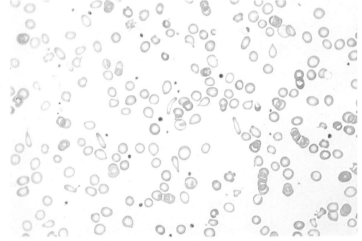

Fig.2.11 Iron deficiency anaemia: low power view of peripheral blood film. The red cells are hypochromic and microcytic. Some poikilocytes are present, including thin elongated ('pencil') cells and occasional target cells. Platelets are plentiful. *Hb:6.4g/dl.*

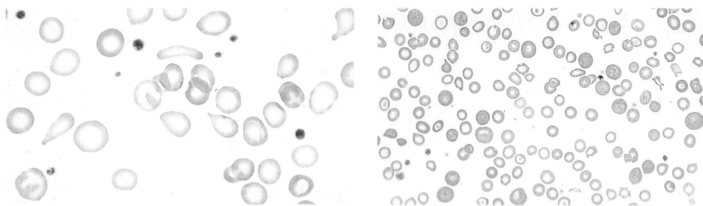

Fig.2.12 Iron deficiency anaemia: high power view of peripheral blood film shows hypochromic microcytic cells and poikilocytes.

Fig.2.13 Iron deficiency anaemia: low power peripheral blood film taken during therapy with oral iron. There is a dimorphic population of hypochromic microcytic cells and well haemoglobinized cells of normal size but with some large polychromatic cells (newly formed well haemoglobinized reticulocytes).

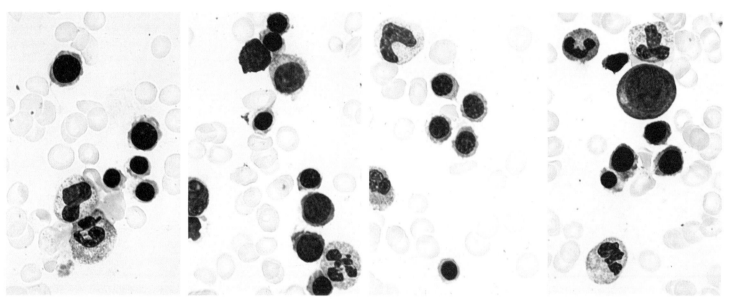

Fig.2.14 Iron deficiency anaemia: bone marrow aspirate. The cytoplasm of polychromatic and pyknotic erythroblasts is scanty, vacuolated and irregular in outline. This type of erythropoiesis has been described as 'micronormoblastic'.

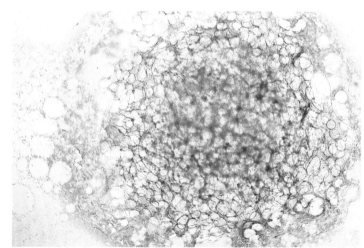

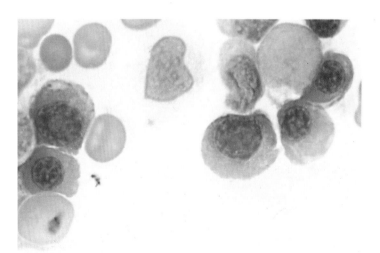

Fig.2.15 Iron deficiency anaemia: bone marrow aspirate showing absence of stainable iron in a bone marrow fragment. The appearances are similar in iron deficiency anaemia and latent iron deficiency (absent iron stores without anaemia). Compare with the appearances of normal iron stores in Fig.1.27. Perls' stain, methyl red counterstain.

Fig.2.16 Iron deficiency anaemia: bone marrow aspirate showing lack of siderotic granules in developing erythroblasts. Compare with the normal appearances of isolated Prussian blue-positive granules in the erythroblast cytoplasm in Fig.1.27. Perls' stain, methyl red counterstain.

Causes of iron deficiency

The causes of iron deficiency anaemia are listed in Fig.2.17. About two-thirds of body iron is circulating in red cells as haemoglobin, one litre of blood containing about 500mg of iron. The next biggest store, which varies between 0–2g, is within the macrophages of the reticuloendothelial system in the form of the storage proteins haemosiderin (visible on light microscopy) and ferritin (seen only by electron microscopy). Absence of iron stores with a fall in serum iron and serum ferritin, but without anaemia and without a fall in red cell indices, is termed 'latent iron deficiency'. Iron in myoglobin and a variety of enzymes make up the rest of body iron.

Daily losses and, thus, requirements for iron in adults, are normally small in relation to body stores, about 1mg daily in males and postmenopausal females, and from 1.5–3.0mg in menstruating females. Requirements are also increased in children (to provide for growth and the increase in red cell mass) and during pregnancy for transfer to the fetus.

Iron deficiency is usually the result of haemorrhage, the most common cause in many countries being hookworm infestation (Fig.2.18); the loss is related to the worm load. In females, menorrhagia or repeated pregnancies without iron supplementation are frequent causes. In men and postmenopausal women, iron deficiency is usually due to chronic gastrointestinal blood

Causes of Iron Deficiency				
Haemorrhage	Gastrointestinal	Pulmonary	Transfer to fetus	Pregnancy
	hiatus hernia	pulmonary haemosiderosis		
	oesophageal varices		Haemosiderinuria	Chronic intravascular haemodialysis
	peptic ulcer	Uterine		paroxysmal nocturnal haemoglobinuria
	aspirin ingestion	menorrhagia		heart valve haemolysis
	hookworm	ante- & postpartum		
	neoplasm		Malabsorption	Atrophic gastritis
	ulcerative colitis	Renal tract		Gluten-induced enteropathy
	telangiectasia	haematuria		Partial gastrectomy
	angiodysplasia	chronic dialysis		
	diverticulosis		Poor diet	Poor quality diet,
	haemorrhoids	Self-induced		especially if mostly vegetable

Fig.2.17 Causes of iron deficiency anaemia.

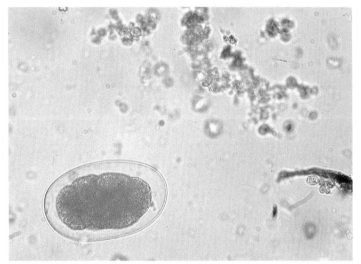

Fig.2.18 Iron deficiency anaemia: ova of *Ancylostoma duodenale* (hookworm). This parasite is a frequent cause of iron deficiency anaemia in many parts of the world. The amount of blood loss and therefore severity of anaemia is related to the degree of parasitization.

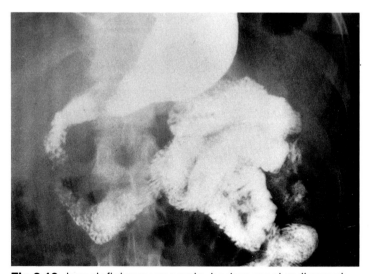

Fig.2.19 Iron deficiency anaemia: barium meal radiograph showing a gross hiatus hernia in a 55-year-old patient. Endoscopy showed a small ulcerated area of bleeding.

loss, which in Western countries is often the result of hiatus hernia (Fig.2.19), peptic ulceration (Fig.2.20), chronic aspirin ingestion, colonic or caecal carcinoma (Fig.2.21), angiodysplasia (Fig.2.22), colonic diverticulosis or haemorrhoids. Rare causes of iron deficiency are pulmonary haemosiderosis (Fig.2.23), chronic intravascular haemolysis as in paroxysmal nocturnal haemoglobinuria, and self-inflicted venesection.

A normal Western diet contains 10-15mg of iron of which five to ten percent is absorbed. Iron absorption is increased in iron deficiency but reduced by some food substances, such as phytates and phosphates. Although

poor dietary intake of iron may be the sole cause of iron deficiency if present for many years, more often it provides a background of reduced iron stores in which other causes of iron deficiency, such as heavy menstrual loss, or increased requirements for pregnancy or for growth in children, may lead to iron deficiency anaemia.

Malabsorption alone is also an unusual cause of iron deficiency. Even in patients with atrophic gastritis or coeliac disease, loss due to increased turnover of cells and exudation of transferrin iron may be as important as the malabsorption. Following gastrectomy, the two main factors are blood loss and malabsorption, more marked for food iron than for inorganic iron.

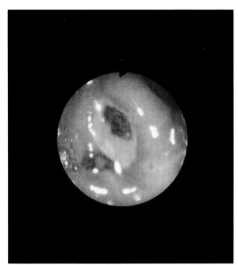

Fig.2.20 Iron deficiency anaemia: endoscopic appearance of a bleeding duodenal ulcer in a 45-year-old male who presented with symptoms of anaemia. Courtesy of Dr. R.E. Pounder.

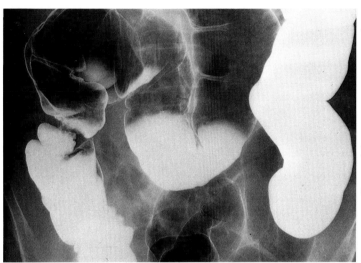

Fig.2.21 Iron deficiency anaemia: barium enema radiograph showing an annular filling defect of the ascending colon due to adenocarcinoma.

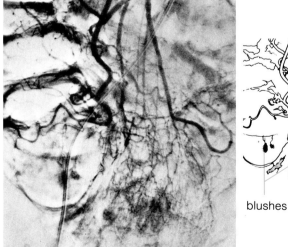

Fig.2.22 Iron deficiency anaemia: angiogram of coeliac axis showing numerous 'blushes' due to angiodysplasia of the terminal ileum and ascending colon. Courtesy of Dr.R. Dick.

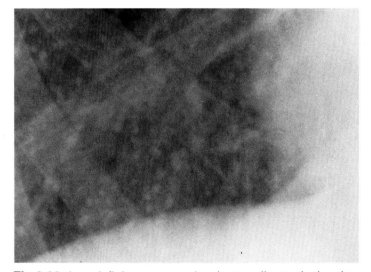

Fig.2.23 Iron deficiency anaemia: chest radiograph showing diffuse mottled appearance due to pulmonary haemosiderosis. The lesions consist of aggregates of iron-laden macrophages with surrounding fibrosis. Courtesy of Dr. R. Dick.

SIDEROBLASTIC ANAEMIA

Sideroblastic anaemia is characterized by the presence of ring sideroblasts in the bone marrow. It is classified into congenital and acquired types; the acquired type is further subdivided into a primary form and secondary types, including some which are associated with other bone marrow disorders (Fig.2.24).

The congenital type usually occurs in males, indicating a sex-linked pattern of inheritance (Fig.2.25); but it is seen, though rarely, in females (Fig.2.26) The blood film is hypochromic and microcytic or dimorphic of varying severity (Fig.2.27). About a third of these cases respond well to pyridoxine (vitamin B$_6$), a greater percentage than in the other types of sideroblastic anaemia.

In primary acquired sideroblastic anaemia, there is usually macrocytosis and gross anisocytosis and poikilocytosis (Fig.2.28). This disease is classified by the French–American–British group as one type of myelodysplasia (see Chapter 9). In a proportion of patients the disease transforms, after a variable number of years, into acute myeloblastic leukaemia. In many cases, careful examination reveals white cell or platelet abnormalities in the peripheral blood or in their precursors in the marrow. These cases with trilineage dysplasia have a much higher incidence of acute myeloblastic leukaemia.

Siderotic granules are frequently seen in the peripheral blood red cells postsplenectomy, but may also be found with the spleen present (Fig.2.29). The bone marrow shows erythroid hyperplasia (Fig.2.30) with vacuolated normoblasts (Fig.2.31).

Causes of Sideroblastic Anaemia
Congenital
Hereditary sex-linked occurring in males
Autosomal
Acquired
Primary
Classified as one of the myelodysplastic syndromes
also termed 'idiopathic acquired sideroblastic anaemia' (see Chapter 9)
Associated with malignant marrow disorders
Acute myeloblastic leukaemia
Polycythaemia vera
Myelosclerosis
Myeloma
Myelodysplastic syndromes
Secondary
Drugs, e.g. isoniazid & cycloserine
Toxins, e.g. lead & alcohol
Megaloblastic anaemia
Haemolytic anaemia
Pregnancy
Rheumatoid arthritis
Carcinoma

Fig.2.24 Causes of sideroblastic anaemia.

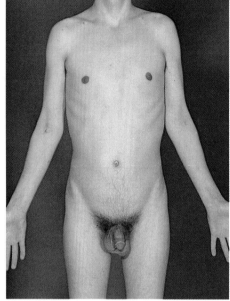

Fig.2.25 Sideroblastic anaemia: an 18-year-old male with hereditary (congenital) sideroblastic anaemia. He presented with symptoms of anaemia at the age of 16 and was found to have a microcytic hypochromic anaemia (*Hb:9.8g/dl; MCV:75fl; MCH:23.1pg*) with many ring sideroblasts in the bone marrow. His height (1.75m) and sexual development are normal. There is pallor of the mucous membranes and early melanin skin pigmentation due to iron overload arising from blood transfusions given over a two-year period, commencing soon after presentation because his haemoglobin had fallen spontaneously to less than 6.0g/dl. He subsequently died of infection with *Yersinia enterocolitica*, having received over 500 units of blood.

The patient's elder brother was also affected, the inheritance being sex-linked recessive. In both cases, the biochemical defect was in haem synthesis in erythroblasts at the level of δ-aminolaevulinic acid synthetase.

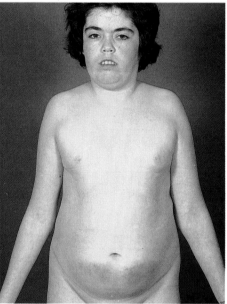

Fig.2.26 Sideroblastic anaemia: 17-year-old female with congenital sideroblastic anaemia, a rare occurrence. Iron overload developed because of the need for regular blood transfusions from the age of 3. She failed to commence menstruation and shows delayed puberty, absence of axillary and pubic hair, and minimal breast development. She also has a thalassaemic facies with a bossed skull, prominent maxilla and abnormally widened spaces between the teeth. The lower abdominal bruising is from the regular insertion of needles for subcutaneous desferrioxamine infusions.

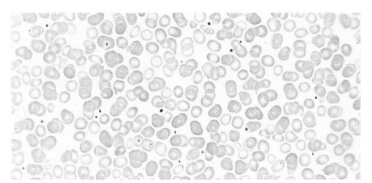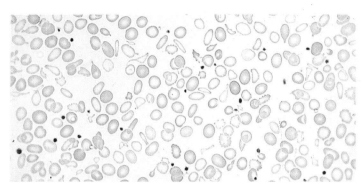

Fig.2.27 Sideroblastic anaemia (hereditary): peripheral blood film from a 19-year-old male shows a dimorphic anaemia with a mixture of poorly haemoglobinized microcytic cells and well haemoglobinized normocytic cells. *Hb:11.5g/dl; MCV:78fl; MCH:25.3pg.*

Fig.2.28 Sideroblastic anaemia (primary acquired): peripheral blood film from a 65-year-old male who presented with a predominantly hypochromic anaemia with numerous poikilocytes. In most cases of this type, the anaemia is dimorphic with an overall increase in MCV to above normal. *Hb:7.2g/dl; MCV:82fl; MCH:26.8pg.*

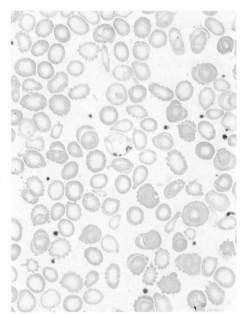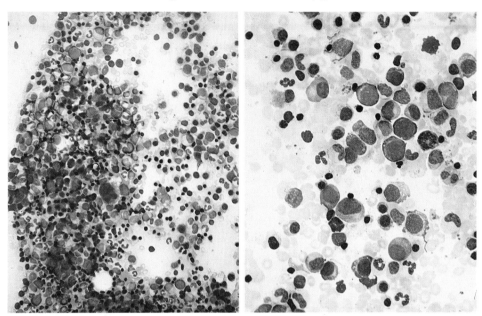

Fig.2.29 Sideroblastic anaemia (primary acquired): peripheral blood film following splenectomy showing abundant Pappenheimer bodies in the red cells. Their iron content is demonstrated by Perls' staining (siderotic granules). In addition, Howell-Jolly bodies (DNA remnants) are present and the platelet count is raised *(652x10⁹/l).*

Fig.2.30 Sideroblastic anaemia (primary acquired): low power view of bone marrow aspirate shows increased cellularity of the fragment and trails (left); at higher power, erythroid hyperplasia is also seen (right).

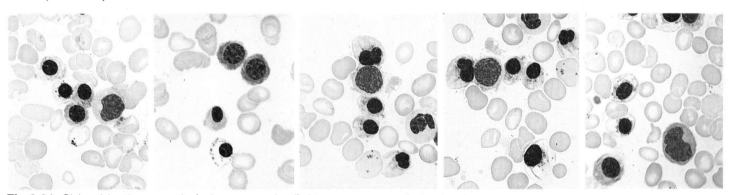

Fig.2.31 Sideroblastic anaemia (primary acquired): bone marrow aspirate showing vacuolation of erythroblasts with intact cytoplasmic margins. In some cells the vacuoles are surrounded by heavily stained cytoplasmic granules (punctate basophilia). Contrast the appearances with those in iron deficiency anaemia (see Fig.2.14) and thalassaemia major (see Fig.5.13).

In contrast to the inherited form, in primary acquired sideroblastic anaemia the erythroblasts are megaloblastic (in about fifty percent of cases; Fig.2.32). Iron staining shows many ring sideroblasts (Fig.2.33) and iron stores may be increased (Fig.2.34). In the primary forms of sideroblastic anaemia, twenty to fifty percent or often more of the normoblasts show partial or complete rings. In the secondary forms, ring sideroblasts are usually less frequent.

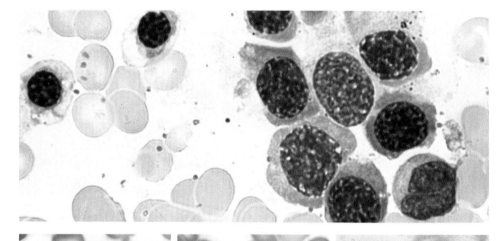

Fig.2.32 Sideroblastic anaemia (primary acquired): bone marrow aspirate showing megaloblastic erythroblasts. In this patient the serum vitamin B$_{12}$ and folate levels were normal; the deoxyuridine suppression test was normal; giant metamyelocytes and hypersegmented polymorphs were absent. Megaloblastic change is found in 50% of patients with this type of anaemia. The biochemical mechanism is uncertain.

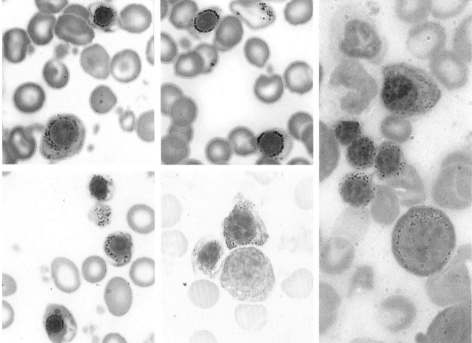

Fig.2.33 Sideroblastic anaemia (primary acquired): bone marrow aspirate showing erythroblasts with complete or nearly complete rings (or collars) of iron granules around their nuclei. The rings are best seen in late erythroblasts but, in severe cases, also occur in the earliest recognizable erythroblasts. Perls' stain.

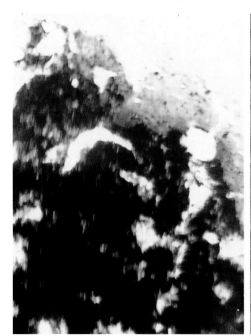
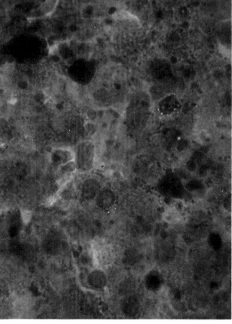

Fig.2.34 Sideroblastic anaemia (hereditary): bone marrow fragment stained for iron shows (left) a gross increase in iron in a patient who had been transfused for many years before the diagnosis was made. Treatment with pyridoxine allowed a satisfactory rise in haemoglobin, enabling subsequent venesections for reduction of iron overload; (right) high power view shows multiple ring sideroblasts and increased iron (haemosiderin) in macrophages.

LEAD POISONING

Clinically this presents with abdominal colic and constipation, a peripheral neuropathy and anaemia. There may be a lead line visible in the gums (Fig.2.35), marked punctate basophilia in the peripheral blood (Fig.2.36), a mild hypochromic anaemia with haemolysis, and ring sideroblasts in the marrow. The punctate basophilia is due to aggregates of undegraded RNA, a result of inhibition of the enzyme pyrimidine 5'nucleotidase.

THE PORPHYRIAS

Two main types of inherited defect of porphyrin synthesis associated with light sensitivity affect the haemopoietic system: congenital erythropoietic porphyria (CEP; Günther's disease); and congenital erythropoietic protoporphyria (CEPP). Although they are not associated with a hypochromic anaemia, they are discussed here for convenience.

CEP is inherited as an autosomal recessive and is characterized by excessive production of uroporphyrinogen I, which forms the pigments uroporphyrin I and coproporphyrin I. There is deficiency of the haem synthetic enzyme uroporphyrin III cosynthase. The plasma cells and erythrocytes contain excessive quantities of uroporphyrin I, coproporphyrin I and protoporphyrin.

The patient has bullous ulcerating lesions on light-exposed skin, hirsutism (Fig.2.37), and a haemolytic anaemia associated with splenomegaly.

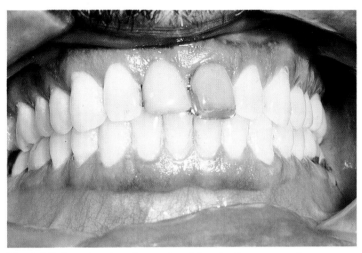

Fig.2.35 Lead poisoning: a lead line in the gums of a young man who presented with abdominal colic. The lead poisoning was from prolonged occupational exposure to molten lead.

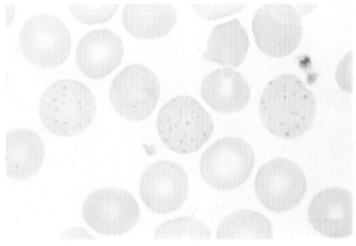

Fig.2.36 Lead poisoning: peripheral blood film showing punctate basophilia. This is due to precipitates of undegraded RNA, the result of inhibition by lead of pyrimidine 5'nucleotidase, one of the enzymes responsible for RNA degradation. Similar appearances occur in hereditary pyrimidine 5'nucleotidase deficiency.

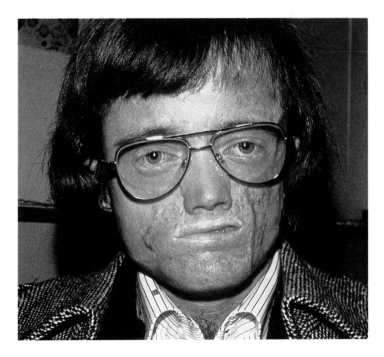

Fig.2.37 Congenital erythropoietic porphyria: this 22-year-old male was first diagnosed to have this condition (Günther's disease) at the age of 6, although skin changes had been noted from the age of 2, especially in the summer. These changes of blistering and susceptibility to mechanical injury were found on exposed areas of skin and led to mutilation of the extremities, including the nose, ears and hands. He has erythrodontia, splenomegaly and increased erythropoiesis with red cells which fluoresce. Haemolysis increased with age and is associated with a reticulocytosis. In this case, increased activity of δ-aminolaevulinate synthase and decreased activity of uroporphyrinogen cosynthase, were demonstrated with increased excretion of uroporphyrin I and coproporphyrin I in the urine, together with increased concentrations of these porphyrins in erythrocytes and plasma cells. Courtesy of Dr. M.R. Moore.

The urine is red and fluorescent (Fig.2.38); the bones and teeth are discoloured and also fluorescent (Fig.2.39). The nucleated red cells fluoresce when exposed to ultraviolet light (Fig.2.40).

CEPP is inherited as an autosomal dominant. The underlying defect is of ferrochelatase (haem synthetase), the final enzyme in haem synthesis. There is excess production of protoporphyrin which accumulates in erythrocytes, the liver and other tissues. The normoblasts fluoresce when exposed to ultraviolet light.

These patients are also light-sensitive and develop pruritus, swelling and reddening of the skin. The urine and teeth are of normal colour and non-fluorescent, and haemolytic anaemia is not present. Cholestasis, hepatitis and cirrhosis may lead to death from liver failure.

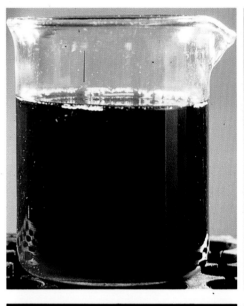
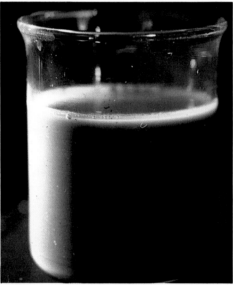

Fig.2.38 Congenital erythropoietic porphyria: urine sample as it appears in (left) daylight and (right) ultraviolet light. Courtesy of Dr. M.R. Moore.

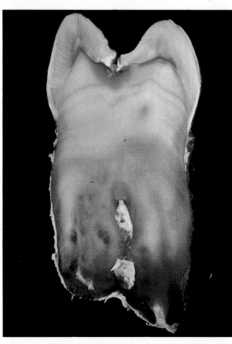
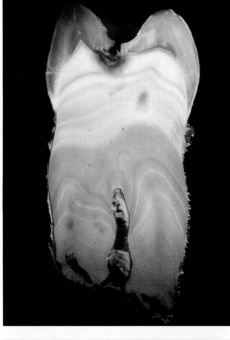

Fig.2.39 Congenital erythropoietic porphyria: molar tooth as it appears in (left) ordinary light, with brown discoloration, and (right) ultraviolet light, with fluorescence most marked in the cortical bone. Courtesy of Dr. M.R. Moore.

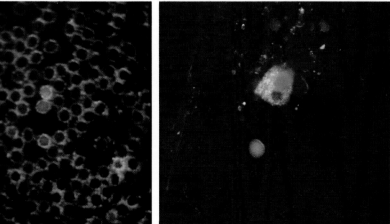

Fig.2.40 Congenital erythropoietic porphyria: peripheral blood film (left) and bone marrow aspirate (right) viewed in ultraviolet light show nuclear fluorescence of erythroblasts due to the presence of large amounts of uroporphyrin I. Courtesy of Dr. I. Magnus.

3
MEGALOBLASTIC ANAEMIAS

The megaloblastic anaemias are a group of disorders characterized by a macrocytic blood picture and megaloblastic erythropoiesis; the causes are listed in Fig.3.1. The underlying biochemical defect appears to be a fault in DNA synthesis. This may be due to a lesion at one or another point in pyrimidine or purine synthesis or to inhibition of DNA polymerization. The anaemia is usually due to deficiency of vitamin B_{12} or folate. In most cases the site of the biochemical defect in DNA synthesis is known. In some types, however, particularly in myeloblastic leukaemia and myelodysplasia in which megaloblastic changes are unresponsive to vitamin B_{12} and folate therapy, the exact site of the defect remains obscure.

The roles of vitamin B_{12} and folate in DNA synthesis are shown in Fig.3.2. Folate deficiency affects thymidylate synthesis, a rate-limiting step in pyrimidine synthesis since a folate coenzyme, 5,10 methylene tetrahydrofolate-polyglutamate, is necessary for this reaction. Folate coenzymes are also required in two reactions in purine synthesis, but these are not thought to be normally rate-limiting for DNA synthesis in humans.

Vitamin B_{12} is not required directly in DNA synthesis. It is needed to convert 5-methyltetrahydrofolate (methyl-THF), which enters cells from plasma, into other folate coenzyme forms (including all the polyglutamate derivatives) through its involvement in the methionine synthetase reaction in which homocysteine is methylated to methionine. In this reaction there is simultaneous removal of the methyl group from methyl-THF to form THF, which can then be converted into other folate coenzymes by the addition of glutamate moieties either before or after formylation.

CLINICAL FEATURES

Megaloblastic anaemia is usually of insidious onset, progressing so slowly that the patient has time to adapt. The patient may therefore not present until the anaemia is quite severe, unless diagnosed early through an incidental blood examination for other reasons. There is jaundice of varying degree in combination with anaemia, giving the patient a lemon-yellow tint (Fig.3.3). The jaundice is caused by unconjugated bilirubin produced in excess because of severe intramedullary death of nucleated red cell precursors ('ineffective erythropoiesis') with reticuloendothelial breakdown of their haemoglobin. There is also a marked rise in serum lactate dehydrogenase concentration due to excessive cell breakdown, and rapid clearance of injected radioiron with poor utilization for red cell formation.

Severe cases show features of intravascular breakdown of haemoglobin with methaemalbuminaemia and haemosiderinuria; pancytopenia often occurs and the patient may present with bruising from thrombocytopenia (Fig.3.4). The white cell and platelet counts are rarely as low as in severe aplastic anaemia.

Causes of Megaloblastic Anaemia I	Causes of Megaloblastic Anaemia II		Causes of Megaloblastic Anaemia III	
Vitamin B_{12} deficiency:	**Folate deficiency:**		**Abnormalities of:**	
Inadequate diet:	Inadequate diet:	Malabsorption:	Vitamin B_{12} metabolism:	DNA synthesis:
veganism	poverty	gluten-induced enteropathy	Congenital:	Congenital:
	institutions	dermatitis herpetiformis	transcobalamin II deficiency	orotic aciduria
Malabsorption:	goat's milk	tropical sprue		Lesch-Nyhan syndrome
Gastric:	special diets	congenital specific	homocystinuria with methylmalonic aciduria	
pernicious anaemia: acquired (autoimmune) & congenital	Excess losses:	Increased utilization:	Acquired:	dyserythropoietic anaemia
partial or total gastrectomy	dialysis	pregnancy	nitrous oxide anaesthesia	thiamine-responsive
Intestinal:	congestive heart failure	prematurity	Folate metabolism:	etc.
stagnant-loop syndrome, e.g. jejunal diverticulosis, ileocolic fistulae	Drugs:	excess marrow turnover, e.g. in haemolytic anaemias	Congenital:	Acquired:
chronic tropical sprue	anticonvulsants	malignancy, e.g. myeloma, carcinoma	inborn errors, e.g. 5-methyltetrahydrofolate transferase deficiency	drugs, e.g. hydroxyurea, cytosine arabinoside, 6-mercaptopurine, 5-azacytidine
ileal resection & Crohn's disease	barbiturates	inflammatory diseases, e.g. Crohn's, rheumatoid arthritis, widespread eczema	Acquired:	
congenital specific malabsorption with proteinuria (Imerslund-Gräsbeck)	Mixed:		antifolate drugs, e.g. methotrexate, pyrimethamine	
fish tapeworm	alcohol			
drugs, e.g. metformin	liver disease			

3.2   **Fig.3.1** Causes of megaloblastic anaemia.

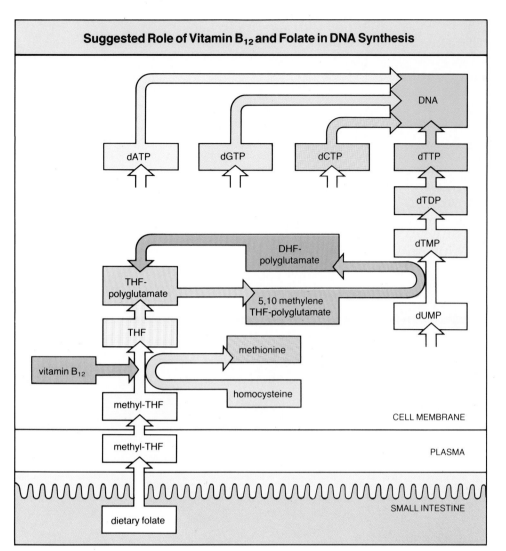

Suggested Role of Vitamin B₁₂ and Folate in DNA Synthesis

Fig.3.2 Megaloblastic anaemia: suggested roles of vitamin B_{12} and folate in DNA synthesis. THF, tetrahydrofolate; DHF, dihydrofolate; B_{12}, vitamin B_{12}; d, deoxyribose; U, uracil; T, thymine; C, cytosine; G, guanine; A, adenine; MP, monophosphate; DP, diphosphate; TP, triphosphate.

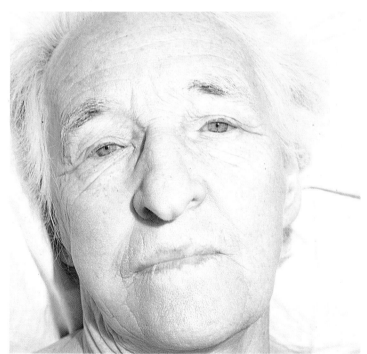

Fig.3.3 Megaloblastic anaemia: typical lemon-yellow appearance of a 69-year-old female with pernicious anaemia and severe megaloblastic anaemia (*Hb:7.0g/dl; MCV:132fl*). The colour is from the combination of pallor due to anaemia and jaundice, the result of the accumulation of unconjugated bilirubin derived from excessive breakdown of haemoglobin in bone marrow macrophages because of ineffective erythropoiesis.

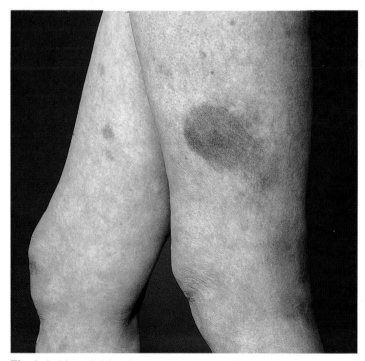

Fig.3.4 Megaloblastic anaemia: spontaneous bruising on the thigh of a 34-year-old female who presented with widespread purpura and menorrhagia. She was found to have megaloblastic anaemia due to nutritional folate deficiency and alcoholism. *Hb:8.1g/dl; MCV:115fl; platelet count:2x10⁹/l.*

Disordered proliferation of the epithelial cell surfaces gives rise to glossitis (Fig.3.5) and angular cheilosis (Fig.3.6), and can also be seen microscopically in the buccal, bronchial, bladder and cervical mucosae.

In a small proportion of cases, melanin pigmentation of skin is present (Fig.3.7). A neuropathy of varying severity may occur with vitamin B_{12} deficiency, such as subacute combined degeneration of the cord which includes posterior and lateral column demyelination (see Fig.3.25), and peripheral or optic neuropathy. The patient presents with bilaterally symmetrical symptoms which are usually most marked in the lower limbs and comprise tingling, unsteadiness of gait, falling over in the dark, altered sensation and reduced strength. Visual and psychiatric disturbances are less frequent.

Blood film appearances
The blood film shows oval macrocytes, fragmented cells, poikilocytes of varying shapes (Figs.3.8–3.11) and hypersegmented neutrophils (showing more than five nuclear lobes; Figs.3.8 & 3.10), some of which may be giant macropolycytes (Fig.3.12). The severity of these changes depends on the degree of anaemia. In the most anaemic patients, megaloblasts may circulate due to extramedullary haemopoiesis in the liver and spleen (Fig.3.13). If the spleen has been removed, as with a gastrectomy, or has atrophied, as in fifteen percent of adult cases with gluten-induced enteropathy, changes due to hyposplenism in the peripheral blood are particularly marked (Fig.3.14). In some extremely anaemic cases, the mean cell volume is normal because of excessive fragmentation of red cells.

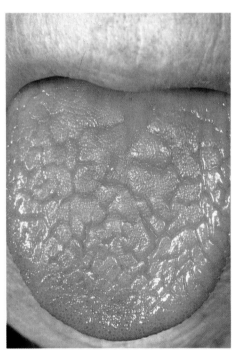

Fig.3.5 Megaloblastic anaemia: glossitis due to vitamin B_{12} deficiency in a 55-year-old female with untreated pernicious anaemia. The tongue is beefy-red and painful, particularly with hot or acidic foods. An identical appearance occurs in folate deficiency because of impaired DNA synthesis in the mucosal epithelium. In some cases with little or no anaemia, symptoms due to the sore tongue may be the presenting feature.

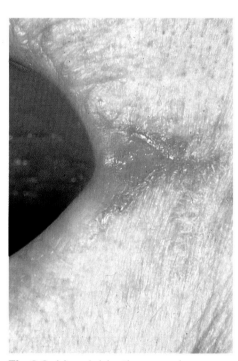

Fig.3.6 Megaloblastic anaemia: angular cheilosis (same patient as in Fig.3.5). This is also thought to be due to impaired proliferation of epithelial cells. It is unusual for this abnormality to be so marked.

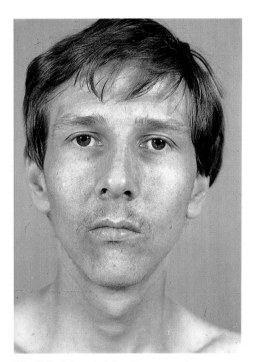

Fig.3.7 Megaloblastic anaemia: melanin pigmentation of the skin in a 24-year-old male with vitamin B_{12} deficiency due to pernicious anaemia. Similar pigmentation affected the nail beds, skin creases, and periorbital and perioral areas. Melanin pigmentation of the skin also occurs in a small percentage of patients with folate deficiency. In both types of megaloblastic anaemia, the pigmentation rapidly disappears with appropriate vitamin therapy. The biochemical basis for the melanin excess is unknown.

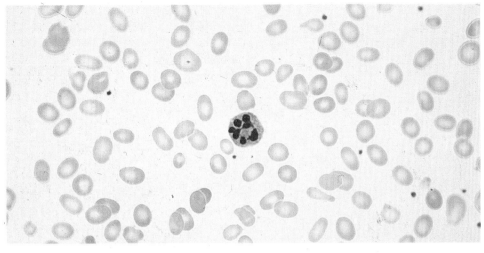

Fig.3.8 Megaloblastic anaemia: peripheral blood film in a severe case showing oval macrocytes, marked anisocytosis and poikilocytosis. There is a neutrophil with a hypersegmented nucleus (more than five lobes). *Hb:5.6g/dl; MCV:127fl; reticulocytes:2.6%; WBC:2.5x10^9/l; platelets:60x10^9/l.*

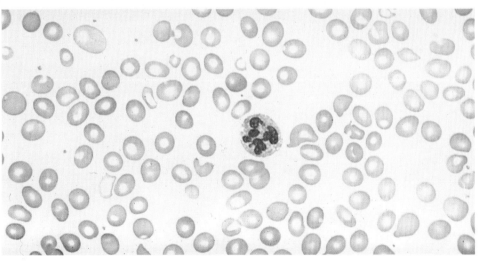

Fig.3.9 Megaloblastic anaemia: peripheral blood film showing marked oval macrocytosis, anisocytosis and poikilocytosis. *Hb:5.4g/dl; MCV:130fl.*

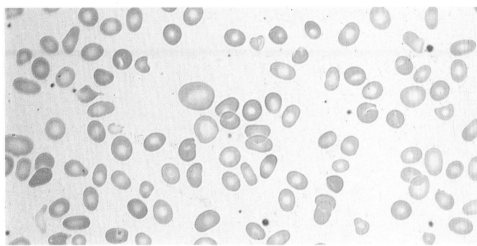

Fig.3.10 Megaloblastic anaemia: peripheral blood film similar to Figs.3.8 & 3.9 but with less severe anaemia. *Hb:7.8g/dl, MCV:119fl.*

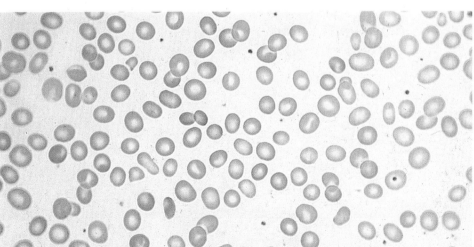

Fig.3.11 Megaloblastic anaemia: peripheral blood film in a mild case showing moderate red cell macrocytosis, anisocytosis and poikilocytosis. *Hb:10.5g/dl; MCV:112fl.*

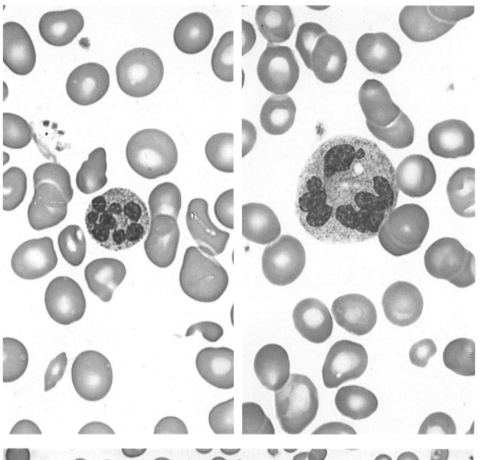

Fig.3.12 Megaloblastic anaemia: higher power views showing (left) a hypersegmented neutrophil and (right) a hyperdiploid neutrophil or 'macropolycyte'.

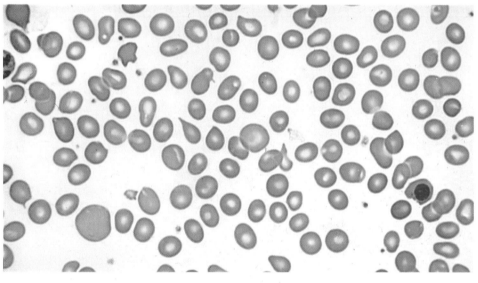

Fig.3.13 Megaloblastic anaemia: peripheral blood film in a severe case showing a circulating orthochromatic nucleated red cell (megaloblast). The presence of circulating megaloblasts may be the result of extramedullary haemopoiesis in the spleen and liver.

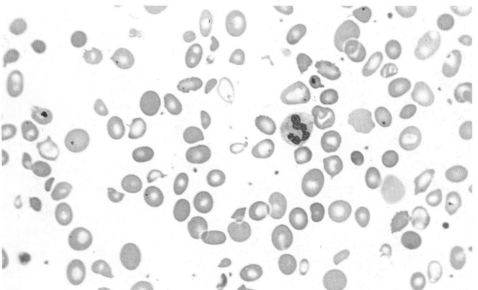

Fig.3.14 Megaloblastic anaemia and splenic atrophy: peripheral blood film showing Howell-Jolly bodies (DNA remnants), and Pappenheimer bodies (iron and protein-containing). The patient had severe folate deficiency and splenic atrophy due to adult coeliac disease.

Bone marrow appearances

In severe cases, the bone marrow is markedly hypercellular with a relative increase in early erythroblasts due to death of later cells (Fig.3.15). The myeloid:erythroid ratio may be reversed with an excess of erythroid precursors. The developing erythroblasts show asynchrony of nuclear and cytoplasmic maturation, the nucleus retaining an open, lacy or stippled appearance while the cytoplasm matures and haemoglobinizes normally. The developing (nucleated) red cells also show a variety of dyserythropoietic features with an excess of multinucleated cells, nuclear bridging and Howell-Jolly bodies; dying cells are also present (Fig.3.16).

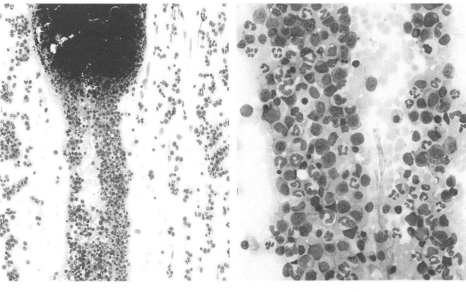

Fig.3.15 Megaloblastic anaemia: (left) low power view of bone marrow fragments showing an increased cellularity with loss of fat spaces; (right) higher power view of cell trails showing accumulation of early cells, an increased proportion of erythroid precursors, and the presence of giant metamyelocytes and hypersegmented neutrophils.

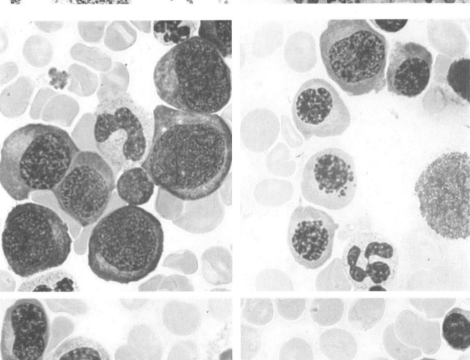

Fig.3.16 Megaloblastic anaemia: high power views showing (upper left) accumulation of early cells, mainly promegaloblasts; (upper right) megaloblasts at all stages. The nuclei have primitive open (lacy) chromatin patterns despite maturation of the cytoplasm with haemoglobinization (pink staining). Two cells have nuclear (DNA) fragments (Howell-Jolly bodies) in their cytoplasm; (lower left) two late megaloblasts with fully orthochromatic (pink-staining) cytoplasm. Two large band-form neutrophils are also present; (lower right) the central orthochromatic cells have karyorrhectic pyknotic nuclei linked by a thin chromatin bridge.

There are giant and abnormally shaped metamyelocytes (Fig.3.17), and the megakaryocytes show hyper-segmented nuclei with an open chromatin network (Fig.3.18).

In milder cases, megaloblastic changes in the red cell precursors are only identified in late erythroblasts with mild asynchrony of nuclear/cytoplasmic development (Fig.3.19). This has been termed 'mild', 'transitional' or 'intermediate' megaloblastic change.

Where iron deficiency and megaloblastic anaemia coexist, there is a dimorphic anaemia with two red cell populations in the peripheral blood, one of well haemoglobinized macrocytes and the other of hypochromic microcytes (Fig.3.20,left). Megaloblastic changes may be masked in the erythroblasts, even though giant metamyelocytes are seen in the bone marrow (Fig.3.20,right). In patients with normal iron stores, there is usually excessive iron granulation of erythroblasts (Fig.3.21) and, in some cases, especially in association with alcohol, ring sideroblasts are frequent but disappear with appropriate therapy. Trephine biopsy confirms the accumulation of early cells and excess mitoses (Fig.3.22). It is of interest that erythropoiesis in early fetal life is also megaloblastic (Fig.3.23).

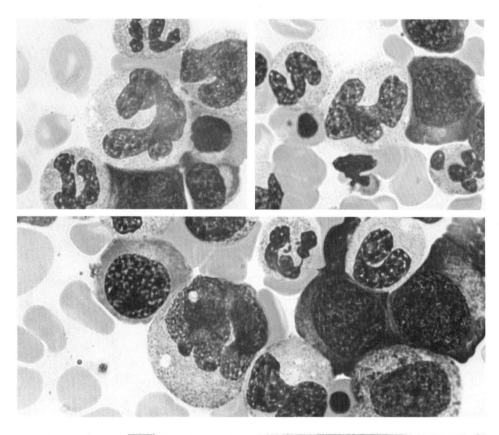

Fig.3.17 Megaloblastic anaemia: high power views showing a number of giant and abnormally shaped metamyelocytes.

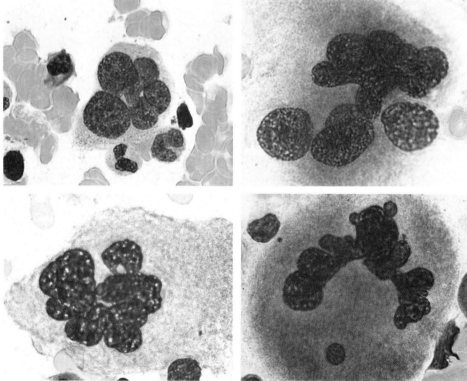

Fig.3.18 Megaloblastic anaemia: megakaryocytes of variable maturity. All show nuclei with abnormal, open chromatin patterns.

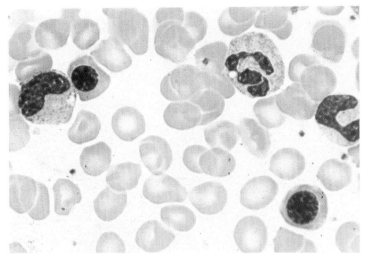

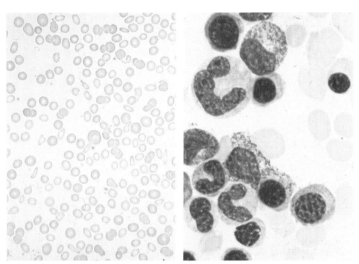

Fig.3.19 Megaloblastic anaemia: mild marrow changes in vitamin B$_{12}$ deficiency following partial gastrectomy. The nucleated red cells show mild asynchrony of nuclear/cytoplasmic development with delay of nuclear maturation (lower right). Iron stores were present. *Hb:12.4g/dl; MCV:105fl; serum vitamin B$_{12}$:80ng/l (normal:160-925ng/l); serum folate:10.3μg/l (normal:6.0-21.0μg/l).*

Fig.3.20 Megaloblastic anaemia: (left) dimorphic peripheral blood film in iron and vitamin B$_{12}$ deficiencies following partial gastrectomy. There is a mixed population of microcytic hypochromic cells and well haemoglobinized macrocytes. *Hb:8.0g/dl; MCV:87fl; MCH:27pg;* (right) bone marrow aspirate (same case). Giant metamyelocytes are present but megaloblastic changes in the erythroblasts are 'masked'.

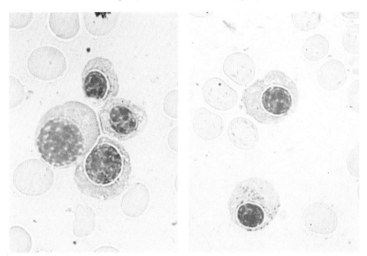

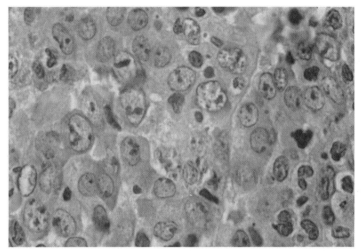

Fig.3.21 Megaloblastic anaemia: bone marrow aspirate in alcoholism and folate deficiency showing partial ring sideroblasts which rapidly disappeared on alcohol withdrawal and folic acid therapy. Perls' stain.

Fig.3.22 Megaloblastic anaemia: trephine biopsy of iliac crest in untreated pernicious anaemia shows many megaloblasts with a fine open chromatin pattern and a number of mitotic figures.

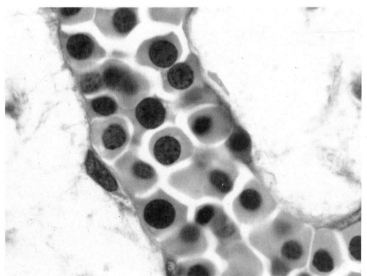

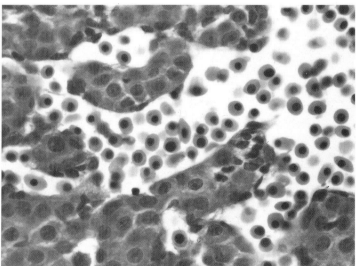

Fig.3.23 Fetal erythropoiesis: sections of (left) placenta showing circulating erythroblasts with a nuclear morphology similar to megaloblasts; (right) liver showing extramedullary megaloblastic erythropoiesis.

CAUSES OF MEGALOBLASTIC ANAEMIA
Vitamin B₁₂ (B₁₂) deficiency

As vitamin B_{12} stores are from 2-3mg, and daily losses and therefore requirements are 1-2µg, it takes two to four years for B_{12} deficiency to develop from dietary lack or malabsorption. Deficiency due to excessive losses or breakdown of vitamin B_{12} have not been described; but the anaesthetic gas, nitrous oxide, may rapidly inactivate body B_{12} from the fully reduced cob(I)alamin state to the oxidized cob(II)alamin and cob(III)alamin forms. If

exposure is prolonged, megaloblastic changes occur (Fig.3.24).

While folate occurs in most foods, including fruit, vegetables and cereals as well as animal products, vitamin B_{12} occurs only in foods of animal origin. Veganism may lead to B_{12} deficiency and this is found most frequently in Hindus. Liver has the highest concentration of both vitamins, since this is the main organ of their storage.

Severe vitamin B_{12} deficiency, assessed by serum B_{12} levels, although not necessarily associated with severe

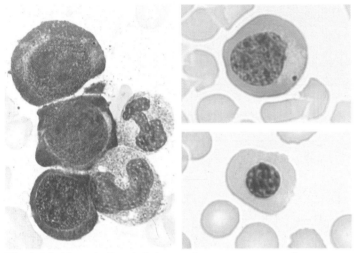

Fig.3.24 Vitamin B_{12} deficiency: bone marrow aspirate showing megaloblasts in a patient receiving prolonged nitrous oxide anaesthesia in intensive care following cardiac surgery.

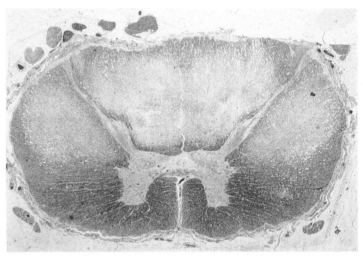

Fig.3.25 Pernicious anaemia: cross-section of spinal cord of a patient who died with severe vitamin B_{12} neuropathy (subacute combined degeneration of the spinal cord). There is demyelination of the lateral (pyramidal) and posterior columns. Weigert-Pal stain.

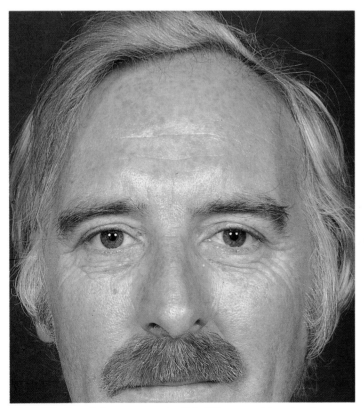

Fig.3.26 Pernicious anaemia: this 38-year-old male shows premature greying and has blue eyes and vitiligo, three features that are more common in patients with pernicious anaemia than in control subjects.

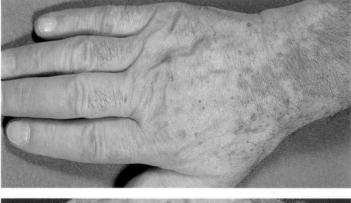

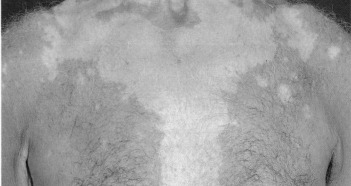

Fig.3.27 Pernicious anaemia: marked vitiligo in a 67-year-old male.

anaemia may cause demyelination of the posterior and lateral columns of the spinal cord (Fig.3.25). It is often associated with a peripheral neuropathy and is found more frequently in males than in females; yet pernicious anaemia, the most common cause of severe B_{12} deficiency, is more common in females.

Addisonian pernicious anaemia is the dominant cause of B_{12} deficiency in Western countries. Although particularly common in Northern Europe, it occurs in all races and countries. It is associated with early greying of the hair (Fig.3.26), vitiligo (Fig.3.27) and thyroid disorders (Fig.3.28) as well as with other organ-specific autoimmune diseases, such as Addison's disease and hypoparathyroidism. There is gastric atrophy (Fig.3.29) with achlorhydria; parietal cell antibodies are present in the serum of ninety percent of patients (Fig.3.30) and intrinsic factor antibodies in fifty percent. Gastric carcinoma develops two to three times more frequently than in control populations (Fig.3.31).

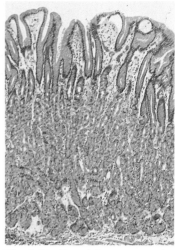

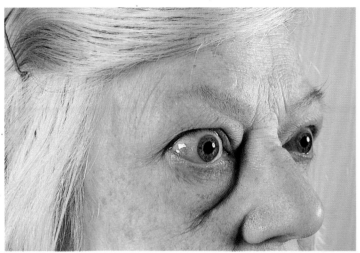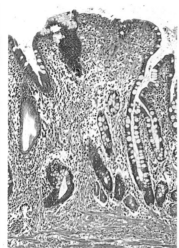

Fig.3.28 Pernicious anaemia: exophthalmic ophthalmoplegia in a patient who developed myxoedema while receiving maintenance vitamin B_{12} therapy, having presented with megaloblastic anaemia six years earlier.

Fig.3.29 Pernicious anaemia: sections of stomach, (left) normal and (right) in pernicious anaemia. There is atrophy of all coats, loss of gastric glands and parietal cells, and infiltration of the lamina propria by lymphocytes and plasma cells. Courtesy of Dr. J.E. McLaughlin.

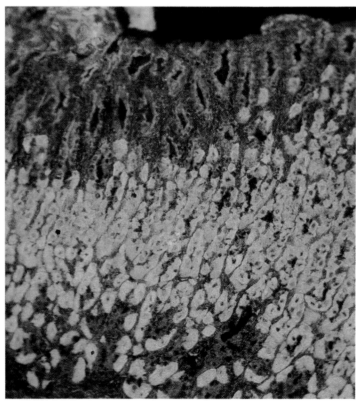

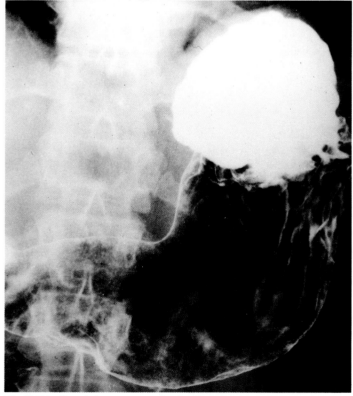

Fig.3.30 Pernicious anaemia: positive indirect immunofluorescent test for parietal cell antibody. A frozen section of gastric mucosa (rat) has been layered with the patient's serum and washed, followed by the addition of rabbit antihuman IgG conjugated with fluorescein.

Fig.3.31 Pernicious anaemia: barium meal radiograph showing gastric atrophy and carcinoma. There is thinning of the gastric wall and lack of mucosal pattern, and an ulcerated filling defect in the horizontal part of the greater curve.

Small intestinal causes of vitamin B$_{12}$ deficiency include the stagnant-loop syndrome, for example, jejunal diverticulosis (Fig.3.32), ileocolic fistula (Fig.3.33) and ileal resection.

Folate deficiency
Since daily requirements of folate are 100–200µg, body stores (10–15mg) are sufficient for only a few months, a period which can be reduced in conditions of increased

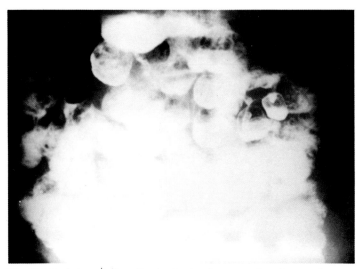

Fig.3.32 Jejunal diverticulosis: barium meal radiograph showing multiple jejunal diverticula in a 71-year-old patient who presented with megaloblastic anaemia due to vitamin B$_{12}$ deficiency. Courtesy of Dr. D. Nag.

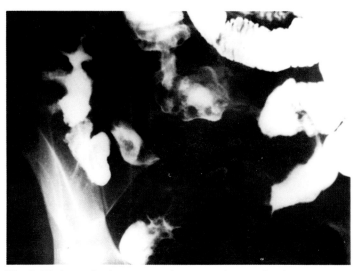

Fig.3.33 Intestinal stagnant-loop syndrome: barium follow-through radiograph in Crohn's disease showing defective filling of the terminal ileum with a blind loop clearly visible. There is early filling of the ascending colon. The patient presented with megaloblastic anaemia due to vitamin B$_{12}$ deficiency. Courtesy of Dr. R. Dick.

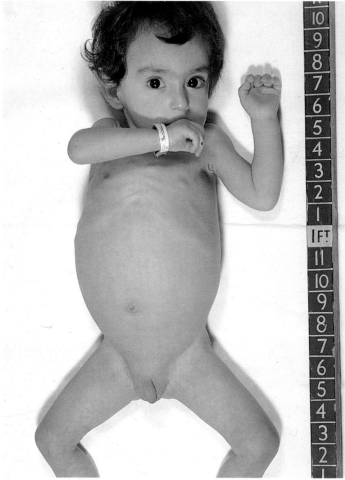

Fig.3.34 Infantile coeliac disease: wasting and abdominal distention in a 2-year-old boy who developed megaloblastic anaemia due to folate deficiency. Coeliac disease was diagnosed by jejunal biopsy.

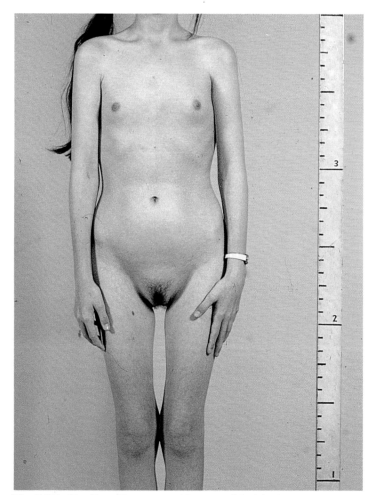

Fig.3.35 Coeliac disease: a 16-year-old girl who presented with severe megaloblastic anaemia due to folate deficiency and on jejunal biopsy was found to have coeliac disease. There was no history of diarrhoea. She had delayed puberty and menarche.

turnover and, hence, breakdown of folates.

Folate deficiency may be due to inadequate dietary intake or to malabsorption, as in gluten-induced enteropathy (Figs.3.34–3.38) and tropical sprue (Fig.3.39).

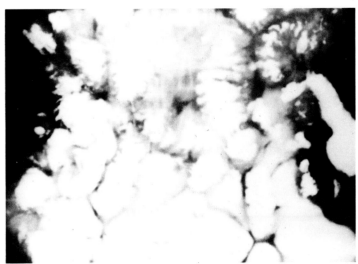

Fig.3.36 Adult coeliac disease: barium follow-through radiograph of the small intestine showing flocculation of barium and lack of the normal fine mucosal pattern. Courtesy of Dr. D. Nag.

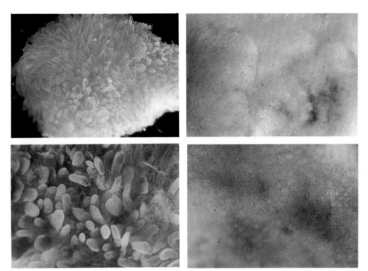

Fig.3.37 Adult coeliac disease: low and medium power views of jejunal biopsies showing (left) normal villi in finger and leaf patterns; (right) mosaic pattern with obvious crypt openings instead of the normal villous pattern. Courtesy of Dr. J.S. Stewart.

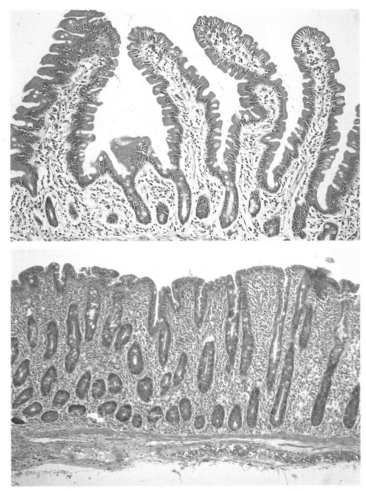

Fig.3.38 Coeliac disease: histological sections of jejunal biopsies showing (upper) normal mucosa with finger-like villi and (lower) subtotal villous atrophy with absence of villi and hypertrophy of the mucosal crypts. Courtesy of Dr. A. Price (lower).

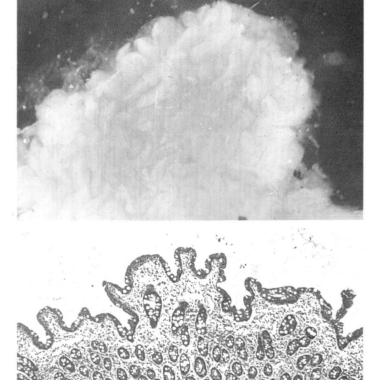

Fig.3.39 Tropical sprue: jejunal biopsy showing (upper) dissecting microscopical appearance with typical convoluted mucosal pattern and (lower) partial villous atrophy. Courtesy of Prof. V. Chadwick.

The skin disease dermatitis herpetiformis is associated with gluten–induced enteropathy and, hence, with folate deficiency (Fig.3.40). The most common cause of deficiency is pregnancy, when folate requirements rise from the normal 100–200μg daily to about 350μg daily. However, the incidence of this complication is now reduced with prophylactic folic acid therapy. Other causes of increased folate utilization include diseases with increased bone marrow or other cell turnover (see Fig.3.1). The excessive demands for folate in these conditions, combined with poor dietary intake, may lead to megaloblastic anaemia.

Abnormalities of vitamin B_{12} or folate metabolism

These may be inherited or acquired. Transcobalamin II deficiency is an autosomal recessive inherited abnormality leading, in the homozygous state, to megaloblastic anaemia due to failure of B_{12} transport into bone marrow and other cells. It presents in the first few months of life (Fig.3.41).

A number or rare abnormalities of folate metabolism have been described, and megaloblastic anaemia may also arise during therapy with the antifolate drugs which inhibit dihydrofolate reductase, such as methotrexate or pyrimethamine.

Other causes

Megaloblastic anaemia as a result of antimetabolite chemotherapy with, for example, hydroxyurea or cytosine arabinoside, shows similar morphological features to those due to vitamin B_{12} or folate deficiencies. However, dyserythropoietic changes are often more marked.

In acute myeloblastic leukaemia of the M_6 type or in myelodysplasia, megaloblastic changes are usually confined to the erythroid series. Giant metamyelocytes, hypersegmented polymorphs and other changes in leucopoiesis, or megakaryocytes seen in vitamin B_{12} or folate deficiency, are not seen.

Rare inborn errors of metabolism other than those affecting vitamin B_{12} or folate metabolism, such as orotic aciduria in which there is a fault in pyrimidine synthesis, may also result in megaloblastic anaemia.

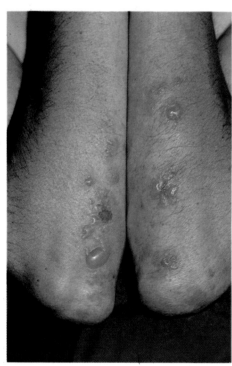

Fig.3.40 Dermatitis herpetiformis: typical appearance of blisters on the extensor surfaces of the arms. This skin condition is associated with gluten-induced enteropathy and folate deficiency. Courtesy of Dr. L. Fry.

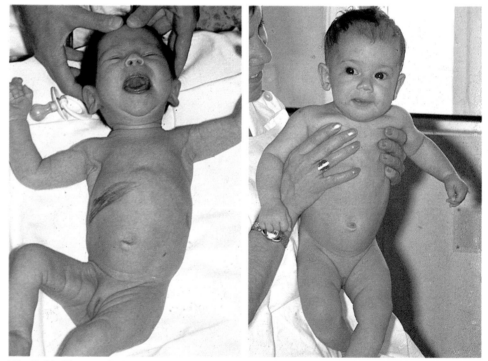

Fig.3.41 Transcobalamin II deficiency: this child, (left) before and (right) 6 months after therapy, presented at 20 days with weight loss, irritability, pallor, glossitis and hepatosplenomegaly. Tests showed a macrocytic anaemia and megaloblastic bone marrow. Serum B_{12} and folate levels were normal but chromatography of serum showed absence of transcobalamin II. Treatment was 1mg hydroxocobalamin intramuscularly twice weekly; the child remains well 3 years later. Courtesy of Dr. M.C. Arrabel.

4

HAEMOLYTIC ANAEMIA

The dominant cause of the anaemia in haemolytic anaemias is an increased rate of red cell destruction. The red cell destruction is usually extravascular in the macrophages of the reticuloendothelial system as in normal individuals but, in some types of acute or chronic haemolysis, red cell destruction occurs intravascularly (Fig. 4.1). The clinical and laboratory features differ according to which of the two is the main site of destruction. In addition to the clinical features of pallor, many patients show mild fluctuating jaundice (Figs.4.2 & 4.3) and splenomegaly (Fig.4.4). Increased bilirubin production may result in pigment gallstones (Figs.4.5 & 4.6).

Laboratory findings in haemolytic anaemia include raised unconjugated serum bilirubin, and increased faecal stercobilinogen and urine urobilinogen from accelerated red cell destruction; serum haptoglobins are absent. A reticulocytosis (Fig.4.7) and bone marrow erythroid hyperplasia (Fig.4.8) are the result of compensatory increases in red cell production. Characteristic changes in red cell morphology occur in a number of haemolytic anaemias and, in the most severe, the peripheral blood film shows red cell polychromasia (due to the reticulocytosis) and occasional erythroblasts (due to extramedullary erythropoiesis; Fig.4.9).

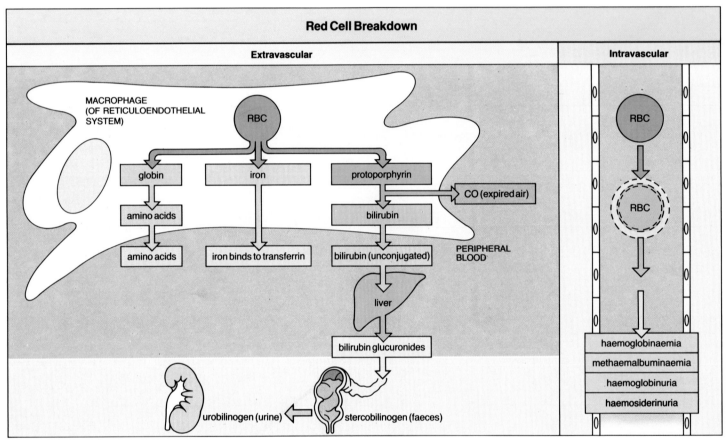

Fig.4.1 Haemolytic anaemia: extravascular and intravascular mechanisms of red cell breakdown.

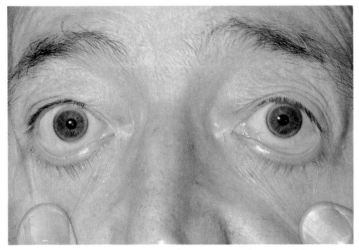

Fig.4.2 Haemolytic anaemia (autoimmune): scleral jaundice.

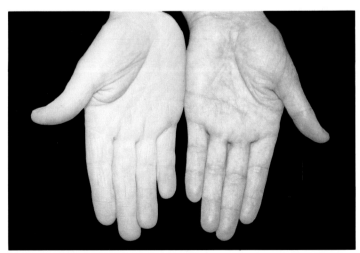

Fig.4.3 Haemolytic anaemia (autoimmune): jaundice of the palmar skin (on the left) contrasted with normal skin colour (on the right).

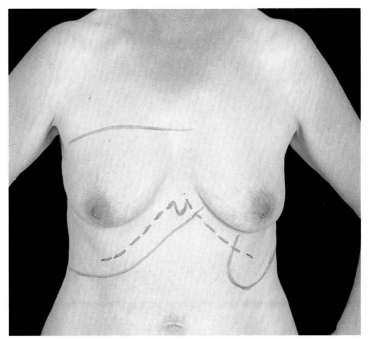

Fig.4.4 Haemolytic anaemia: mild splenomegaly and jaundice in a delayed haemolytic transfusion reaction.

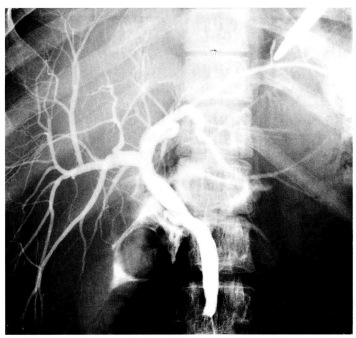

Fig.4.5 Thalassaemia major: operative cholangiogram shows a distended biliary tree and failure of contrast to pass gallstone obstruction at the lower part of the common bile duct. Courtesy of Dr. R. Dick.

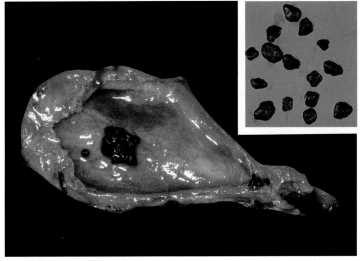

Fig.4.6 Thalassaemia major: opened gallbladder and its bilirubin gallstones (inset).

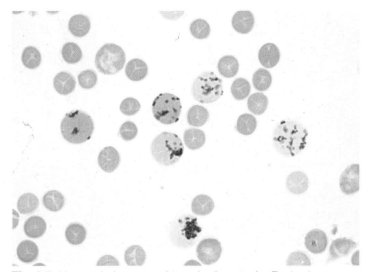

Fig.4.7 Haemolytic anaemia: reticulocytosis. Reticular (precipitated RNA) material is seen in the larger cells. New methylene blue stain, Giemsa counterstain.

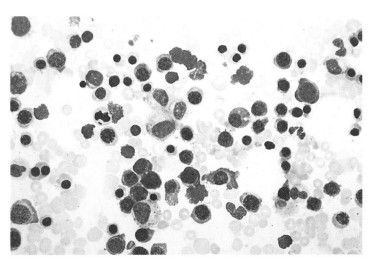

Fig.4.8 Haemolytic anaemia: bone marrow cell trail with erythroid hyperplasia shows a dominance of erythroblasts.

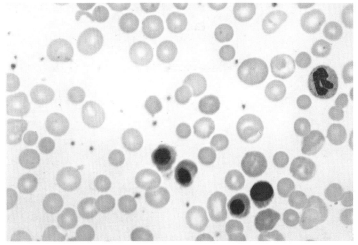

Fig.4.9 Haemolytic anaemia (autoimmune): peripheral blood film showing erythroblasts, red cell polychromasia and spherocytosis.

In those anaemias caused by oxidant damage to haemoglobin and to other red cell proteins, Heinz bodies may be found in reticulocyte preparations (Fig.4.10). Intravascular red cell destruction is accompanied by haemoglobinaemia, haemoglobinuria (Fig.4.11), plasma methaemoglobinaemia, methaemalbuminaemia and haemosiderinuria (Fig.4.12). Jaundice is less common.

HEREDITARY HAEMOLYTIC ANAEMIA

The hereditary haemolytic anaemias are usually the result of intrinsic red cell defects. A simplified classification is shown in Fig.4.13; thalassaemia and haemoglobinopathy are discussed in Chapter 5.

Normal red cell membrane

This consists of a lipid bilayer with polar phospholipids on the external and inner surfaces, with one or two non-polar fatty-acid side chains towards the centre (Fig.4.14). The bilayer also contains a variable proportion of cholesterol. Proteins may be either transmembrane integral proteins, for example, band 3 and glycophorins A or B, or peripheral (extrinsic) proteins, such as spectrin, actin, bands 2.1 (ankryn), 4.1 and 4.2. The band numbers refer to the Commassie blue bands on SDS–PAGE electrophoresis.

The lipids or proteins on the external surface may carry sugars which determine blood groups or act as viral receptors at the head ends. Spectrin consists of two

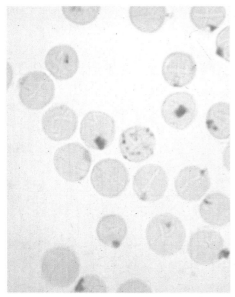

Fig.4.10 Deficiency of glucose 6-phosphate dehydrogenase: peripheral blood film showing Heinz bodies in red cells and a single reticulocyte. Supravital new methylene blue stain.

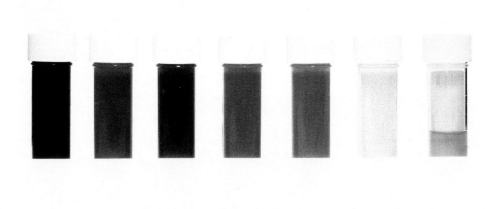

Fig.4.11 Glucose 6-phosphate dehydrogenase deficiency: urine samples showing haemoglobinuria of decreasing severity following an episode of acute intravascular haemolysis.

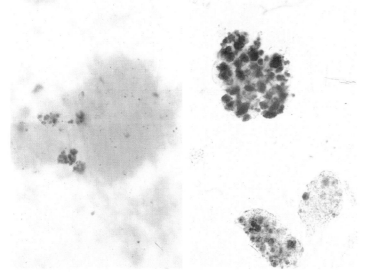

Fig.4.12 Intravascular haemolysis in paroxysmal nocturnal haemoglobinuria: haemosiderinuria. Prussian-blue positive material seen in urinary deposit (left) and at higher magnification, in individual renal tubular cells (right). Perls' stain.

Hereditary Haemolytic Anaemia		
Membrane defects	Metabolic defects	Haemoglobin defects
hereditary spherocytosis	deficiency of:	defective synthesis, e.g. thalassaemia (α or β)
hereditary elliptocytosis	pyruvate kinase	
	triose phosphate isomerase	abnormal variants, e.g. Hb S, Hb C, unstable
hereditary stomatocytosis	pyrimidine-5-nucleotidase	
etc.	glucose-6-phosphate dehydrogenase	
	glutathione synthetase	
	etc.	

Fig.4.13 Causes of hereditary haemolytic anaemia.

forms, α and β, which are joined at the head ends to form a heterodimer with a hairpin structure. The protein ankryn binds the spectrin α–chains to band 3, a large integral membrane protein, while the tail end of spectrin binds to protein 4.1, thus forming spectrin oligomers. Protein 4.1 also binds to glycophorin A or aminophospholipids to serve as secondary attachment sites of the skeleton to the bilayer.

Hereditary spherocytosis
This condition may be due to a variety of abnormalities of the cytoskeletal proteins of the red cell membrane. Defects of spectrin or protein 4.1 have been described in various kindreds. The cells are excessively permeable to sodium influx; glycolysis is increased as is ATP turnover. The marrow produces red cells of normal biconcave shape but these lose membrane during passage through the spleen and the rest of the reticuloendothelial system. The resultant rigid and spherical cells have a shortened lifespan, the spleen being the principal organ of red cell destruction.

The condition is characterized by a dominant inheritance pattern. Typically there is anaemia, jaundice and splenomegaly. A blood film shows microspherocytes (Fig.4.15); red cell osmotic fragility is characteristically increased (Fig.4.16), and tests for autohaemolysis show increased lysis of red cells at least partly corrected by glucose (Fig.4.17).

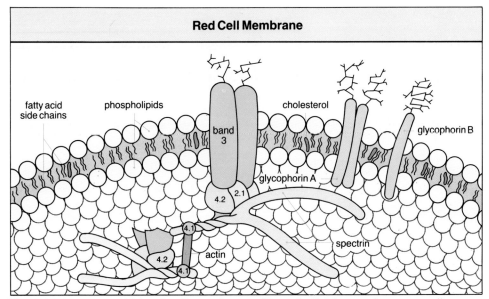

Fig.4.14 Human red blood cell membrane. Phospholipids are shown as yellow balls attached to hydrophobic fatty-acid side chains. The orange ellipses within the lipid bilayer represent cholesterol. Modified from S.L. Schrier, *Recent Advances in Haematology*, 3, p 77. Churchill Livingstone: Edinburgh.

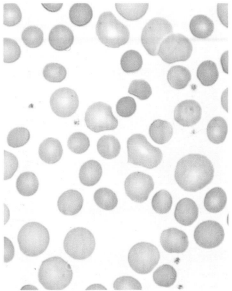

Fig.4.15 Hereditary spherocytosis: peripheral blood film showing smaller spherocytes among larger polychromatic red cells.

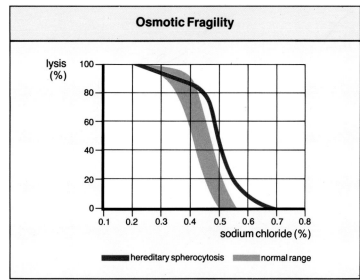

Fig.4.16 Osmotic fragility test: graph comparing red cell lysis in severe hereditary spherocytosis and in normal blood. The curve is shifted to the right of the normal range but a tail of osmotically resistant cells (reticulocytes) is present.

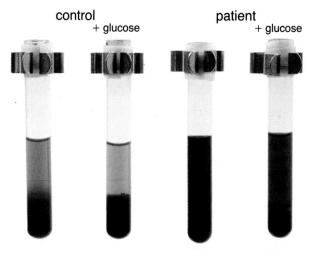

Fig.4.17 Autohaemolysis test: red cells are incubated in saline at 37°C for 48 hours with and without additional glucose. The amount of lysis is determined. Autohaemolysis, particularly in the absence of an energy supply (glucose), is markedly increased in hereditary spherocytosis.

Splenectomy produces a considerable improvement in red cell survival and is associated with a rise in haemoglobin levels to normal. Sections of splenic tissue reveal gross entrapping of the spherocytic red cells in the splenic cords (Fig.4.18).

Hereditary elliptocytosis
The characteristic feature in this disorder is the presence of elongated red cells in the peripheral blood (Fig.4.19). It appears likely that a number of inherited protein defects may produce this condition. A common defect is defective spectrin dimer–dimer interaction resulting in an increased proportion of dimers in relation to spectrin tetramers. The clinical expression in heterozygotes (elliptocytosis trait) is variable; while some have anaemia

and splenomegaly, the majority have only minimal or no reduction in red cell survival with little or no anaemia. In rare homozygous patients, there is severe anaemia with marked haemolysis and splenomegaly (Fig.4.20) and bizarre red cell morphology (Fig.4.21).

Other rare inherited defects of red cell membrane
These include hereditary stomatocytosis (Fig.4.22) and acanthocytosis associated with the McLeod blood group (Fig.4.23).

Normal red cell metabolism
Normal red cells maintain themselves in a physiological state for about one hundred and twenty days by metabolizing glucose through the glycolytic

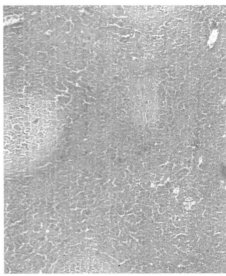

Fig.4.18 Hereditary spherocytosis: section of spleen showing marked hyperplasia of reticuloendothelial cordal tissue and entrapment of large numbers of red cells.

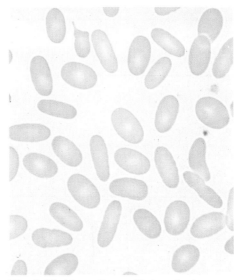

Fig.4.19 Hereditary elliptocytosis: blood film showing characteristic elliptical red cells.

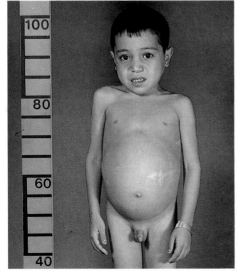

Fig.4.20 Hereditary elliptocytosis: abdominal swelling due to massive splenomegaly in a homozygous patient. The facies indicates expansion of haemopoietic tissue in the skull bones, particularly in the maxillae.

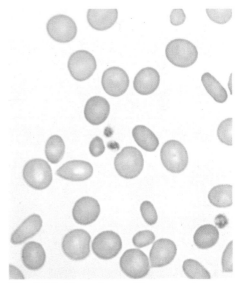

Fig.4.21 Hereditary elliptocytosis: peripheral blood film from the child in Fig.4.20 shows red cell anisocytosis and poikilocytosis with elliptocytes and microspherocytes.

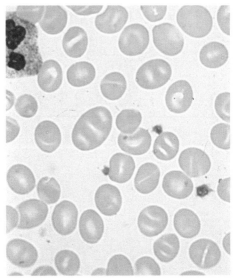

Fig.4.22 Hereditary stomatocytosis: peripheral blood film showing many cells with the characteristic loosely folded appearance of the membrane. The membrane has increased passive permeability, allowing excess sodium.

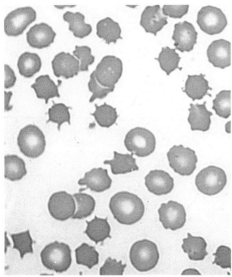

Fig.4.23 McLeod phenotype: peripheral blood film showing marked acanthocytosis of red cells associated with the rare McLeod blood group. There is lack of the Kell antigen precursor (Kx).

(Embden-Meyerhof) and pentose-phosphate (hexose-monophosphate shunt) pathways (Fig.4.24). In this way the cells are able to generate energy as ATP which is needed for maintaining cell shape and flexibility as well as cation and water content through the action of sodium and calcium pumps. ATP may also act as a substitute for 2,3-diphosphoglycerate (2,3-DPG) in maintaining the position of the oxygen dissociation curve. 2,3-DPG, the most abundant red cell phosphate, is generated by the Rapoport-Luebering shunt of the glycolytic pathway (Fig.4.25). The higher the 2,3-DPG content of red cells, the more easily oxygen is liberated from haemoglobin. Reducing power is also generated as NADH, NADPH and reduced glutathione (GSH) which protect the membrane, haemoglobin and other cell structures from oxidant damage.

Glucose 6-phosphate dehydrogenase deficiency

There are numerous inherited variants of the enzyme glucose 6-phosphate dehydrogenase which show much less activity than normal. The most frequent clinical syndrome is acute intravascular haemolysis due to oxidant stress (drugs, fava beans) or during severe infection, diabetic ketoacidosis or hepatitis. There are marked changes in red cell morphology (Fig.4.26), Heinz bodies (see Fig.4.10) and haemoglobinuria (see Fig.4.11). Neonatal jaundice may also occur and the most severe defects result in a chronic non-spherocytic haemolytic anaemia. The inheritance is sex-linked.

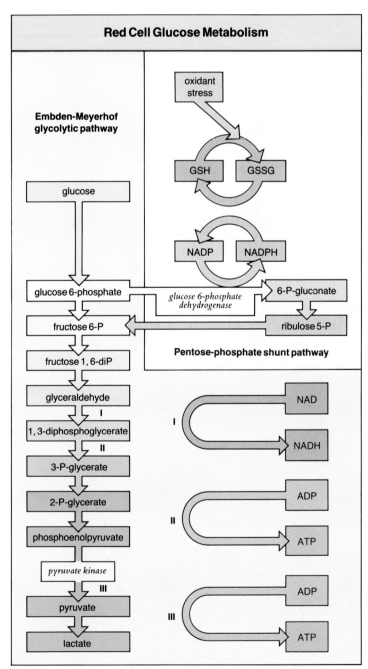

Fig.4.24 Normal red cell metabolism: Embden-Meyerhof glycolytic and pentose-phosphate (hexose-monophosphate) shunt pathways.

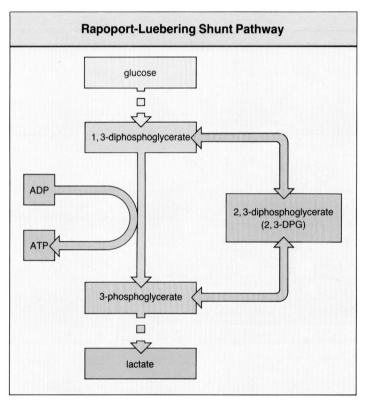

Fig.4.25 Normal red cell metabolism: the Rapoport-Luebering shuttle pathway for maintenance of red cell 2,3-DPG levels.

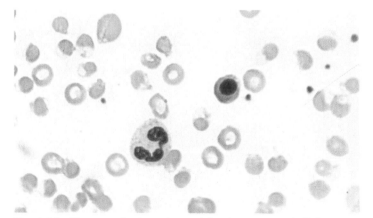

Fig.4.26 Glucose 6-phosphate dehydrogenase deficiency: peripheral blood film following acute oxidant drug-induced haemolysis shows an erythroblast and damaged red cells, including irregularly contracted 'blister' and 'bite' cells.

Pyruvate kinase deficiency

This is the most frequently encountered haemolytic anaemia due to an inherited enzyme defect in the glycolytic pathway. The majority have red cells which show no particular diagnostic features (Fig.4.27), although 'prickle' cells may be found, especially following splenectomy (Fig.4.28). The postsplenectomy reticulocyte count is often very high (Fig.4.29). There is an abnormal autohaemolysis test not corrected by glucose, and diagnosis is made by a specific enzyme assay.

Pyrimidine 5-nucleotidase deficiency

This rare congenital haemolytic anaemia is associated with basophilic stippling of the red cells (Fig.4.30) caused by abnormal residual RNA. This enzyme normally catalyzes the hydrolytic dephosphorylation of pyrimidine 5'-ribose monophosphates to freely diffusible pyrimidine nucleosides, an important step in the breakdown of RNA at the reticulocyte stage. It is also inhibited by lead.

ACQUIRED HAEMOLYTIC ANAEMIA

The majority of acquired haemolytic anaemias are caused

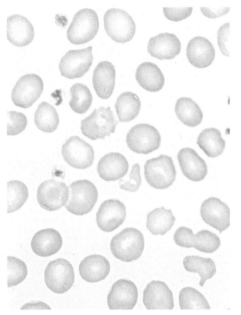

Fig.4.27 Pyruvate kinase deficiency: peripheral blood film presplenectomy shows red cell anisocytosis and poikilocytosis.

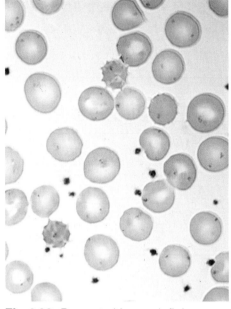

Fig.4.28 Pyruvate kinase deficiency: peripheral blood film postsplenectomy with two small acanthocytes or 'prickle' cells.

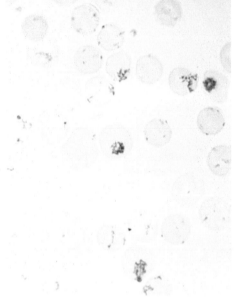

Fig.4.29 Pyruvate kinase deficiency: gross reticulocytosis (over 90%) postsplenectomy. Supravital new methylene blue stain.

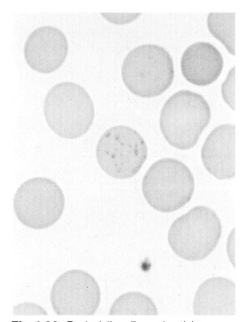

Fig.4.30 Pyrimidine 5-nucleotidase deficiency: peripheral blood film showing basophilic stippling in the central red cell.

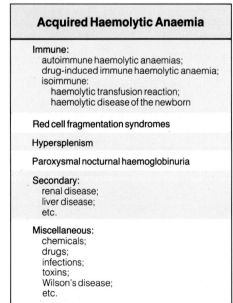

Acquired Haemolytic Anaemia

Immune:
  autoimmune haemolytic anaemias;
  drug-induced immune haemolytic anaemia;
  isoimmune:
    haemolytic transfusion reaction;
    haemolytic disease of the newborn

Red cell fragmentation syndromes

Hypersplenism

Paroxysmal nocturnal haemoglobinuria

Secondary:
  renal disease;
  liver disease;
  etc.

Miscellaneous:
  chemicals;
  drugs;
  infections;
  toxins;
  Wilson's disease;
  etc.

Fig.4.31 Causes of acquired haemolytic anaemia.

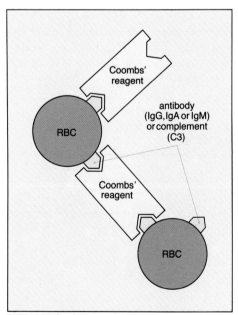

Fig.4.32 Direct antiglobulin (Coombs') test: the Coombs' reagent may be broad spectrum or specifically directed against IgG, IgM, IgA or complement (C3d). The test is positive if the red cells agglutinate.

by extracorpuscular or environmental changes. A simplified classification appears in Fig.4.31.

Autoimmune haemolytic anaemias

These anaemias are characterized by a positive direct Coombs' (antiglobulin) test (Fig.4.32) and are divided into 'warm' and 'cold' types, according to whether the antibody reacts better with red cells at 37°C or at 4°C. These acquired disorders occur at any age and produce haemolytic anaemias of varying severity, often with associated disease (Fig.4.33). In the warm type, usually the peripheral blood shows marked red cell spherocytosis (Figs.4.34 & 4.35). In the cold type, the antibodies are usually IgM and may be associated with intravascular haemolysis. Marked autoagglutination of red cells may be seen in the blood film (Fig.4.36). In many patients the haemolysis is aggravated by cold weather and often associated with Raynaud's phenomenon (Fig.4.37). Rarely, the blood films show neutrophil/red cell rosetting (Fig.4.38).

Autoimmune Haemolytic Anaemia	
Warm Type	**Cold Type**
Idiopathic	Idiopathic
Secondary:	Secondary:
systemic lupus erythematosus, other connective tissue disorders	*Mycoplasma* pneumonia
	infectious mononucleosis
chronic lymphocytic leukaemia	malignant lymphoma
malignant lymphoma	paroxysmal cold haemoglobinuria: rare; may be primary or associated with infection
ulcerative colitis	
ovarian teratoma	
drugs, e.g. methyldopa	

Fig.4.33 Causes of autoimmune haemolytic anaemia.

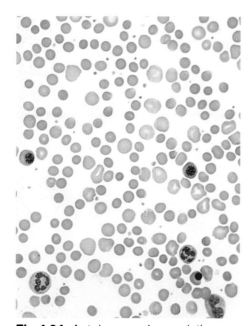

Fig.4.34 Autoimmune haemolytic anaemia: peripheral blood film showing erythroblasts, polychromatic macrocytes and marked spherocytosis.

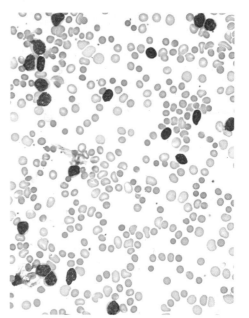

Fig.4.35 Autoimmune haemolytic anaemia with associated chronic lymphocytic leukaemia: peripheral blood film shows red cell polychromasia, spherocytosis and increased numbers of lymphocytes.

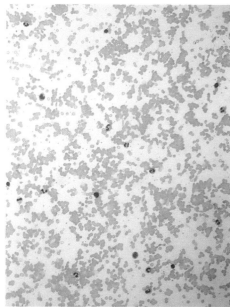

Fig.4.36 Autoimmune haemolytic anaemia: peripheral blood film showing autoagglutination of red cells in the 'cold' type.

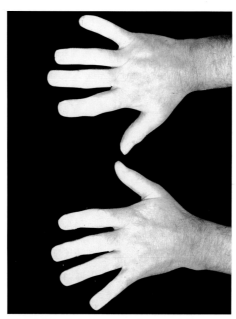

Fig.4.37 Autoimmune haemolytic anaemia: Raynaud's phenomenon manifested by marked pallor of the fingers, in the 'cold' type.

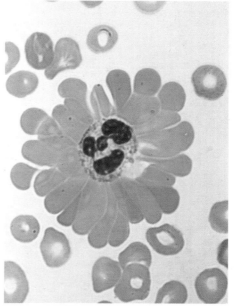

Fig.4.38 Autoimmune haemolytic anaemia: peripheral blood film showing a neutrophil/red cell rosette.

Drug-induced immune haemolytic anaemia

Drugs cause immune haemolytic anaemia by three mechanisms: antibodies are directed against a red cell membrane/drug complex, for example, penicillin; there is deposition of a protein/antibody/drug complex on the red cell surface, for example, phenacetin; or occasionally an autoimmune process is involved, for example, methyldopa.

Isoimmune haemolytic anaemia

Severe haemolysis follows transfusion of incompatible blood, particularly if the blood is of the wrong ABO group. There may be massive intravascular haemolysis and the blood film usually shows both autoagglutination and spherocytosis (Fig.4.39). The other major cause of this condition is haemolytic disease of the newborn, which may be due to a number of different blood group incompatibilities between the fetus and mother (Figs.4.40–4.42).

Red cell fragmentation syndromes

Fragmentation arises from direct damage to red cells, either on abnormal surfaces, such as artificial heart valves, or when red cells pass through fibrin strands deposited in the microcirculation due to disseminated intravascular coagulation, as in mucin-secreting adeno-carcinomas (Fig.4.43), thrombotic thrombocytopenic purpura (Fig.4.44) or in the haemolytic-uraemic syndrome (Fig.4.45). Other causes of microangiopathic haemolytic anaemia include gram-negative septicaemia (Fig.4.46) and malignant hypertension.

Secondary haemolytic anaemias

In a number of systemic disorders, haemolysis may contribute to observed anaemia. In renal failure there may be crenated cells ('echinocytes'), including 'burr' cells and acanthocytes (Fig.4.47; see also Fig.6.33). Red cell targetting is a feature of the haemolysis associated with liver disease; with severe liver failure there is often marked haemolysis with prominent red cell acanthocytosis (see Fig.6.32).

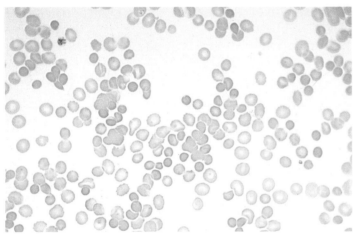

Fig.4.39 ABO-incompatibility transfusion reaction: peripheral blood film showing red cell autoagglutination and spherocytosis.

Blood group system	Frequency of antibodies	Haemolytic disease of newborn
ABO	very common	causal
Rhesus	common	causal
Kell	occasional	causal
Duffy	occasional	causal
Kidd	occasional	causal
Lutheran	rare	causal
Lewis	rare	not causal
P	rare	not causal
MNSs	rare	not causal
Ii	rare	not causal

Fig.4.40 Isoimmune haemolytic anaemia: the main blood group systems and their association with haemolytic disease of the newborn.

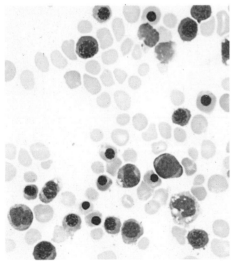

Fig.4.41 Rhesus D haemolytic disease of the newborn (erythroblastosis fetalis): peripheral blood film from an infant born with severe anaemia showing large numbers of erythroblasts and microspherocytes.

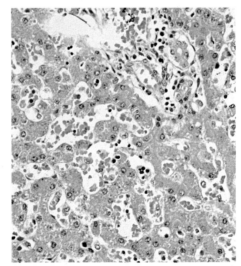

Fig.4.42 Rhesus D haemolytic disease of the newborn: histological section of liver from a fatal case shows extramedullary haemopoiesis in the hepatic venous sinuses.

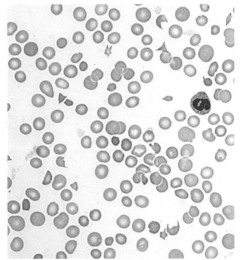

Fig.4.43 Red cell fragmentation syndrome: peripheral blood film in widespread metastatic mucin-secreting adenocarcinoma showing red cell fragments ('schistocytes') and anisocytosis.

Paroxysmal nocturnal haemoglobinuria (PNH)

In this acquired disorder, the bone marrow produces red cells with defective cell membranes which are particularly sensitive to lysis by complement. There is chronic intravascular haemolysis (see Fig.4.11) and many patients develop recurrent venous thromboses. Occasional patients present with the Budd–Chiari syndrome (Fig.4.48). PNH is diagnosed by finding positive acid (Fig.4.49) and sucrose lysis tests.

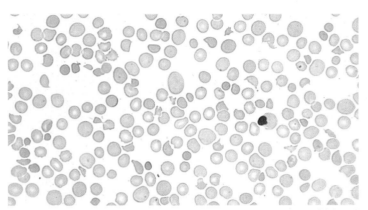

Fig.4.44 Red cell fragmentation syndrome: peripheral blood film showing polychromatic and fragmented red cells in thrombotic thrombocytopenic purpura.

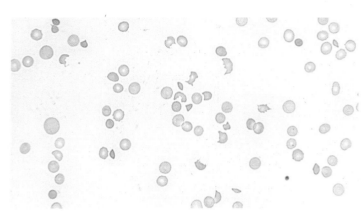

Fig.4.45 Red cell fragmentation syndrome: peripheral blood film in haemolytic-uraemic syndrome.

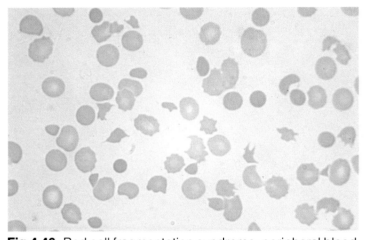

Fig.4.46 Red cell fragmentation syndrome: peripheral blood film showing red cell polychromasia and fragmentation in gram-negative septicaemia.

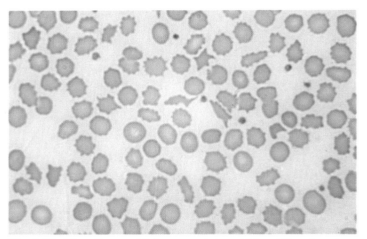

Fig.4.47 Chronic renal failure: peripheral blood film showing red cell changes, including 'burr' cells and acanthocytes (coarse crenated cells).

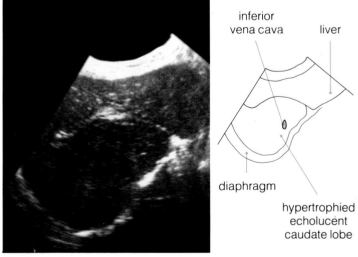

inferior vena cava   liver

diaphragm

hypertrophied echolucent caudate lobe

Fig.4.48 Paroxysmal nocturnal haemoglobinuria: ultrasound study of the liver in Budd-Chiari syndrome. The caudate lobe is hypertrophied and spongy, and the inferior vena cava is compressed in its passage through it. Courtesy of Dr. L.Berger.

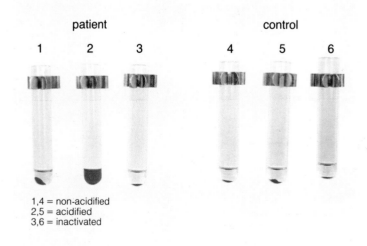

patient   control

1   2   3   4   5   6

1,4 = non-acidified
2,5 = acidified
3,6 = inactivated

Fig.4.49 Paroxysmal nocturnal haemoglobinuria: acid lysis test. The affected red cells (on left) show marked complement-dependent lysis in acidified fresh serum at 37°C. Preheating the acidified serum inactivates complement, preventing lysis of the affected cells.

Other haemolytic anaemias

Severe haemolytic anaemia may be found during clostridial septicaemia (Fig.4.50) and in other infections including malaria and bartonellaemia (see Chapter 16). Haemolytic anaemias may also be caused by extensive burns (Figs.4.51 & 4.52), chemical poisoning, and snake and spider bites. Overdose with oxidizing drugs, such as sulphasalazine (Fig.4.53) or dapsone (Fig.4.54), may also cause severe haemolysis. Wilson's disease is also a cause of haemolysis thought to be due to oxidant damage to red cells caused by excess copper (Fig.4.55).

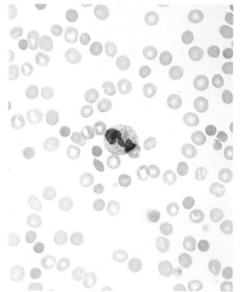

Fig.4.50 Haemolytic anaemia in clostridial septicaemia: peripheral blood film showing red cell spherocytosis.

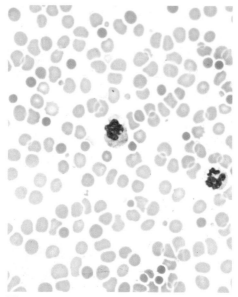

Fig.4.51 Haemolytic anaemia following extensive burns: peripheral blood film showing marked spherocytosis, including microspherocytic cells.

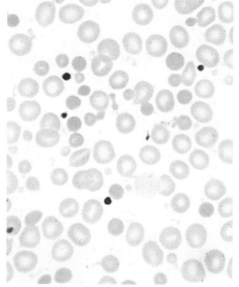

Fig.4.52 Haemolytic anaemia following extensive burns: peripheral blood film showing microspherocytes, ghost cells, cells with membrane projections and 'dumb-bell' forms.

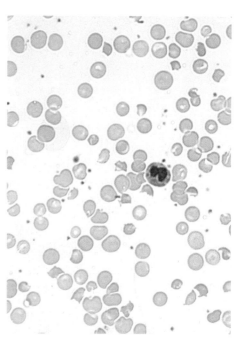

Fig.4.53 Drug-induced haemolytic anaemia: peripheral blood film associated with overdose of sulphasalazine. The red cells show polychromasia, irregular contraction and some fragmentation.

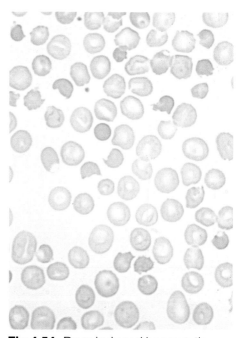

Fig.4.54 Drug-induced haemolytic anaemia: peripheral blood film in a case associated with high dosage dapsone therapy for dermatitis herpetiformis. The red cells show irregular contraction, target cells and cells with 'bites' out of the membrane. There is a single 'blister' cell in the lower central area of the field.

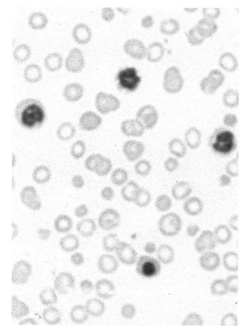

Fig.4.55 Acute haemolytic anaemia in Wilson's disease: peripheral blood film in a 14-year-old girl who presented with severe anaemia (Hb:5.4g/dl) and reticulocytosis (reticulocytes: 30%). She had Kayser-Fleischer rings in the eyes, disturbed liver function, and raised liver and urine copper levels. The red cells show micro-spherocytosis, fragmentation and irregular gaps or 'bites' in the membrane; normoblasts are present.

5

THALASSAEMIA AND THE HAEMOGLOBINOPATHIES

THALASSAEMIA

Globin synthesis depends on two gene clusters situated on chromosomes 11 and 16 (Fig.5.1,upper). Globin molecules are synthesized from the appropriate genes via an RNA transcript. Following transcription, the RNA is processed to remove redundant RNA derived from introns situated within the coding part of each gene (Fig.5.1,middle). Each molecule of haemoglobin consists of four globin chains (Fig.5.1,lower). In normal adults, haemoglobin (Hb) A ($\alpha_2\beta_2$) forms ninety-six to ninety-seven percent of the haemoglobin. The thalassaemias are a group of disorders in which the underlying abnormality is reduced synthesis of either the α or β chains of haemoglobin A (Fig.5.2). The global distribution of thalassaemia and the more common haemoglobinopathies is shown in Fig.5.3.

The α–thalassaemias are classified according to the number of α genes affected. There is duplication of the α–globin genes. In the α_0 lesion, both α genes on one

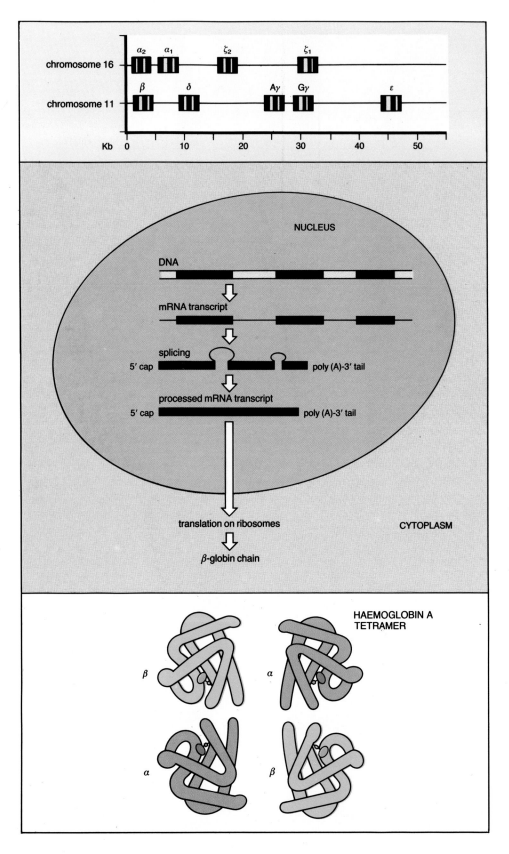

Fig.5.1 Synthesis of haemoglobin: (upper) organization of the clusters of genes and their coding regions (exons, in black) for globin-chain synthesis on chromosomes 11 and 16. Non-coding regions (introns) occur between the exons; (middle) stages in the synthesis of β-globin from DNA to the final polypeptide chain; (lower) the haemoglobin tetramer, in this example, Hb A.

chromosome are deleted or ineffective whereas, in the milder α_+ lesion, only one of the two genes is deleted or defective.

β-thalassaemia is divided into: a homozygous (major) form, in which there is complete or almost complete absence of β-chain synthesis; a heterozygous (minor) or trait form, in which synthesis of only one β-chain is reduced; and a clinically intermediate form, which can be a mild form of homozygous β-thalassaemia, the result of interaction of β-thalassaemia with other haemoglobinopathies, or an unusually severe form of β-thalassaemia trait.

In general, β-thalassaemias are the result of point mutations in or near the globin genes causing, for example, defective splicing, premature stop codons, nonsense lesions and frameshift changes. Gene deletions are more common in the α-thalassaemias. Over forty different genetic lesions have already been detected in the α- and β-thalassaemias.

Classification of Thalassaemias I	Classification of Thalassaemias II				
Clinical	**α-thalassaemias**				
Thalassaemia major:	Designation	Haplotype	Heterozygous	Homozygous	
transfusion-dependent homozygous β_0-thalassaemia	α_1-thalassaemia	$--/$	α_0-thalassaemia; MCH, MCV low	hydrops fetalis	
homozygous β_+-thalassaemia (some types)	dysfunctional α-thalassaemia	$-\alpha_0/$	α_0-thalassaemia; MCH, MCV low	hydrops fetalis	
	α_2-thalassaemia	$-\alpha/$	α_+-thalassaemia; minimal, if any, haematological abnormality	as heterozygous α_1-thalassaemia	
Thalassaemia intermedia:	non-deletion α-thalassaemia	$\underline{\alpha}\,\underline{\alpha}/$	variable	Hb H disease in some cases	
haemoglobin Lepore syndromes	Hb-Constant Spring (CS)	$-$	0.5-1% Hb CS	more severe than hetero-zygous α_1-thalassaemia	
homozygous $\delta\,\beta$-thalassaemia and hereditary persistence of fetal haemoglobin	The combination of α_1-thalassaemia (or dysfunctional α-thalassaemia), and α_2-thalassaemia gives rise to Hb H disease.				
combinations of α- & β-thalassaemias	**Classification of Thalassaemias III**				
haemoglobin H disease	**β-thalassaemias**				
Thalassaemia minor:	Type	Heterozygous		Homozygous	
β_0-thalassaemia trait	β_0	thalassaemia minor; Hb A_2:>3.5%		thalassaemia major; Hb F: 98%; Hb A_2:2%; no Hb A	
$\delta\,\beta$-thalassaemia trait					
hereditary persistence of fetal haemoglobin	β_+	thalassaemia minor; Hb A_2:>3.5%		thalassaemia major; Hb F: 70-80% Hb A: 10-20%; Hb A_2: variable	
β_+-thalassaemia trait	$\delta\,\beta$ and hereditary persistence of fetal haemoglobin	thalassaemia minor; Hb F:5-20%; Hb A_2:normal or low		thalassaemia intermedia; Hb F:100%	
α_1 (α_0)-thalassaemia trait	Hb Lepore	thalassaemia minor; Hb A:80-90%; Hb Lepore:10%; Hb A_2:reduced		thalassaemia major or intermedia; Hb F:80%; Hb Lepore:10-20%; Hb A, Hb A_2:absent	
α_2 (α_+)-thalassaemia trait					

Fig.5.2 Classification of the thalassaemia disorders: (left) clinical; (upper right) α-thalassaemias; (lower right) β-thalassaemias.

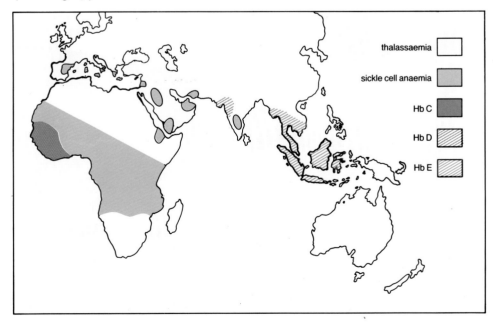

Fig.5.3 The geographical distribution of thalassaemia, sickle cell anaemia and the other common haemoglobin disorders. It is likely that the carriers of these disorders have a selective advantage against malaria compared to normal individuals. The disorders are also found in other parts of the world where emigrants from areas of high incidence have settled.

thalassaemia
sickle cell anaemia
Hb C
Hb D
Hb E

β-thalassaemia major

The clinical features of β-thalassaemia major are due to a severe anaemia combined with an intense increase in erythropoiesis, largely ineffective with excessive bone marrow activity and extramedullary haemopoiesis. In the poorly transfused patient, there is expansion of the flat bones of the face and skull (Figs.5.4–5.7) and expansion of the marrow in all bones (Fig.5.8). Spontaneous fractures may occur.

Another feature is enlargement of the liver and spleen (Figs.5.9 & 5.10), mainly because of extramedullary erythropoiesis but also from excessive breakdown of red cells and iron overload. The peripheral blood in the

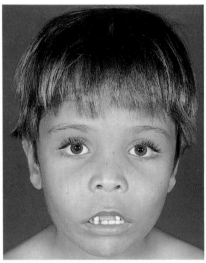

Fig.5.4 β-thalassaemia major: characteristic facies of a 7-year-old Middle Eastern boy includes prominent maxillae and widening of the bridge of the nose. There is also marked bossing of the frontal and parietal bones.

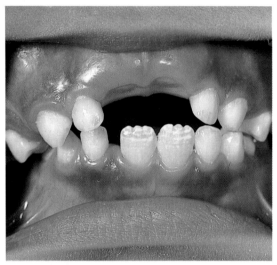

Fig.5.5 β-thalassaemia major: the teeth (same case as in Fig.5.4) are splayed due to widening of the maxilla and mandible.

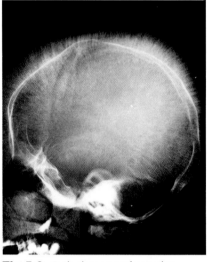

Fig.5.6 β-thalassaemia major: lateral radiograph of the skull (same case as in Fig.5.4) shows the typical 'hair-on-end' appearance, with thinning of the cortical bone and widening of the marrow cavity.

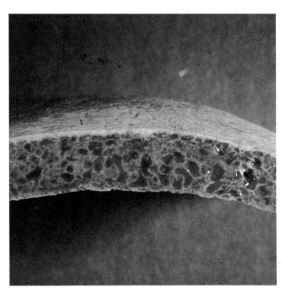

Fig.5.7 β-thalassaemia major: section through the skull at necropsy shows marked thinning of the cortices and an open porotic cancellous bone. The mahogany-brown colour is the result of extensive iron deposition as haemosiderin in the marrow. Courtesy of Drs. P.G. Bullough and V.J. Vigorita.

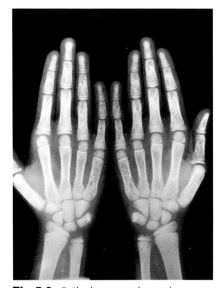

Fig.5.8 β-thalassaemia major: radiograph of the hands of an undertransfused 7-year-old child. There is thinning of the cortical bone due to expansion of the marrow space.

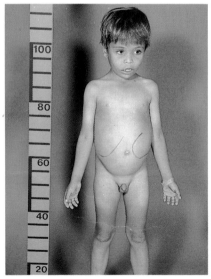

Fig.5.9 β-thalassaemia major: overall view of the boy in Fig.5.4 shows enlargement of the liver and spleen, and stunted growth. The child had been inadequately transfused since presenting with anaemia at the age of 4 months.

poorly transfused patient shows the presence of hypochromic cells, target cells and nucleated red cells (Fig.5.11). Postsplenectomy there are increased red cell inclusions (for example, iron granules and Howell-Jolly bodies) and a high platelet count (Fig.5.12). The bone marrow shows red cell hyperplasia with pink-staining inclusions of precipitated α-globin chains in the cytoplasm of erythroblasts (Fig.5.13). Many of the erythroblasts die in the marrow and are digested by macrophages. There is increased iron in the macrophages and increased iron granules in developing erythroblasts (Fig.5.14).

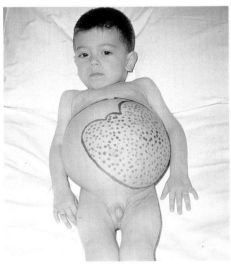

Fig.5.10 β-thalassaemia major: this 4-year-old inadequately transfused Cypriot boy has enlargement of the spleen to an unusual degree. It may be partly reversed by adequate transfusion. Splenectomy is usually required but should usually be delayed until the child is over 6 years old to reduce the incidence of postoperative fatal infection.

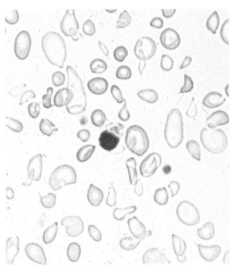

Fig.5.11 β-thalassaemia major: peripheral blood film showing prominent hypochromic microcytic cells, target cells and a normoblast. Some normochromic cells are present from a previous blood transfusion.

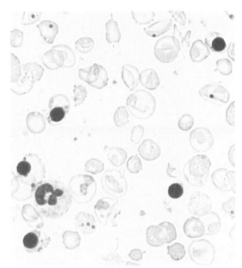

Fig.5.12 β-thalassaemia major: peripheral blood film postsplenectomy in which hypochromic cells, target cells and normoblasts are prominent. Pappenheimer and Howell-Jolly bodies are also seen and the platelet count is raised.

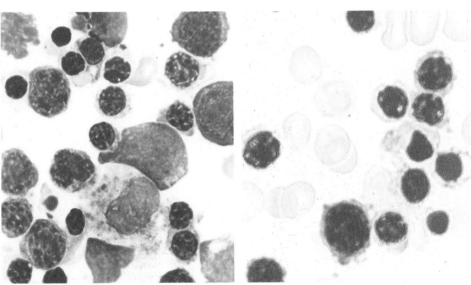

Fig.5.13 β-thalassaemia major: bone marrow aspirates showing (left) marked erythroid hyperplasia and normoblasts with vacuolated cytoplasm. Degenerate forms are present and a macrophage containing pigment; (right) normoblasts with pink-staining cytoplasmic inclusions ('haemoglobin lakes'), precipitates of excess α-globin chains.

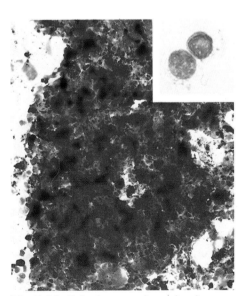

Fig.5.14 β-thalassaemia major: low power view of bone marrow fragment showing grossly increased iron stores, largely contained in macrophages as haemosiderin and, on electron microscopy, as ferritin. Bone marrow normoblasts show prominent coarse iron granules (inset). Perls' stains.

5.5

Much of the bone abnormality can be prevented by regular transfusions from the age of presentation (usually six months) to maintain the haemoglobin at all times at a level above 9–10g/dl. However, these regular transfusions, together with increased iron absorption, lead to iron overload. Each unit of blood contains 200–250mg iron. After 50–100 units have been transfused, siderosis develops with increased pigmentation of skin exposed to light (Figs.5.15 & 5.16) and susceptibility to

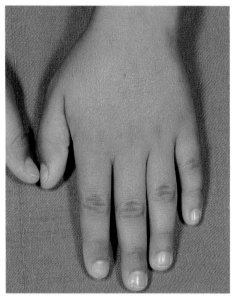

Fig.5.15 β-thalassaemia major: the hands of a 9-year-old girl show marked melanin skin pigmentation, particularly in the skin creases and nail beds, due to iron overload.

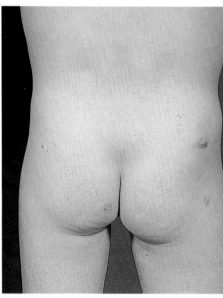

Fig.5.16 β-thalassaemia major: buttocks and lower back of an 18-year-old male show melanin pigmentation except on the parts not exposed to light.

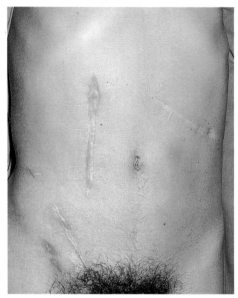

Fig.5.17 β-thalassaemia major: 21-year-old male with multiple scars of operative incisions. The patient presented with features similar to those of acute appendicitis but had infection with *Yersinia enterocolitica*, particularly common in patients with transfusional iron overload. Susceptibility may also be increased by desferrioxamine therapy. There was subsequent formation of a psoas abscess.

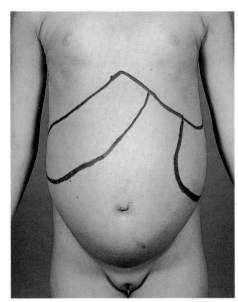

Fig.5.18 β-thalassaemia major: abdominal appearance of an 18-year-old girl with enlarged liver and spleen. There is a lack of secondary sexual development, mainly because of iron damage to the hypothalamus-pituitary system. In some cases, iron overload in the gonads also causes lack of sexual development.

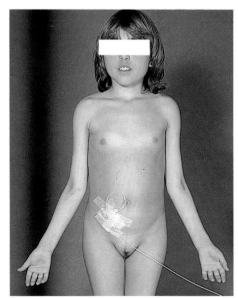

Fig.5.19 β-thalassaemia major: this 17-year-old girl shows reduced stature (height:134cm) and delayed pubertal development. Since circulating growth hormone levels are usually normal, the lack of growth is due to 'end-organ' failure. Subcutaneous infusion of desferrioxamine is in progress.

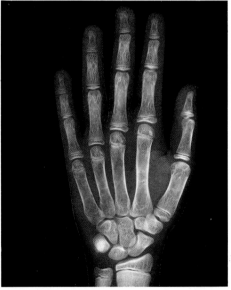

Fig.5.20 β-thalassaemia major: radiograph of the hand of a 19-year-old male. The estimated bone age is 14 years and there is failure of epiphyseal closure. Widening of the marrow cavity and thinning of trabeculae and cortex are also seen.

infection (Fig.5.17), reduced growth, and delayed sexual development and puberty (Figs.5.18 & 5.19).
There is delayed and abnormal bone development (Figs.5.20 & 5.21), damage and iron overloading in the pancreas (Fig.5.22) often with diabetes mellitus, liver (Fig.5.23) and myocardium (Figs.5.24 & 5.25) as well as damage to the other endocrine organs, particularly the hypothalamus and pituitary. Iron deposition may occur in bone (Fig.5.26). Liver damage may also be due to viral hepatitis from repeated transfusions.

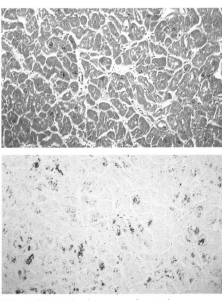

Fig.5.21 β-thalassaemia major: radiograph of the knee (same case as in Fig.5.20) shows the same characteristic features of delayed and abnormal development.

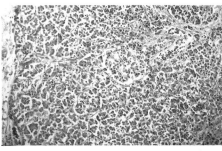
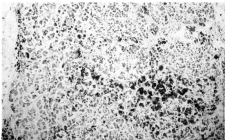

Fig.5.22 β-thalassaemia major: post-mortem sections of pancreas showing (upper) pigment (haemosiderin and lipofuscin) in acinar cells, macrophages and connective tissue, with less obvious pigment in the islet cells; and (lower) gross iron (haemosiderin) deposits in all cell types, particularly marked in the acinar cells. H & E (upper), Perls' (lower) stains.

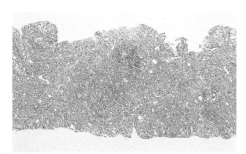
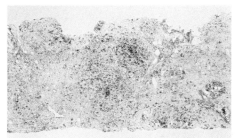

Fig.5.23 β-thalassaemia major: needle biopsy of liver showing (upper) disturbances of normal architecture with increased mixed inflammatory cells, fibrosis in portal tracts and nodular regeneration of hepatic paren-chymal cells; and (lower) Grade IV siderosis with iron deposition in the hep-atic parenchymal cells, bile duct epi-thelium, macrophages and fibroblasts. H & E (upper), Perls' (lower) stains.

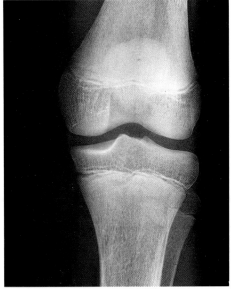

Fig.5.24 β-thalassaemia major: post-mortem sections of myocardium seen by (upper) H & E and (lower) Perls' staining. The individual muscle fibres contain heavy deposits of iron pigment. In transfusional iron overload, iron deposition is most marked in the left ventricle (shown here) and interventricular septum.

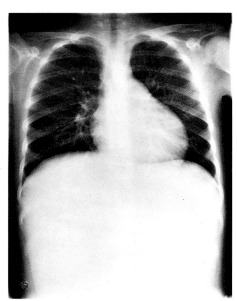

Fig.5.25 β-thalassaemia major: chest radiograph showing cardiomegaly due to chronic anaemia and iron overload. Enlargement occurs mainly in the ventricles and interventricular septum.

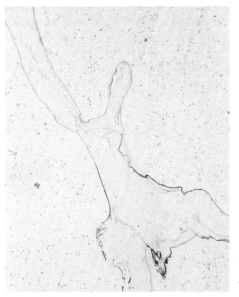

Fig.5.26 β-thalassaemia major: section of bone showing iron deposition in the cement lines of the trabecula and in macrophages (as haemosiderin) throughout the bone marrow. Courtesy of P.G. Bullough and V.J. Vigorita.

Iron overload may, however, be substantially reduced by daily subcutaneous desferrioxamine infusions (see Fig.5.19). The iron is then excreted as ferrioxamine in the urine, which appears red, and in the bile. Thalassaemia major may be cured by marrow transplantation (Fig.5.27).

Thalassaemia intermedia

Thalassaemia intermedia is compatible with normal growth and development (Fig.5.28) but is characterized by bone deformities, extramedullary haemopoiesis (Fig.5.29) and iron overload. Ankle ulcers (Fig.5.30), probably the result of anoxia due to anaemia and stasis of the local circulation, may arise as in thalassaemia major, sickle cell anaemia and other haemolytic anaemias.

β-thalassaemia trait

In β-thalassaemia trait there is a hypochromic microcytic blood picture with a high red cell count (greater than $5.5 \times 10^{12}/1$; Fig.5.31).

Antenatal diagnosis

If both parents are carriers, fetal diagnosis is carried out using fetoscopy to obtain blood (Fig.5.32, left) and measurement of the α/β-chain synthesis ratio or by amniocentesis or trophoblast biopsy (Fig.5.32, right) to obtain DNA for hybridization with relevant DNA probes (Fig.5.33). A homozygous fetus can then be aborted.

α-thalassaemia

In its most severe form, in which all four genes are deleted, α-thalassaemia is incompatible with life; and the fetus is stillborn or critically ill with hydrops fetalis (Fig.5.34). The blood shows gross hypochromia and erythroblastosis (Fig.5.35).

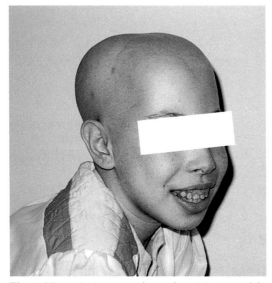

Fig.5.27 β-thalassaemia major: 14-year-old girl, after marrow transplantation from an HLA-matching sibling, shows hair loss due to chemotherapy, and bossing of the skull. Courtesy of Prof. G. Luccarelli.

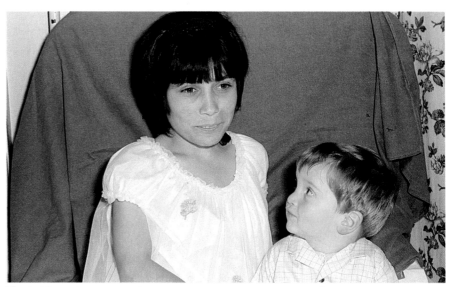

Fig.5.28 β-thalassaemia intermedia: this 29-year-old Cypriot patient had received occasional blood transfusions with her haemoglobin ranging between 6.5-9.0g/dl. She displays a thalassaemic facies with marked maxillary expansion, and had also developed pigment gallstones. She has normal sexual development and fertility, as witnessed by her 2-year-old son.

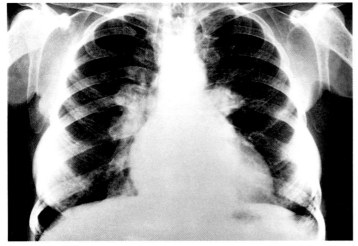

Fig.5.29 β-thalassaemia intermedia: chest radiograph of the patient in Fig.5.28 shows hilar shadows due to paravertebral extramedullary haemopoietic deposits. There is also marked medullary expansion within the ribs, clavicles and humeri, with thinning of cortical bone, and kyphosis of the spine.

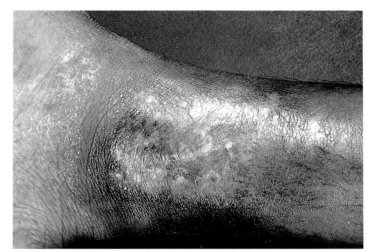

Fig.5.30 β-thalassaemia intermedia: healed ankle ulcer in a normally developed 28-year-old female who required occasional blood transfusions until the age of 22 with increasing blood requirements subsequently, necessitating splenectomy. There is residual local scarring and irregular pigmentation above the medial malleolus.

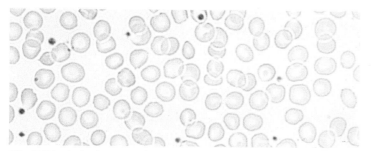

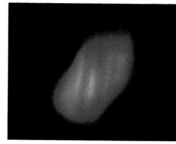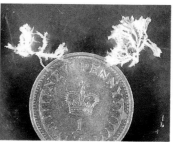

Fig.5.31 β-thalassaemia trait: peripheral blood film from a 20-year-old Cypriot female shows microcytic hypochromic red cells with occasional target cells and poikilocytes. The red cell indices show a much reduced MCV (67fl) and MCH (18.3pg), despite the levels of haemoglobin (10.2g/dl) and PCV (37.3%) being only slightly below normal. The red cell count was raised to 5.6×10^{12}/l and haemoglobin electrophoresis showed a raised haemoglobin A_2 (4.5%) with a normal haemoglobin F (0.9%).

Fig.5.32 Antenatal diagnosis: (left) fetal veins at 14 weeks, as seen through a fetoscope; (right) chorionic villus biopsy from a 12-week-old fetus (size compared with a half-penny coin). Courtesy of Mr. C. Rodeck (left) and Mr. J.W. Keeling (right).

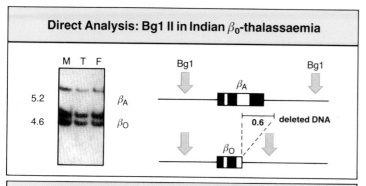

Direct Analysis: Bg1 II in Indian β_0-thalassaemia

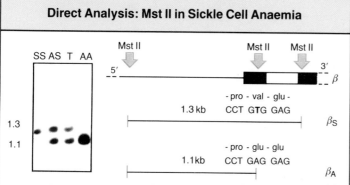

Direct Analysis: Mst II in Sickle Cell Anaemia

Fig.5.33 Antenatal diagnosis: restriction enzyme analysis of trophoblast DNA in (upper) Indian β_0-thalassaemia. After digestion of DNA by the restriction enzyme Bg1 II, the fragments are separated according to size by electrophoresis in agarose gel, transferred to nitrocellulose, and a radioactive β-gene probe added. Autoradiography shows hybridization to a 5.2 kilobase (kb) fragment when the chromosome contains a normal β_A gene but to a 4.6 kb fragment on a chromosome carrying Indian β_0 gene because of deletion of an 0.6 kb fragment. M, mother; T, trophoblast; F, father; (lower) Southern blot analysis in sickle cell anaemia. DNA has been digested by Mst II. An adenine base in the normal β-globin gene is replaced by a thymine base in the sickle β-globin gene, removing a normal restriction site for Mst II and producing a larger 1.3 kb fragment which hybridizes with the β-globin gene probe. In this case, as the trophoblast (T) DNA shows both normal (A) and sickle (S) restriction fragments, the fetus is AS (in other words, a sickle carrier). Courtesy of Dr. J. Old and The Royal College of Obstetrics and Gynaecology.

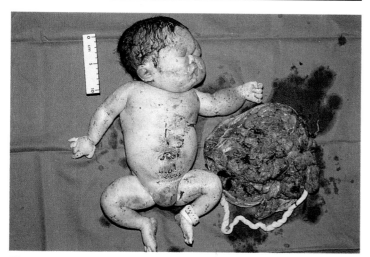

Fig.5.34 α-thalassaemia: hydrops fetalis, the result of deletion of all four α-globin genes (homozygous α_0-thalassaemia). The main haemoglobin present is Hb Bart's (γ_4). The condition is incompatible with life beyond the fetal stage. Courtesy of Prof. D. Todd.

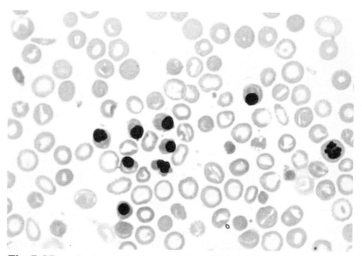

Fig.5.35 α-thalassaemia: peripheral blood film in homozygous α_0-thalassaemia (hydrops fetalis) at birth shows marked hypochromasia, polychromasia and many circulating normoblasts.

Deletion of three genes (haemoglobin H disease) presents as a moderately severe anaemia *(Hb:7.0-11.0g/dl)* with splenomegaly and a hypochromic, microcytic blood film appearance (Fig.5.36). Haemoglobin H (β_4) is demonstrable by special staining (Fig.5.37) or haemoglobin electrophoresis.

α-thalassaemia trait may be caused by deletion of two genes (α_0 trait) or of one gene (α_+ trait), and shows a hypochromic, microcytic blood appearance of varying severity. Haemoglobin electrophoresis gives a normal pattern in adults; but, at birth, as much as five to fifteen percent of Hb Barts (γ_4) may be detected in α_0 trait, and up to two percent in α_+ trait. In α_0 trait an occasional cell in the adult blood film may show Hb H bodies after incubation with a dye such as brilliant cresyl blue.

THE HAEMOGLOBINOPATHIES
Sickle cell anaemia

This is the most common of the severe haemo-globinopathies. It is the result of substitution of valine for glutamic acid in the sixth position of the β-chain due to a single base change in the corresponding portion of DNA (see Fig.5.33,lower). Sickle haemoglobin (Hb S) is insoluble at low oxygen tensions and tends to crystallize, causing the red cells to assume a sickle–like appearance. The oxygen dissociation curve is shifted to the right so that oxygen is given up relatively easily to tissues. The patient has few symptoms of anaemia, despite an haemoglobin in the steady state of 6-8g/dl, and has a chronic haemolytic anaemia punctuated by sickle crises. Typically the patient is of asthenic build (Fig.5.38), and is mildly jaundiced. Ulcers around the ankle are common (Fig.5.40). There may be bone deformities due to infarcts (Fig.5.41). If the small bones of the hands and feet are affected, there may be unequal growth of the digits ('hand-foot' syndrome; Figs.5.42-5.45).

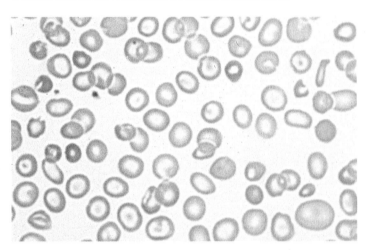

Fig.5.36 α-thalassaemia: peripheral blood film in haemoglobin H disease (three α-globin gene deletion or α_0/α_+ thalassaemia) shows marked hypochromic and microcytic cells with target cells and poikilocytes. The patient was a normally developed 23-year-old male with a spleen enlarged to 6cm below the costal margin, moderate anaemia, *(Hb:9.2g/dl)* and grossly reduced red cell indices (*MCV:59fl; MCH:15.2pg*). Electrophoresis showed Hb:A,76.6%; A_2,2.5%; F,0.9%; H (β_4),20%.

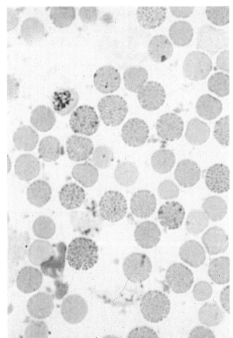

Fig.5.37 α-thalassaemia: peripheral blood film in haemoglobin H disease stained supravitally with brilliant cresyl blue. Some of the cells show multiple fine, deeply staining, deposits which are precipitated aggregates of β-globin chains ('golf-ball' cells). Reticulocytes are also stained.

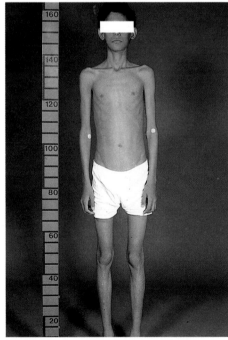

Fig.5.38 Sickle cell anaemia: this patient of Middle Eastern origin is tall with long thin limbs, a large arm span, and narrow pectoral and pelvic girdles. Sexual development is normal.

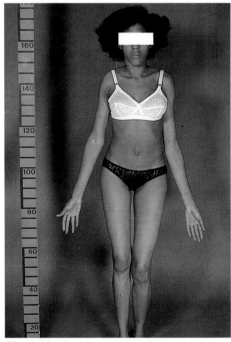

Fig.5.39 Sickle cell anaemia: this patient of West Indian origin is also of asthenic build. She has deformities of both hips due to previous avascular necroses which required total replacement of the hip joints.

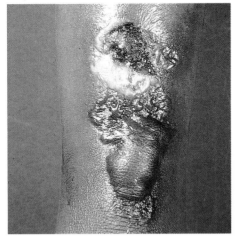

Fig.5.40 Sickle cell anaemia: anterior aspect of the calf of a 12-year-old Nigerian boy shows necrosis and ulceration.

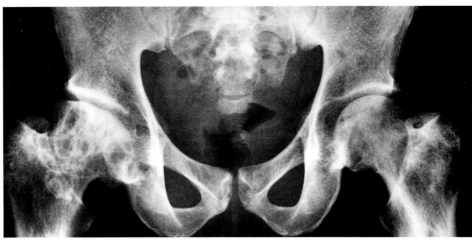

Fig.5.41 Sickle cell anaemia: radiograph of the pelvis of the patient in Fig.5.39 shows avascular necrosis with flattening of the femoral heads, more marked on the right, coarsening of the bone architecture and cystic areas in the right femoral neck due to previous infarcts.

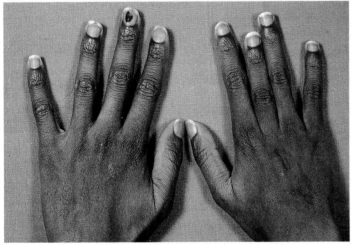

Fig.5.42 Sickle cell anaemia: hands of an 18-year-old Nigerian boy with the 'hand-foot' syndrome. There is marked shortening of the right middle finger because of dactylitis in childhood affecting the growth of the epiphysis.

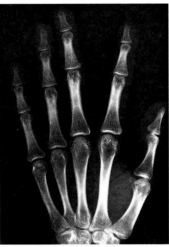

Fig.5.43 Sickle cell anaemia: radiograph of the hands shown in Fig.5.42. There is shortening of the right middle metacarpal bone due to infarction of the growing epiphysis during childhood. The patient was receiving intravenous rehydration during a painful crisis.

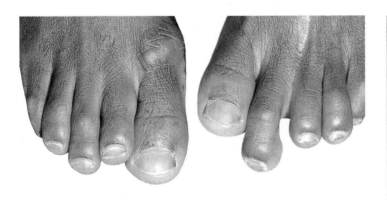

Fig.5.44 Sickle cell anaemia: the toes of the patient shown in Fig.5.42 show irregularities in length.

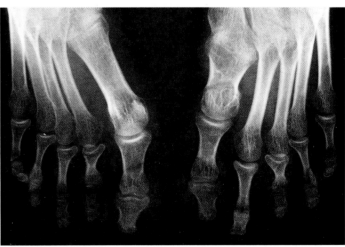

Fig.5.45 Sickle cell anaemia: radiograph of the toes shown in Fig.5.44. The unequal growth of the metatarsal bones are due to infarcts of the growing epiphyses in childhood.

As a result of infections together with infarcts, pneumonia (Figs.5.46 & 5.47) and osteomyelitis, usually from *Salmonella* (Figs.5.48 & 5.49) but sometimes from other organisms, may occur.

Following occlusion of small vessels in the retina during sickle cell crises, there may be characteristic regrowth of blood vessels at the affected sites (Fig.5.50). Infarction and atrophy of the spleen are usual after childhood (Fig.5.51).

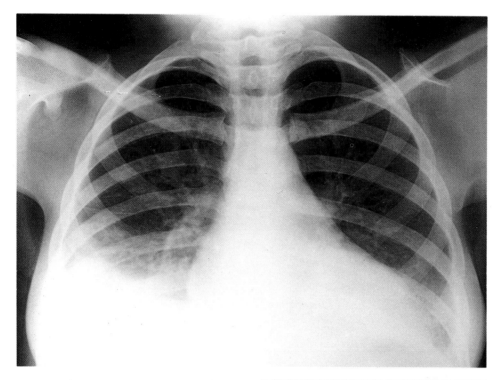

Fig.5.46 Sickle cell anaemia: chest radiograph of an 18-year-old female admitted in crisis with a pulmonary syndrome. There is generalized cardiomegaly and increased vascularity of the lungs, typical of a chronic haemolytic anaemia. In addition, there is shadowing, particularly in the right lower and middle lobes, which resolved slowly on antibiotic therapy and was considered to be due to infection and small vessel obstruction.

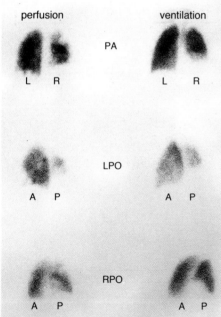

Fig.5.47 Sickle cell anaemia: ventilation-perfusion lung scan of the patient shown in Fig.5.46 shows (left) perfusion measured with technetium Tc 99m aggregated albumin (50μ particles); (right) ventilation using krypton 81m. The ventilation defect at the base of the right lung suggests infection only, but the multiple perfusion defects apparent in other areas of both lungs suggest blockage of segmental and subsegmental arteries. Courtesy of Dr. A. Hilson.

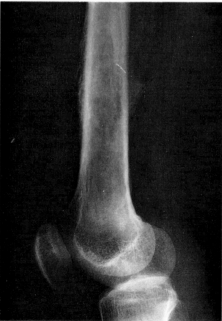

Fig.5.48 Sickle cell anaemia: lateral radiograph of the lower limb and knee in *Salmonella* osteomyelitis. The periosteum is irregularly raised in the lower third of the femur.

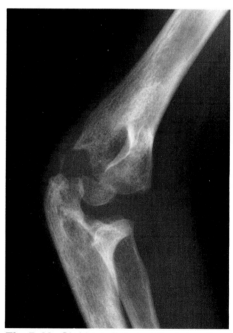

Fig.5.49 Sickle cell anaemia: lateral radiograph of the elbow joint in staphylococcal osteomyelitis shows destructive changes in the humerus and ulna.

The blood film shows the presence of sickle cells, target cells (Fig.5.52) and, in most adult cases, features of splenic atrophy (Fig.5.53). The haemopoietic marrow expands down the long bones (Fig.5.54) and the myeloid:erythroid ratio is reversed.

The different types of haemoglobin may be separated and quantitated by electrophoresis in cellulose acetate (Fig.5.55) or agar gel.

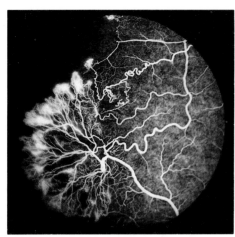

Fig.5.50 Sickle cell anaemia: fluorescein angiogram of the retina shows abnormal vessels and retinitis proliferans (leaking fluorescein) at the junction of the vascularized and ischaemic areas. The vessels are unusually tortuous with arteriovenous anastomoses. Courtesy of Dr. G. Serjeant.

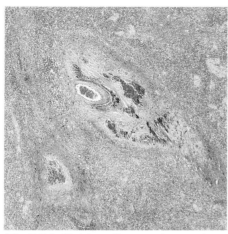

Fig.5.51 Sickle cell anaemia: section of atrophied spleen showing deposits of haemosiderin in nests of macrophages (gamma-Gandy bodies) around the vessels. There is severe reduction of both red and white pulp. H & E stain.

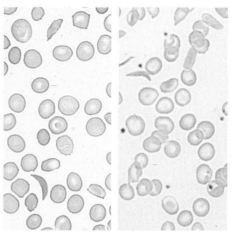

Fig.5.52 Sickle cell anaemia: peripheral blood films showing (left) deeply staining sickle cells with target cells and polychromasia; (right) sickle, hypochromic and target cells.

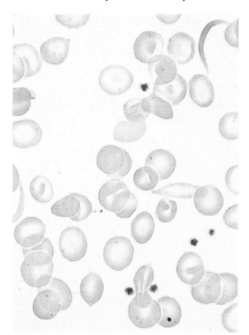

Fig.5.53 Sickle cell anaemia: peripheral blood film in a patient with splenic atrophy. Howell-Jolly and Pappenheimer bodies are seen in addition to the sickle cells and target cells.

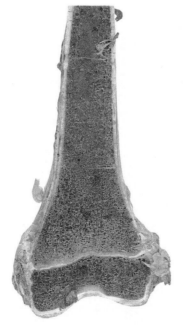

Fig.5.54 Sickle cell anaemia: post-mortem longitudinal section of femur showing expansion of red (haemopoietic) marrow down the shaft towards the knee with thinning of cortical bone. Courtesy of Dr. J.E. McLaughlin.

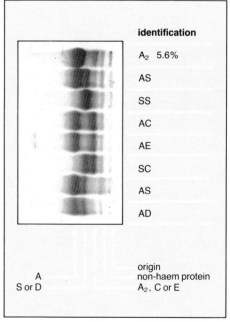

Fig.5.55 Sickle cell anaemia: haemoglobin electrophoresis on cellulose acetate, Ponceau S stain. S and D, and A_2, C and E, run together. Agar gel separation is usually used to distinguish them. The uppermost lane shows the raised Hb A_2 level of β-thalassaemia trait.

Sickle cell trait gives a normal blood appearance, possibly with an occasional sickle cell present, unless a crisis is induced, for example, by anoxia or severe infection. Recurrent haematuria due to renal papillary necrosis is an occasional problem. Combinations of sickle trait with other haemoglobin defects, such as thalassaemia trait (Fig.5.56) or C trait (Fig.5.57), give rise clinically to mild forms of sickle cell disease.

Other haemoglobinopathies

Other common haemoglobinopathies include haemoglobin C (Fig.5.58), haemoglobin D and haemoglobin E diseases (Fig.5.59). Rare syndromes produced by haemoglobin abnormalities include haemolytic anaemia because of an unstable haemoglobin (Fig.5.60), hereditary polycythaemia and hereditary methaemoglobinaemia.

Fetal haemoglobin

Fetal haemoglobin (haemoglobin F; $\alpha_2\gamma_2$) forms 0.3–1.2% of circulating haemoglobin in normal adults. It is demonstrated in a very minor proportion of the red cells using the Kleihauer (acid elution) technique (Fig.5.61), but is detected in up to seven percent of red cells using more sensitive immunological methods. Fetal haemoglobin is the dominant haemoglobin in fetal life but a switch from γ to β–chain production occurs at about three months of postnatal life.

In the β-thalassaemia syndromes, fetal haemoglobin production may be increased; this is particularly the case in $\delta\beta$-thalassaemia when the haemoglobin is heterogeneously distributed. It is also increased in a variety of disorders termed 'hereditary persistence of fetal haemoglobin' when the haemoglobin is homogeneously distributed throughout the red cells. There is a slight increase of fetal haemoglobin in adult blood in a variety of acquired blood disorders, such as megaloblastic anaemia, acute leukaemia and paroxysmal nocturnal haemoglobinuria.

Fetal red cells may circulate postnatally in maternal blood due to a fetal to maternal bleed at delivery; such cells may be detected by the Kleihauer technique (Fig.5.61).

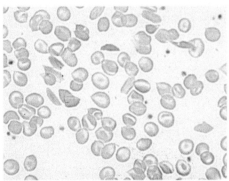

Fig.5.56 Sickle cell/β-thalassaemia: peripheral blood film showing sickle cells, target cells and normoblasts as well as microcytic hypochromic cells, punctate basophilia and polychromasia.

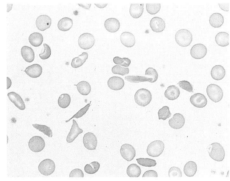

Fig.5.57 Sickle cell/haemoglobin C disease: peripheral blood film in which sickle cells and target cells are prominent.

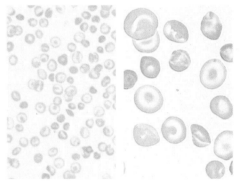

Fig.5.58 Homozygous haemoglobin C disease: peripheral blood films in low (left) and high (right) power views. Many target cells are seen without obvious microcytic hypochromic cells.

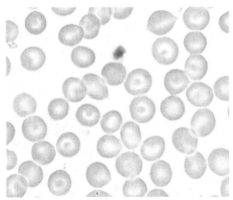

Fig.5.59 Homozygous haemoglobin E disease: peripheral blood film showing target cells with an absence of hypochromic or microcytic cells.

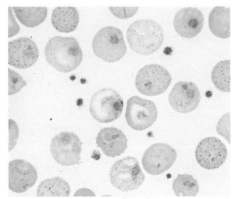

Fig.5.60 Unstable haemoglobin (Hb Hammersmith): peripheral blood film postsplenectomy shows many cells with punctate basophilia, or containing single or multiple inclusion bodies composed of precipitated, denatured haemoglobin (seen as Heinz bodies on special staining). The underlying lesion is substitution of the amino acid phenylalanine by serine at position 42 in the β-chain.

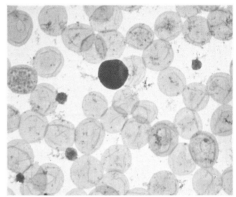

Fig.5.61 Fetal haemoglobin: acid elution (Kleihauer) technique showing a fetal red cell in maternal blood. The darkly staining fetal cell contains fetal haemoglobin which has resisted elution at low pH. The adult cells appear as 'ghosts' because the adult haemoglobin has been leeched out of the cells.

6

Aplastic, Dyserythropoietic and Secondary Anaemias, and Bone Marrow Transplantation

APLASTIC ANAEMIA

Aplastic (hypoplastic) anaemia consists of pancytopenia due to hypoplasia of the marrow. It may be transient, for example, following cytotoxic therapy, but the term is usually used to denote the chronic forms of the condition. The condition may be congenital or acquired (Fig.6.1).

In about half of the acquired cases, no cause can be found. The response to antilymphocyte globulin in a substantial proportion of these 'idiopathic' cases, however, suggests that an immune mechanism may be involved. The success of bone marrow transplantation implies that the haemopoietic microenvironment of the marrow is intact, at least in the majority of cases.

The cause of the anaemia in about a third of the patients appears to be damage by a drug or toxin to the haemopoietic stem cells which are then reduced in

Causes of Aplastic Anaemia	
Congenital	**Acquired**
Fanconi	Idiopathic
Non-Fanconi	Secondary:
Associated with dyskeratosis congenita	drugs: hypersensitivity (phenylbutazone, chloramphenicol, gold, sulphonamides, etc.); cytotoxics (busulphan, cyclophosphamide, etc.)
	irradiation
	infection: postviral hepatitis
	toxins: insecticides; benzene; etc.

Fig.6.1 Causes of aplastic anaemia.

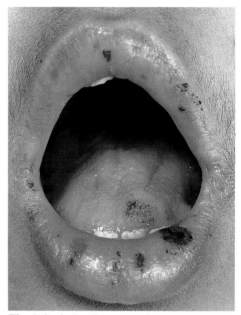

Fig.6.2 Aplastic anaemia: spontaneous mucosal haemorrhages in a 10-year-old boy with severe congenital (Fanconi) anaemia. *Hb:7.3g/dl; WBC:1.1x10^9/l (neutrophils:21%; lymphocytes:77%); platelets:<5.0x10^9/l.*

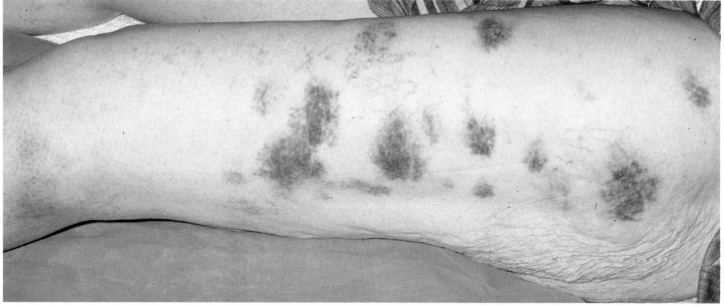

Fig.6.3 Aplastic anaemia: spontaneous bruising over the thigh and leg of a 57-year-old female with idiopathic acquired aplastic anaemia. *Hb:8.9g/dl; WBC:1.7x10^9/l; platelets:12x10^9/l.*

number as they lose their ability to self-renew and proliferate. The drugs most frequently associated with aplastic anaemia are the sulphonamides, chloramphenicol, phenylbutazone and its derivatives, and gold; but a wide range of drugs has been implicated. In some patients these drugs give rise to only a selective neutropenia or thrombocytopenia. Aplastic anaemia may also be caused by radiation or infection, particularly viral hepatitis.

The anaemia is mildly macrocytic or normocytic. The clinical features are those of anaemia, haemorrhage due to thrombocytopenia or infections because of neutropenia. Bleeding is usually into the skin as petechiae or ecchymoses, or into or from mucosal surfaces (Figs.6.2 & 6.3), but may also occur into internal organs (Fig.6.4), cerebral haemorrhage being the major risk. Infections are usually bacterial (Fig.6.5) but may also be viral (Fig.6.6), fungal (Fig.6.7) or protozoal, particularly later in the disease.

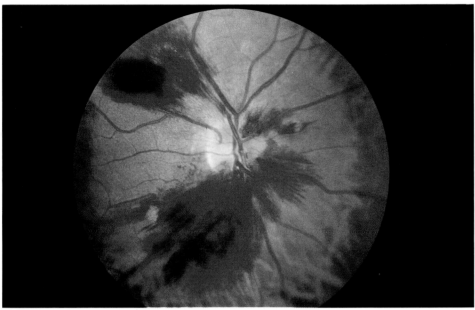

Fig.6.4 Aplastic anaemia: retinal haemorrhages in a patient with acquired disease and profound thrombocytopenia.

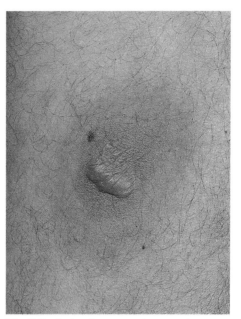

Fig.6.5 Aplastic anaemia: purple discoloration and blistering of the skin due to infection with *Pseudomonas pyocyanea*.

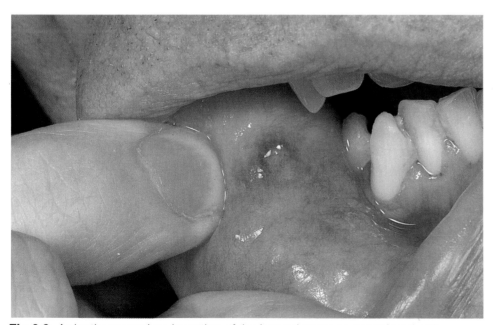

Fig.6.6 Aplastic anaemia: ulceration of the buccal mucosa associated with severe neutropenia. Herpes simplex virus was grown from the ulcers. *Total leucocyte count:0.8x10^9/l; neutrophils:20%*.

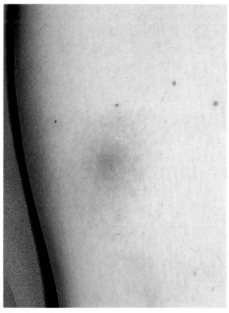

Fig.6.7 Aplastic anaemia: raised, erythematous skin nodule due to infection with *Candida albicans* which was also present in the bloodstream. The patient, a 27-year-old female, had previously been treated with antibacterial agents for prolonged periods of fever due to bacterial infections.

Congenital aplastic anaemia

The congenital forms of aplastic anaemia may be associated with other congenital defects as in the Fanconi syndrome, an autosomal recessive inherited disease in which random chromosomal breaks with endoreduplication and chromatid exchange can be demonstrated in peripheral lymphocytes; skeletal, renal and other defects may be present as well as hyperpigmentation, small stature from birth and hypogonadism (Figs.6.8–6.11).

A less common association of the congenital form of aplastic anaemia is dyskeratosis congenita in which skin, nails and hair are abnormal (Figs.6.12 & 6.13). There may also be telangiectasia, alopecia and abnormal sweating as well as mental retardation, growth failure and hypogonadism but, in contrast to Fanconi anaemia, the chromosomal pattern is normal.

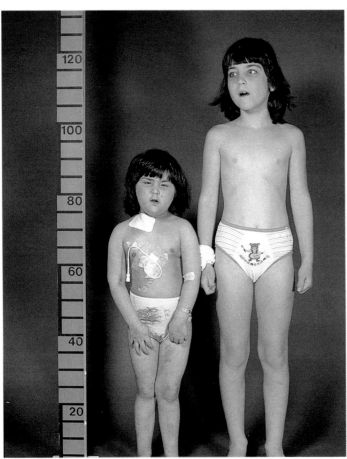

Fig.6.8 Fanconi anaemia: the patient, aged six, shows short stature and a minor degree of microcephaly compared with her normal older sister who was HLA-identical and the donor for bone marrow transplantation.

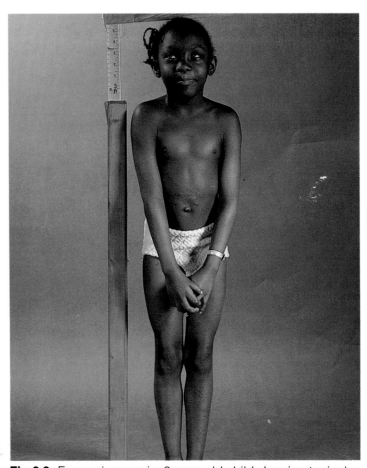

Fig.6.9 Fanconi anaemia: 9-year-old child showing typical short stature (height:42 inches or 1.06m). Courtesy of Dr. B. Wonke.

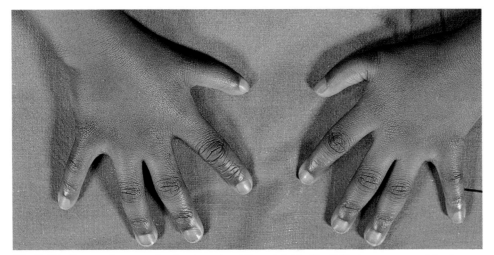

Fig.6.10 Fanconi anaemia: the hands of the child in Fig.6.9 show symmetrical abnormalities of the thumbs, resulting in their resemblance to fingers. Courtesy of Dr. B. Wonke.

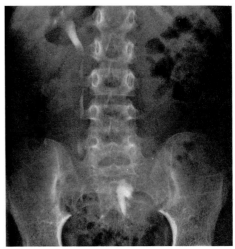

Fig.6.11 Fanconi anaemia: intravenous pyelogram of the child in Fig.6.9 shows a normal right kidney but a left kidney which is abnormally placed in the pelvis.

Bone marrow appearances

The bone marrow fragments show reduced cellularity (Fig.6.14), fat spaces occupying more than seventy-five percent of the marrow. The trails are also reduced in cellularity with particularly low numbers of megakaryocytes and often a predominance of lymphocytes and plasma cells. The hypoplasia is best shown by trephine biopsy (Fig.6.15). There may be areas of normal cellularity despite the overall hypocellularity (Fig.6.16), and lymphoid follicles may be prominent (Fig.6.17).

Because therapy differs according to the degree of aplasia, a standard classification of severity has been adopted. Criteria for severe disease are: less than $50 \times 10^5/l$ reticulocytes, $10 \times 10^9/l$ platelets and $0.5 \times 10^9/l$ granulocytes in peripheral blood; and more than eighty percent of the remaining cells in the marrow are non-myeloid. Any three of these four conditions persisting for more than two weeks classifies the patient as having severe aplastic anaemia.

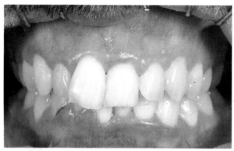

Fig.6.12 Dyskeratosis congenita: 24-year-old male with longstanding aplastic anaemia and dyskeratosis congenita. There are irregularities of the teeth in size and shape and of the gum margins.

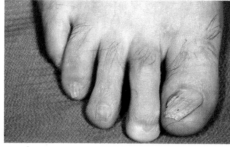

Fig.6.13 Dyskeratosis congenita: the feet of the patient in Fig.6.12 shows grossly abnormal nails and excessive hair over the toes and feet in an abnormal distribution.

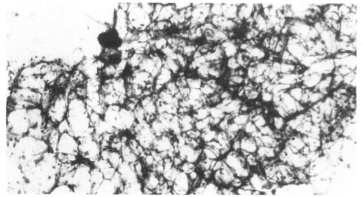

Fig.6.14 Aplastic anaemia: low power view of bone marrow fragment shows severe reduction of haemopoietic cells with an increase in fat spaces.

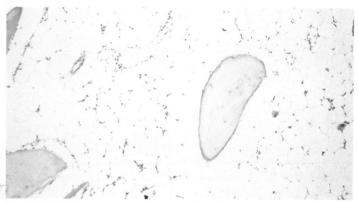

Fig.6.15 Aplastic anaemia: trephine biopsy of posterior iliac crest shows gross hypocellularity with replacement by fat.

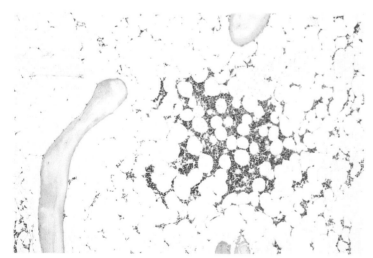

Fig.6.16 Aplastic anaemia: trephine biopsy shows some haemopoietic cellular foci in an otherwise grossly hypocellular marrow.

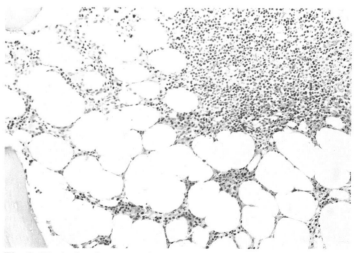

Fig.6.17 Aplastic anaemia: higher power view of the same biopsy as in Fig.6.16 shows grossly hypocellular marrow with a remaining lymphoid follicle in the upper right field.

During the recovery phase, cellularity increases to normal (Fig.6.18); the platelet count is usually the last of the blood cells to recover completely. Paroxysmal nocturnal haemoglobinuria (PNH) or a PNH defect may develop transiently or chronically, and some of these patients may have aplasia of the marrow.

Ferrokinetics

Ferrokinetic studies show a slow clearance of transferrin-bound radioiron with predominant uptake in the liver and reduced incorporation into circulating red cells. Scanning studies show absence of iron uptake by the bone marrow with accumulation of iron in the liver (Fig.6.19).

RED CELL APLASIA

The causes of pure red cell aplasia are listed in Fig.6.20. Like aplastic anaemia it may also be a congenital disease and may be familial or acquired. In the congenital Diamond-Blackfan syndrome (Figs.6.21 & 6.22) there are skeletal defects but without renal and chromosomal abnormalities. The exact pattern of inheritance is unclear. The acquired form may be idiopathic or appear in conjunction with another disease, such as a thymoma (Fig.6.23).

A transient form of red cell aplasia occurs in the course of chronic and other haemolytic anaemias but is best recognized in sickle cell anaemia. In nearly all cases this form is the result of parvovirus infection with selective damage by the virus to bone marrow red cell progenitors. It is likely that a similar red cell aplasia occurs in normal subjects with this infection but is not clinically apparent because of the longer red cell lifespan. In all forms the bone marrow is of normal cellularity but there is a relative absence of erythroid precursors (Fig.6.24).

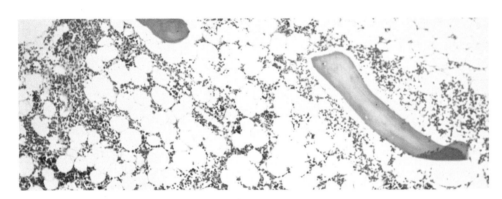

Fig.6.18 Aplastic anaemia: trephine biopsy (same case as in Fig.6.16) shows partial recovery of cellularity four weeks after treatment with antilymphocyte globulin. There was also a modest rise in peripheral blood cell counts.

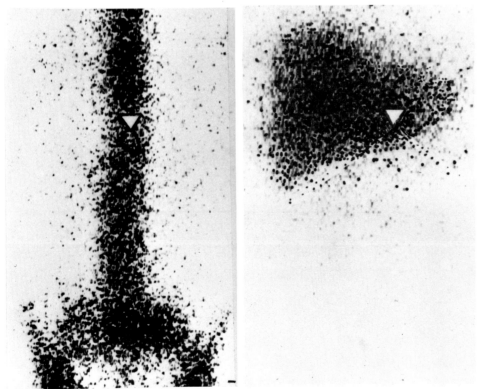

Fig.6.19 Aplastic anaemia: iron-52 (^{52}Fe) scans showing (left) normal concentration of isotope in the bones of the spine and pelvis and (right) accumulation of iron isotope only in the liver in aplastic anaemia. The triangle marks the position of the xiphisternum.

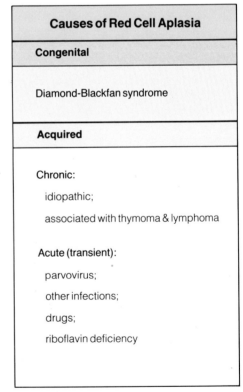

Causes of Red Cell Aplasia
Congenital
Diamond-Blackfan syndrome
Acquired

Chronic:
  idiopathic;
  associated with thymoma & lymphoma
 	
Acute (transient):
  parvovirus;
  other infections;
  drugs;
  riboflavin deficiency

Fig.6.20 Causes of red cell aplasia.

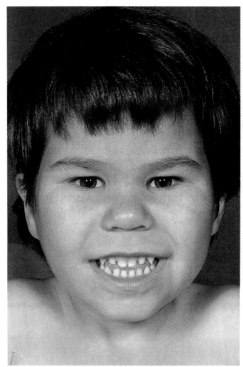 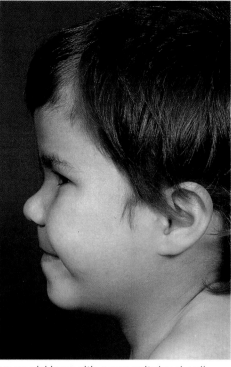 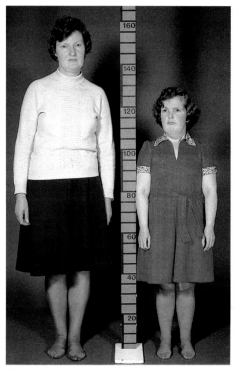

Fig.6.21 Diamond-Blackfan syndrome: 3-year-old boy with congenital red cell aplasia shows the typical facies with a sunken bridge of nose. This child was treated with blood transfusions and subsequently corticosteroids to which he made a partial response and became transfusion-independent. His mental development is normal but his growth has been partly retarded because of the steroid therapy. *Hb:6.1g/dl; WBC:7.2×10⁹/l; neutrophils:55%; lymphocytes:41%; monocytes:4%; platelets:289×10⁹/l.*

Fig.6.22 Diamond-Blackfan syndrome: this 24-year-old female (on the right) had received corticosteroid therapy as an infant and child in order to reduce the need for blood transfusions. This led to stunted growth (compare with her normal mother). The patient had received over 100 units of blood and developed transfusional haemosiderosis with enlargement of the liver and spleen.

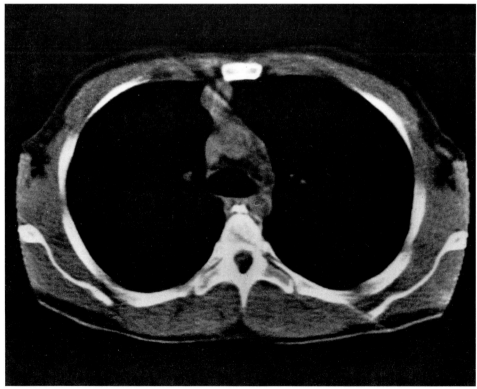 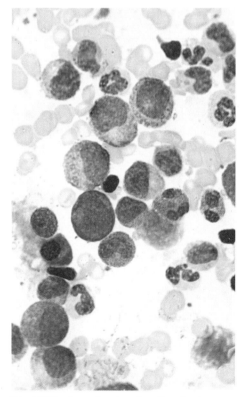

Fig.6.23 Acquired red cell aplasia: upper mediastinal computerized tomographic scan shows a thymoma as a retrosternal mass of irregular outline. The patient, a 62-year-old male, had developed myasthenia gravis and pure red cell aplasia which required regular blood transfusions. Courtesy of Dr. R. Dick.

Fig.6.24 Acquired red cell aplasia: bone marrow aspirate cell trail shows normal numbers of granulocytes and their precursors but an absence of normoblasts.

6.7

CONGENITAL DYSERYTHROPOIETIC ANAEMIAS (CDA)

These rare autosomal recessive diseases are characterized clinically by anaemia, often with jaundice due to ineffective erythropoiesis and shortened red cell survival, and morphologically by abnormal red cell precursors in the bone marrow. The anaemia is usually macrocytic, and the reticulocyte count may be raised but is low relative to the degree of anaemia.

The diseases are divided into three main groups according to the appearance of the bone marrow. In CDA I (Figs.6.25 & 6.26), megaloblastic changes and internuclear chromatin bridges are prominent. In CDA II (Figs.6.27 & 6.28), the most frequent type (also known as HEMPAS), there are bi- and multinucleated erythroblasts, pluripotent mitoses and a positive acidified serum lysis test. CDA III (Figs.6.29 & 6.30) is characterized by multinuclearity and gigantoblasts.

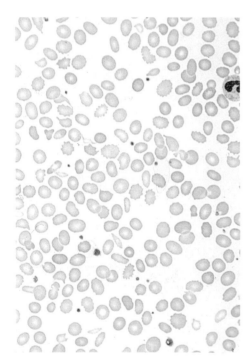

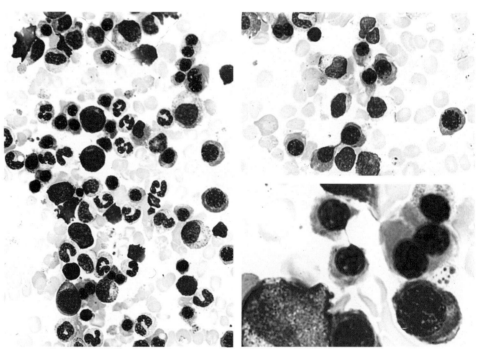

Fig.6.25 Congenital dyserythropoietic anaemia (Type I): peripheral blood film showing oval macrocytes, poikilocytes and small fragmented cells. The platelets and granulocytes are normal.

Fig.6.26 Congenital dyserythropoietic anaemia (Type I): bone marrow aspirate showing (left) erythroid hyperplasia, megaloblastic erythropoiesis and binucleate erythroblasts; (right) higher power view showing two examples of cells with internuclear bridges.

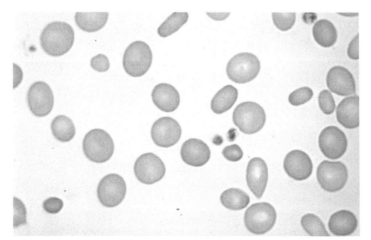

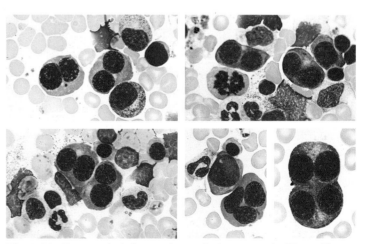

Fig.6.27 Congenital dyserythropoietic anaemia (Type II): peripheral blood film shows marked red cell anisocytosis and poikilocytosis.

Fig.6.28 Congenital dyserythropoietic anaemia (Type II): selected high power views of bone marrow aspirate show multinucleated erythroblasts.

SECONDARY ANAEMIAS

Many anaemias are not part of a primary blood disorder but occur in patients with other systemic disease. In these anaemias there are often a number of contributing factors, such as iron and folate deficiencies, haemolysis, marrow infiltration or marrow suppression by therapy.

In chronic inflammatory or malignant conditions usually with a raised erythrocyte sedimentation rate, there is also a mild (*Hb:>9.0g/dl*) normochromic or hypochromic anaemia associated with low serum iron, reduced total iron binding capacity and normal or raised serum ferritin. The severity of this anaemia is related to the severity of the underlying disease. Bone marrow iron stores are normal or increased, but siderotic granules are not seen in developing erythroblasts (Fig.6.31). This 'anaemia of chronic disorders' is thought to arise as a result of a combination of failure of iron release from reticuloendothelial cells, reduced red cell survival and an inadequate erythropoietin response.

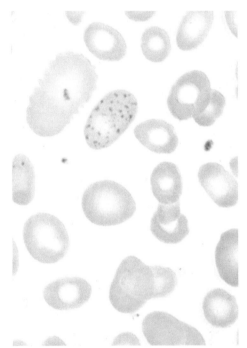

Fig.6.29 Congenital dyserythropoietic anaemia (Type III): peripheral blood film shows gross macrocytosis, anisocytosis, poikilocytosis and punctate basophilia. Courtesy of Dr. I.M. Hann.

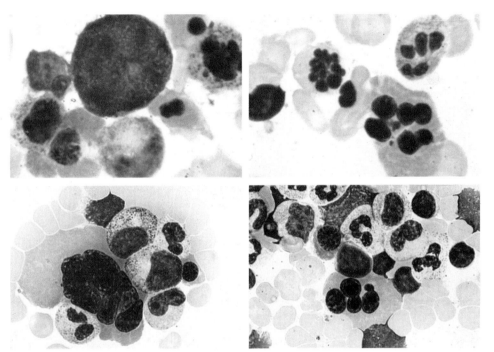

Fig.6.30 Congenital dyserythropoietic anaemia (Type III): selected high power views of bone marrow aspirate show multinucleated erythroblasts and karyorrhexis. Courtesy of Dr. I.M. Hann.

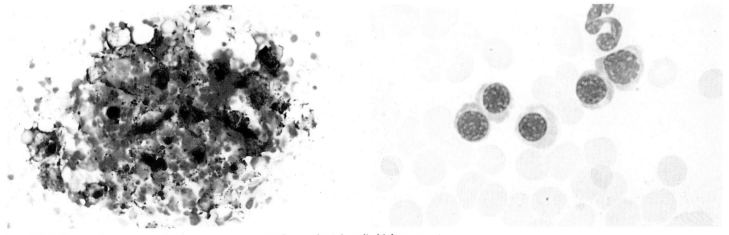

Fig.6.31 Secondary anaemia: bone marrow aspirate showing (left) fragments containing adequate iron in the reticuloendothelial cells and (right) no siderotic granules in the developing erythroblasts. Perls' stains.

In the majority of patients with systemic disease and anaemia, no particular morphological features are seen in the blood other than mild hypochromasia. However, in liver disease there is frequently red cell macrocytosis, acanthocytosis and target cell formation (Fig.6.32). The mean cell volume is particularly raised when alcohol is the underlying cause. Bleeding due to oesophageal or gastric varices, peptic ulceration, folate deficiency, haemolysis especially in Zieve's syndrome (jaundice, hyperlipidaemia, hypercholesterolaemia and haemolytic anaemia with excess alcohol intake) may complicate the picture. In chronic renal failure, 'burr' cells and other bizarre poikilocytes are characteristic (Fig.6.33). In disseminated adenocarcinoma, microangiopathic haemolytic anaemia (Fig.6.34; see Fig.4.40) may occur. Small acanthocytic forms are found in some patients with hypothyroidism (Fig.6.35).

Connective tissue diseases are also important causes of anaemia in which haemolysis, renal failure and the anaemia of chronic disorders may all play a part. The lupus erythematosus (LE) cell test (Fig.6.36), used to diagnose systemic lupus erythematosus, has now been replaced by tests for antinuclear factor and DNA binding.

BONE MARROW TRANSPLANTATION (BMT)
This is usually carried out between siblings who are human leucocyte antigen (HLA)-identical and mixed lymphocyte culture unreactive (allogeneic transplantation). Syngeneic (twin), haploidentical and HLA-matched but unrelated donors may also be used in appropriate cases. The recipient has severe aplastic anaemia or poor prognosis leukaemia (for example, acute myeloblastic leukaemia in first remission; acute lymphoblastic leukaemia in second or subsequent remission or in first remission with poor prognostic features; or chronic granulocytic leukaemia in chronic phase).

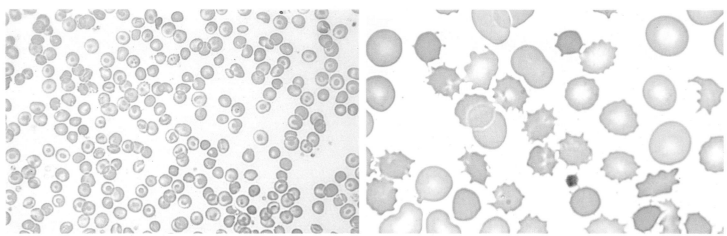

Fig.6.32 Liver disease: peripheral blood films showing (left) marked target cell formation and (right) at higher magnification, marked red cell acanthocytosis.

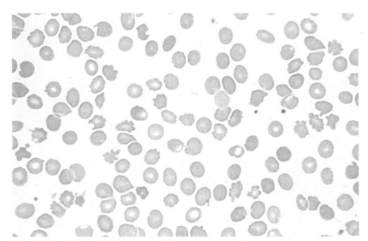

Fig.6.33 Renal failure: peripheral blood film showing coarse acanthocytes and 'burr' cells.

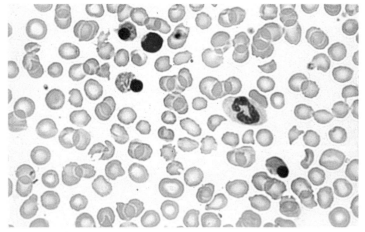

Fig.6.34 Carcinomatosis: peripheral blood film of microangiopathic haemolytic and leucoerythroblastic anaemias in a 52-year-old man who presented with severe anaemia (Hb:4.1g/dl; reticulocytes:18%) associated with widespread adenocarcinoma in the bone marrow. The primary site was unknown. There are deeply staining fragmented red cells, polychromasia and circulating normoblasts. Platelets were severely reduced (32x10⁹/l) and fibrin degradation products were present in serum.

Bone marrow transplantation has also been carried out for certain benign congenital or acquired abnormalities of the marrow (for instance, thalassaemia major or paroxysmal nocturnal haemoglobinuria), of the lymphoid system (as in severe combined immune deficiency) or of the macrophage system (as in Hurler's disease).

Failure of engraftment is unusual in well-matched transplants for leukaemia but is more common when the recipient has aplastic anaemia or when donor and recipient are not fully matched.

Complications of BMT

Transplantation is not usually carried out for patients over forty-five years of age because of the increased incidence of complications. The recipient's marrow is first eliminated by intensive chemotherapy which is usually combined in the case of leukaemia with total body irradiation. There is a period of at least two weeks of pancytopenia before the infused donor marrow pluripotential stem cells, having seeded the recipient's bone marrow, proliferate and differentiate sufficiently to produce new mature red cells, leucocytes and platelets.

Infections are a major hazard during the post-transplant period. Attempts at prevention include reverse-barrier or laminar-flow nursing, prophylactic non-absorbable antibiotics and antifungal agents, and early use of systemic antibiotics for febrile episodes. Prolonged antibiotic therapy, however, increases the likelihood of fungal infections (Figs.6.37 & 6.38).

Cytomegalovirus may arise from reactivation of previous infection or transmission of the virus in blood products and may result in severe pneumonitis (Figs.6.39 & 6.40).

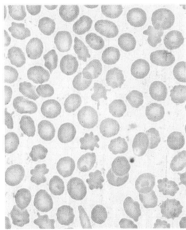

Fig.6.35 Hypothyroidism: peripheral blood film showing mild macrocytosis, poikilocytosis and irregular acanthocytosis.

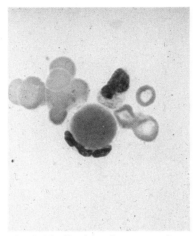

Fig.6.36 Positive lupus erythematosus (LE) cell test: the amorphous purple-staining nucleus has been phago-cytosed by a neutrophil.

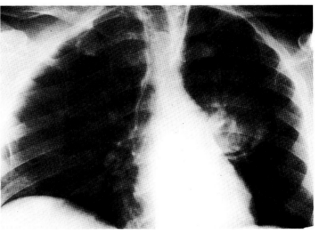

Fig.6.37 Bone marrow transplantation: chest radiograph showing an opacity in the upper left zone with a cystic centre containing a dense central zone. This was found to be due to aspergillosis.

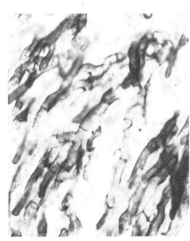

Fig.6.38 Bone marrow transplantation: cytology of sputum from the case in Fig.6.37 shows the typical branching septate hyphae of *Aspergillus*. Methenamine silver stain. Courtesy of Dr. Y.S. Erosan.

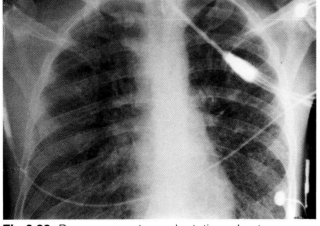

Fig.6.39 Bone marrow transplantation: chest radiograph showing widespread interstitial pneumonia. Sputum cultures and indirect immunofluorescence showed the presence of cytomegalovirus.

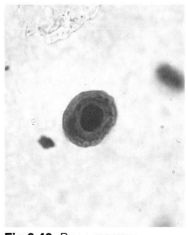

Fig.6.40 Bone marrow transplantation: sputum cytology shows a pulmonary cell with degenerative changes and a large intranuclear inclusion body typical of cytomegalovirus infection. Papanicolaou stain. Courtesy of Dr. Y.S. Erosan.

Herpes simplex is a frequent viral complication which tends to become generalized and may cause pneumonia, encephalitis or skin lesions (Fig.6.41). Infection can be prevented by the use of prophylactic intravenous acyclovir. Pneumonia due to *Pneumocystis carinii* is another frequent complication of the immuno-suppression and neutropenia (Figs.6.42 & 6.43).

Total body irradiation itself may cause side effects involving epithelial structures; there is damage to the nails and nail beds (Fig.6.44) and temporary complete alopecia (Fig.6.45).

Graft-versus-host disease (GvHD)

Another major post-transplant development is reaction of the immunocompetent cells in the graft against the tissues of the host, causing graft-versus-host disease which may be acute (occurring in the first one hundred days post-transplant) or chronic. There is a triad of skin,

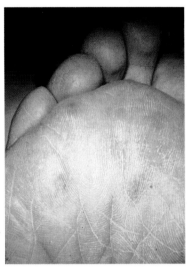

Fig.6.41 Bone marrow transplantation: herpes simplex infection with multiple widespread lesions on the skin of the sole of the foot. Courtesy of Dr. H.G. Prentice.

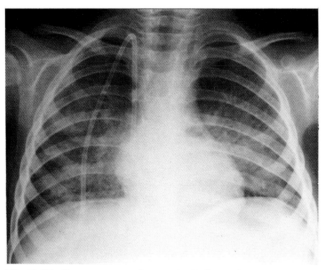

Fig.6.42 Bone marrow transplantation: chest radiograph showing typical 'bat wing' shadowing of both lung fields due to *Pneumocystis carinii* infection.

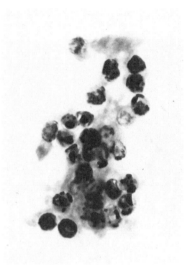

Fig.6.43 Bone marrow transplantation: high power view of concentrated bronchial washings showing typical appearance of *Pneumocystis carinii*. Gram/Weigert stain. Courtesy of Dr. Y.S. Erosan.

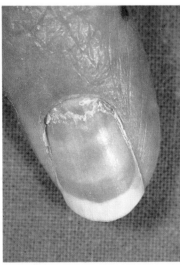

Fig.6.44 Bone marrow transplantation: this nail shows horizontal ridges and atrophy of the nail bed as a result of total body irradiation. Courtesy of Dr. H.G. Prentice.

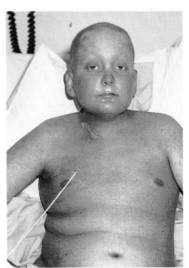

Fig.6.45 Bone marrow transplantation: widespread erythematous skin rash in acute GvHD. An indwelling central Hickman catheter is in place. Courtesy of Dr. H.G. Prentice.

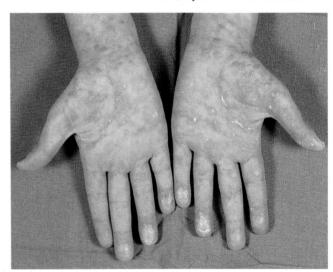

Fig.6.46 Bone marrow transplantation: the palmar surfaces of these hands show an erythematous maculopapular eruption with bullous ulceration and denudation in GvHD. Courtesy of Dr. H.G. Prentice.

mucous membrane and gut, and liver involvement which is graded according to severity into Grades I, II, III or IV.

In acute cases of GvHD there is a widespread erythematous itchy skin rash (Fig.6.45) which tends to be particularly severe on the hands and feet. In severe cases there may be a bullous eruption and subsequent widespread exfoliation (Fig.6.46).

In chronic cases the lesions tend to be firm, red and plaque-like (Fig.6.47) and ultimately may, in some patients, form a scleroderma-like picture with contractures and ulceration (Fig.6.48). The hands and feet may continue to exfoliate (Fig.6.49). The mucous membranes may also be affected with formation of lichen planus-like lesions in the mouth and pharynx (Fig.6.50).

The histological appearances of GvHD are normally seen in life after skin or rectal biopsy. In acute GvHD the skin shows inflammatory changes with death of epidermal cells and a lymphoid infiltrate (Fig.6.51) leading, in severe cases, to denudation.

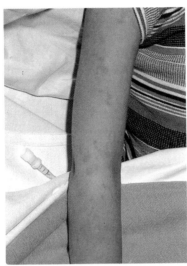

Fig.6.47 Bone marrow transplantation: these patchy raised erythematous skin lesions are characteristic of chronic GvHD. Courtesy of Dr. H.G. Prentice.

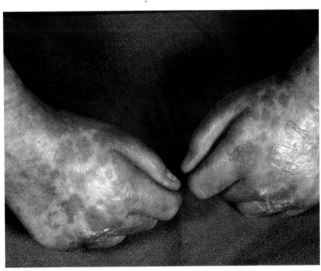

Fig.6.48 Bone marrow transplantation: chronic GvHD may result in scleroderma-like contractions of the hands with thickening of the skin and marked pigmentation. Courtesy of Dr. H.G. Prentice.

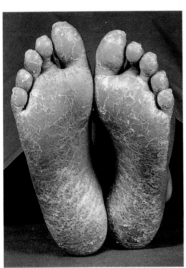

Fig.6.49 Bone marrow transplantation: erythema and exfoliation of the epidermis of the soles of the feet in chronic GvHD. Courtesy of Dr. H.G. Prentice.

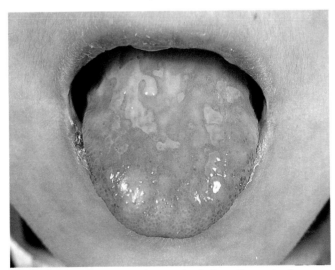

Fig.6.50 Bone marrow transplantation: these lesions of the tongue and lips in chronic GvHD are similar to those of lichen planus. Courtesy of Dr. H.G. Prentice.

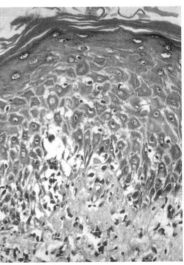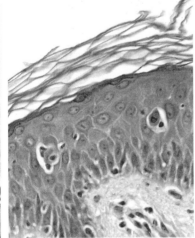

Fig.6.51 Bone marrow transplantation: histological sections of skin in moderately severe (Grade II) acute GvHD of the skin showing (left) vacuolation of the basal epidermal cells with inflammatory changes in the superficial dermis; (right) prominent vacuoles containing necrotic epidermal cells and lymphocytes, from a black patient.

The rectal mucosa also shows death of epithelial (crypt) cells and inflammatory changes (Fig.6.52). When severe there is loss of small and large intestinal mucosa (Fig.6.53).

Liver function is abnormal in acute and chronic GvHD except in mild cases. The histological appearances include damage to bile duct epithelial cells, inflammatory changes and cholestasis (Fig.6.54).

Graft-versus-host disease now can largely be prevented in HLA-matched allogeneic transplantation if T-lymphocytes are completely removed *in vitro* from donor bone marrow.

A frequent post-transplantation complication is an interstitial pneumonia (Fig.6.55) which is more common in patients with GvHD but may also be related to lung irradiation and to infection, particularly with cytomegalovirus.

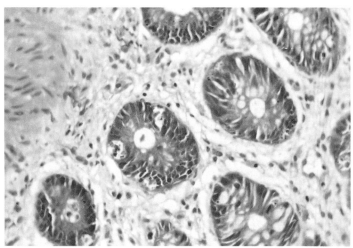

Fig.6.52 Bone marrow transplantation: high power view of rectal biopsy in Grade I acute GvHD shows individual crypt cell necrosis and oedema of the lamina propria.

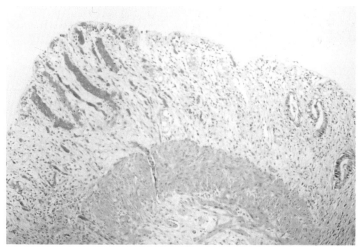

Fig.6.53 Bone marrow transplantation: post mortem section of colon in Grade IV acute GvHD shows almost complete denudation of the epithelium with oedema and lymphocytic infiltration of the submucosa.

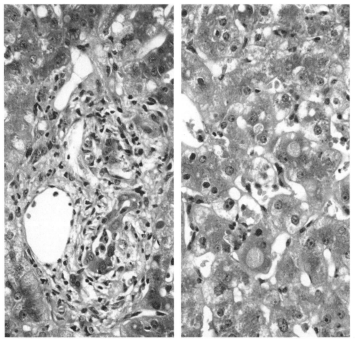

Fig.6.54 Bone marrow transplantation: high power views of liver biopsy in acute GvHD showing (left) damaged, irregular and elongated bile duct epithelial cells with occasional pyknotic nuclei in the portal tract. There is a moderate infiltration of lymphocytes and neutrophils; (right) cholestatic changes include dilated bile canaliculi and pigmented hepatocytes. Courtesy of Prof. P.J. Scheuer.

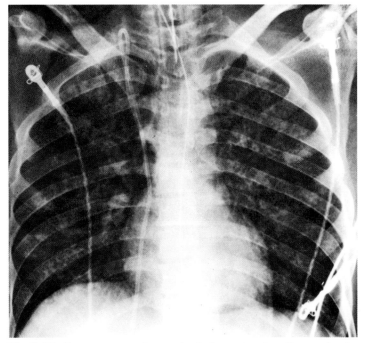

Fig.6.55 Bone marrow transplantation: chest radiograph of interstitial pneumonitis shows widespread diffuse mottling. The patient had received total body irradiation and had Grade III GvHD. No infective cause of the pneumonitis was identified.

7
LEUCOCYTES

Normal white cell appearances and production have been discussed in Chapter 1. This chapter is concerned with conditions which may be associated with abnormal white cell morphology, only some of which are associated with clinical problems. Also included here is some of the more recent information on lymphocyte development, including gene rearrangements. The acquired immune deficiency syndrome (AIDS) is dealt with in this chapter. The acute and chronic lymphoid leukaemias, lymphomas and myeloma are discussed in Chapters 8 to 11.

HEREDITARY VARIATION IN WHITE CELL MORPHOLOGY
Pelger-Huët anomaly
In this condition, characteristic bilobed neutrophils are found in the peripheral blood. Occasional unsegmented neutrophils with round nuclei are also seen, particularly during infection (Fig.7.1). The inheritance is autosomal dominant. The condition appears to be of no clinical significance and the affected cells have not been shown to be functionally abnormal.

May-Hegglin anomaly
In this rare condition, which has a dominant inheritance pattern, abnormal condensations of ribonucleic acid (RNA) appear as mildly basophilic inclusions in the neutrophil cytoplasm (Fig.7.2). The majority of patients also have thrombocytopenia and giant platelets. Athough most affected individuals have no clinical abnormality, in some there are haemorrhagic manifestations. Similar cytoplasmic inclusions, which are termed Döhle bodies, may be seen in neutrophils during severe infections (see Fig.7.10) and occasionally in normal pregnancy.

Chédiak-Higashi syndrome
This severe anomaly is associated with giant neutrophil granules. Similar granular abnormality is seen in granulopoietic cells in the marrow and in eosinophils, monocytes and lymphocytes (Fig.7.3). The inheritance is autosomal recessive. Affected children usually have

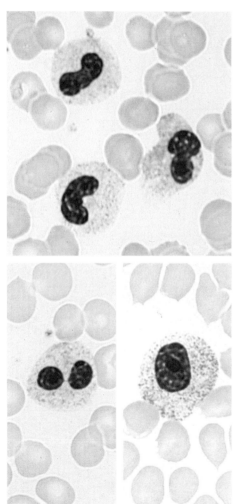

Fig.7.1 Pelger-Huët anomaly: coarse clumping of the chromatin in neutrophils (heterozygous; upper) and 'pince-nez' configurations (lower left); a single rounded nucleus (lower right) seen mostly in rare homozygous patients. 'Pseudo-Pelger' neutrophils can be seen in myeloid leukaemias and the myelodysplastic syndromes.

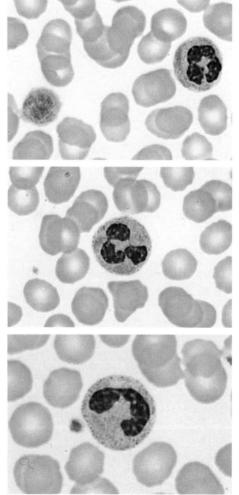

Fig.7.2 May-Hegglin anomaly: the neutrophils contain basophilic inclusions 2-5μm in diameter. These inclusions are similar to Döhle bodies (see Fig.7.10) but are not related to infection. There is an associated mild thrombocytopenia with giant platelets (upper).

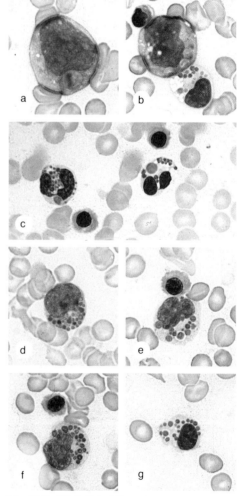

Fig.7.3 Chédiak-Higashi syndrome: bizarre giant granules are found in the cytoplasm of all types of leucocytes and their precursors: (a) promyelocyte; (b) promonocyte and lymphocyte; (c) neutrophils; (d) early eosinophil; (e & f) monocytes; and (g) lymphocyte.

associated neutropenia and thrombocytopenia, and suffer from recurrent severe infections. Clinical examination frequently reveals partial albinism and marked hepatosplenomegaly. The majority die in childhood from infection or haemorrhage.

Alder's (Alder–Reilly) anomaly

This anomaly gives rise to deep purple-coloured granules in neutrophils (Fig.7.4). Similar abnormal granules are found in other granulocytes, monocytes and lymphocytes. The inheritance is autosomal recessive and the majority of affected individuals have no clinical problems. However, similar leucocyte abnormalities are seen in patients with mucopolysaccharide storage disorders, such as Hurler's and Maroteaux–Lamy syndromes, and occasionally in amaurotic family idiocy, for instance, Spielmeyer–Vogt syndrome (see below).

Mucopolysaccharidoses VI and VII

Abnormal granulation of blood granulocytes and monocytes, together with lymphocyte vacuolation, is found in the Maroteaux–Lamy syndrome which is also known as mucopolysaccharidosis VI (Fig.7.5). The striking white cell abnormality may also be seen in patients with mucopolysaccharidosis VII. These lysosomal storage disorders are caused by inherited deficiency of enzymes related to the breakdown of acid mucopolysaccharides. Storage-related abnormalities of connective tissue, the heart, the bony skeleton and the central nervous system, produce clinical disabilities similar to, but milder than, those found in classical Hurler's syndrome (mucopolysaccharidosis I-H).

Other causes of lymphocyte vacuolation

Similar lymphocyte vacuoles may be found in rare patients with inherited defects of enzymes which are involved in the catabolism of oligosaccharide components of glycoproteins, for example, mannosidosis, and in the rare Spielmeyer–Vogt syndrome (Fig.7.6).

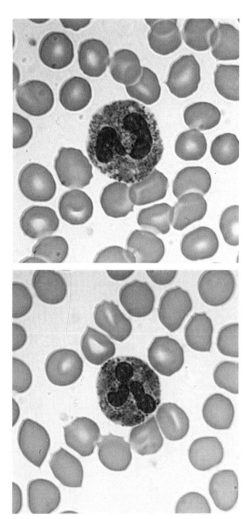

Fig.7.4 Alder's anomaly: coarse red-violet granules in neutrophils. In this case there was no associated clinical abnormality.

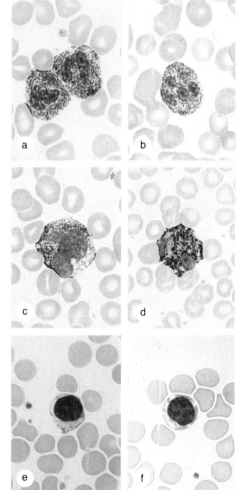

Fig.7.5 Maroteaux-Lamy syndrome: coarse red-violet granules in neutrophils (a & b), monocyte (c), basophil (d) and prominent vacuolation of lymphocytes (e & f). In this variant of Hurler's syndrome, there are severe skeletal abnormalities and clouding of the cornea.

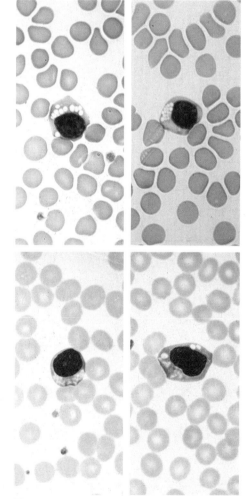

Fig.7.6 Lymphocyte vacuolation: further examples of prominent cytoplasmic vacuolation in lymphocytes in mannosidosis (upper) and in the Spielmeyer-Vogt syndrome (juvenile onset amaurotic idiocy; lower).

LEUCOCYTOSIS

The term 'leucocytosis' refers to an increase in white blood cells (usually to above $12 \times 10^9/l$). The most frequent cause is an increase in blood neutrophils. Other leucocytoses involve a predominance of one of the other white cell types found in the blood.

Neutrophil leucocytosis (neutrophilia)

An increase in neutrophils in the blood greater than $7.5 \times 10^9/l$ is one of the most frequent abnormalities found in blood counts and blood films (Fig.7.7). Clinically there is often fever due to the release of leucocyte pyrogen. In most neutrophilias there is an increase in the number of band forms; occasionally, more primitive cells such as metamyelocytes and myelocytes appear in the peripheral blood (the so-called shift to the left). In most causes of reactive neutrophil increases (Fig.7.8), toxic changes appear in the neutrophil cytoplasm and on

occasions there are Döhle bodies (Figs.7.9 & 7.10). The neutrophil alkaline phosphatase score (Fig.7.11) is characteristically elevated.

Eosinophil leucocytosis (eosinophilia)

Eosinophilia is the term applied to an increase in blood eosinophils above $0.400 \times 10^9/l$ (Fig.7.12). Its causes are listed in Fig.7.13.

There are a number of pulmonary eosinophilic syndromes of varying severity, characterized by transient pulmonary infiltrates (Fig.7.14, left), cough, low fever and peripheral eosinophilia. Steroid treatment usually results in resolution of symptoms and prompt clearing of the infiltrates (Fig.7.14, right). Similar changes may occur in some parasitic infestations when circulating parasites lodge in the lungs.

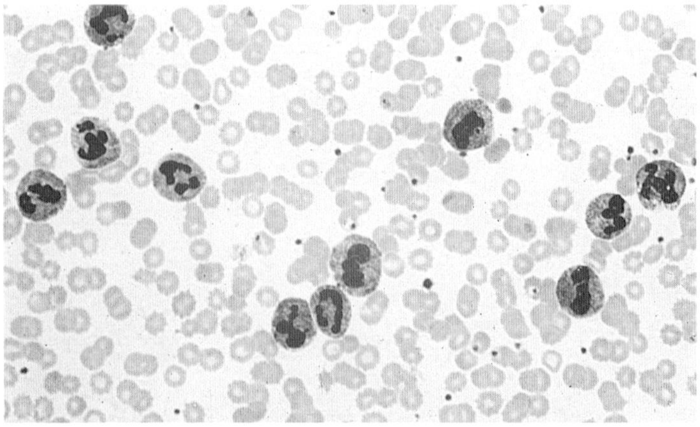

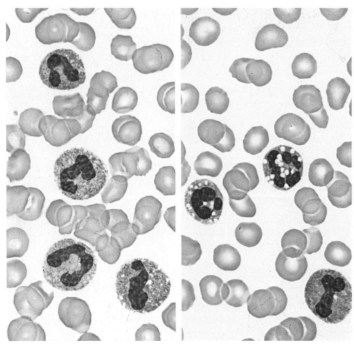

Fig.7.7 Neutrophil leucocytosis: large numbers of band-form and segmented neutrophils in the peripheral blood. The patient had abdominal sepsis. *WBC:45x10⁹/l; neutrophils:41x10⁹/l.*

Causes of Neutrophil Leucocytosis	

Bacterial infections
  pyogenic: localized
          or generalized
	Corticosteroid therapy

	Acute haemorrhage and haemolysis

Inflammation necrosis:
  cardiac infarct; ischaemia;
  trauma; vasculitis
	Myeloproliferative disorders:
	  polycythaemia vera;
	  myelofibrosis;
	  chronic granulocytic leukaemia

Metabolic disorders:
  uraemia; acidosis;
  gout; poisoning;
  eclampsia
	Chronic myelomonocytic leukaemia

	Malignant neoplasms

Fig.7.8 Causes of neutrophil leucocytosis.

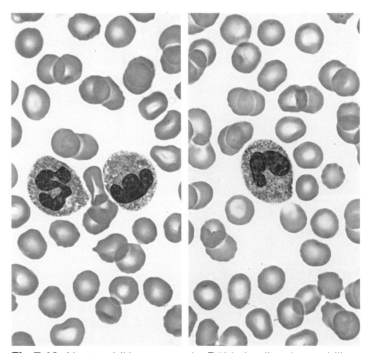

Fig.7.9 Neutrophil leucocytosis: toxic changes in neutrophils include the presence of red-purple granules in the band-form neutrophils (left) and cytoplasmic vacuolation (right).

Fig.7.10 Neutrophil leucocytosis: Döhle bodies, basophilic inclusions of denatured RNA, can be seen in the cytoplasm of these neutrophils.

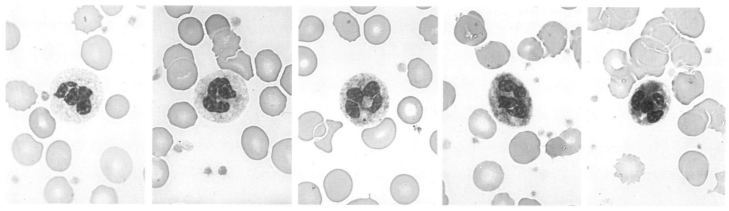

Fig.7.11 Neutrophil alkaline phosphatase score: after cytochemical staining for alkaline phosphatase activity, 100 neutrophils are assessed for intensity of staining reaction of enzyme activity. From left to right, the cells score 0, 1, 2, 3 and 4. High scores are found typically in reactive neutrophil leucocytoses, polycythaemia vera and myelofibrosis. Very low scores are found in chronic granulocytic leukaemia.

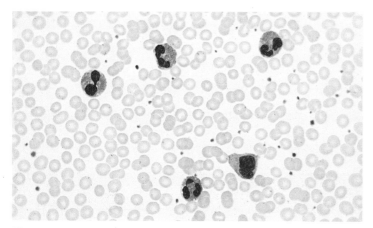

Fig.7.12 Eosinophilia: four eosinophils and a monocyte in dermatitis herpetiformis. *Total WBC:20x10⁹/l; eosinophils:16.5x10⁹/l.*

Causes of Eosinophilia	

Allergies:
    asthma; hayfever;
    urticaria; drugs
 	
Parasites:
    ancylostomiasis; ascariasis;
    filariasis; trichinosis;
    toxocariasis
 	
Skin diseases:
    eczema; psoriasis;
    dermatitis herpetiformis
 	
Neoplastic disease:
    Hodgkin's disease & others
	Eosinophilic leukaemia
	
	Miscellaneous:
	    eosinophilic granuloma;
	    erythema multiforme;
	    polyarteritis nodosa;
	    sarcoidosis;
	    hypereosinophilic syndrome;
	    post-irradiation;
	    pulmonary eosinophilia
	        (including Löffler's syndrome);
	    tropical eosinophilia

Fig.7.13 Causes of eosinophilia.

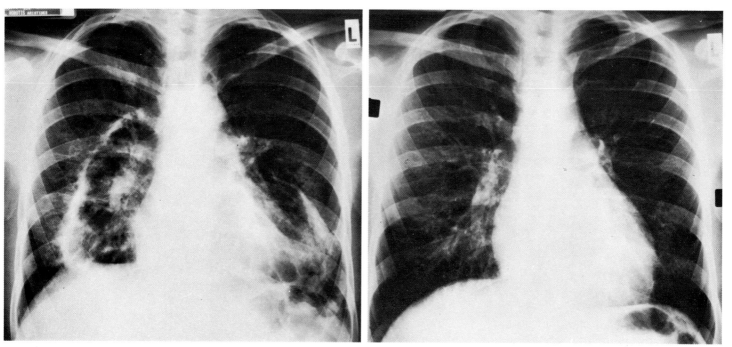

Fig.7.14 Pulmonary eosinophilia: chest radiographs showing (left) diffuse infiltrates in the right middle and lower, and left lower zones. Prominent band shadows suggest areas of collapse. The patient had been taking sulphasalazine for ulcerative colitis. This drug was stopped and prednisolone commenced; (right) same patient 3 weeks later. There is almost complete resolution of the pulmonary changes.

Monocytosis and basophil leucocytosis

Conditions associated with monocytosis (Fig.7.15) are listed in Fig.7.16. A basophil leucocytosis is seen most frequently in patients with chronic granulocytic leukaemia (Fig.7.17) or polycythaemia vera. Moderate increases in blood basophils also occur in myxoedema, chicken pox, smallpox and ulcerative colitis.

LEUKAEMOID REACTION

The leukaemoid reaction is a benign but excessive leucocytosis characterized by the presence of immature cells (blasts, promyelocytes and myelocytes) in the peripheral blood. Whereas most leukaemoid reactions involve blood granulocytes (Fig.7.18), lymphocytic reactions also occur. The majority of these reactions occur in association with severe or chronic infections. They are also sometimes a feature of widespread metastatic cancer or severe haemolysis. Leukaemoid reactions occur more frequently in children.

From the diagnostic point of view, the main problem is to distinguish these reactions from chronic granulocytic leukaemia. Changes such as toxic granulation, Döhle bodies and a high neutrophil alkaline phosphatase score are characteristically found in leukaemoid reactions while large numbers of myelocytes and the presence of the Philadelphia chromosome indicate chronic granulocytic leukaemia.

LEUCOERYTHROBLASTIC REACTION

In this blood cell variation, erythroblasts as well as primitive white cells are found in the peripheral blood (Figs.7.19 & 7.20). This reaction is most frequently found when there is a distortion of marrow architecture either due to proliferative disorders of the marrow or marrow infiltrations, or when there is extramedullary erythropoiesis. The principal causes of the leucoerythroblastic reaction are listed in Fig.7.21.

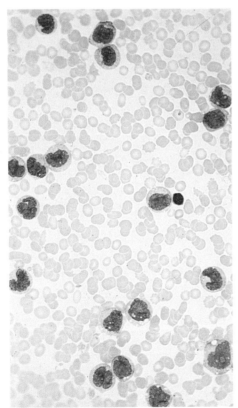

Fig.7.15 Monocytosis: in this peripheral blood film of myelodysplastic syndrome type V, with the exception of a single lymphocyte (centre), all of the nucleated cells shown are monocytes. *Total WBC:36×10⁹/l; monocytes:30×10⁹/l.*

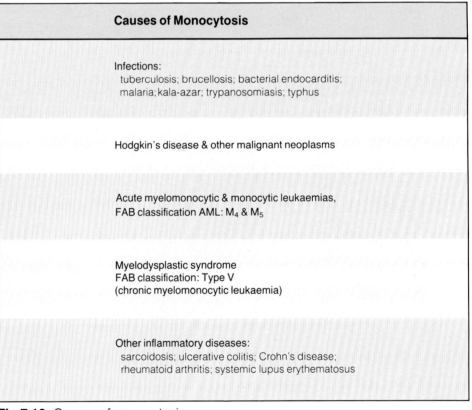

Causes of Monocytosis

Infections:
   tuberculosis; brucellosis; bacterial endocarditis;
   malaria; kala-azar; trypanosomiasis; typhus

Hodgkin's disease & other malignant neoplasms

Acute myelomonocytic & monocytic leukaemias,
FAB classification AML: M₄ & M₅

Myelodysplastic syndrome
FAB classification: Type V
(chronic myelomonocytic leukaemia)

Other inflammatory diseases:
   sarcoidosis; ulcerative colitis; Crohn's disease;
   rheumatoid arthritis; systemic lupus erythematosus

Fig.7.16 Causes of monocytosis.

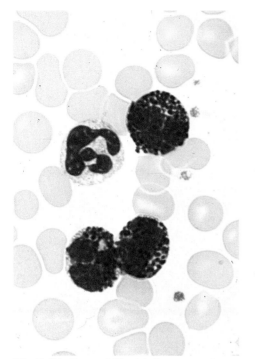

Fig.7.17 Basophilia: high power view of three basophils and a neutrophil in a peripheral blood film of chronic granulocytic leukaemia. *Total WBC:73×10⁹/l; basophils:7.3×10⁹/l.*

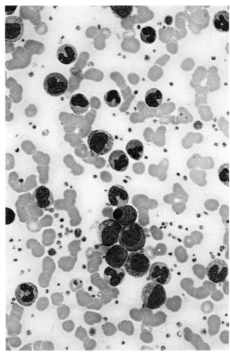

Fig.7.18 Leukaemoid reaction: neutrophils, stab forms, metamyelocytes, myelocytes and a single necrobiotic neutrophil (centre) in staphylococcal pneumonia. *WBC:94×10⁹/l.*

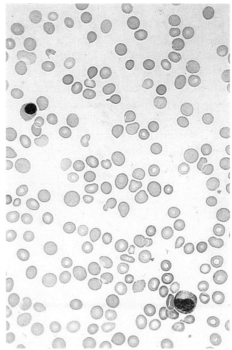

Fig.7.19 Leucoerythroblastic change: an erythroblast, a myelocyte, red cell polychromasia, anisocytosis and poikilocytosis including 'tear-drop' forms, in myelofibrosis. *Hb:9.5g/dl; WBC:5×10⁹/l; 6 erythroblasts per 100 WBC; platelets:45×10⁹/l.*

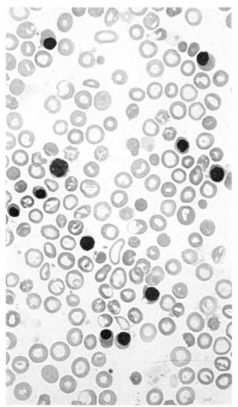

Fig.7.20 Leucoerythroblastic change: erythroblasts, two lymphocytes, red cell polychromasia, hypochromia, poikilocytosis, acanthocytosis and spherocytosis. The differential white cell count included metamyelocytes and myelocytes. This is a case of homozygous α-thalassaemia (Hb Bart's disease).

Causes of Leucoerythroblastic Change
Metastatic carcinoma in the marrow
Myelofibrosis
Leukaemia
Multiple myeloma
Hodgkin's disease
Non-Hodgkin's lymphoma & histiocytic tumours
Miliary tuberculosis
Severe megaloblastic anaemia
Severe haemolysis, particularly in the young
Osteopetrosis (Albers-Schönberg disease)

Fig.7.21 Causes of leucoerythroblastic change.

NEUTROPENIA

Neutropenia is defined by a blood neutrophil count of less than $2.5 \times 10^9/l$. However, it should be noted that many African and Middle Eastern populations have normal ranges with significantly lower limits that this. Clinical problems related to recurrent infections are associated with absolute levels below $1 \times 10^9/l$, and neutrophil counts of less than $0.2 \times 10^9/l$ carry very grave risks. Neutropenia may be selective or part of a general pancytopenia (Fig. 7.22). The majority of neutropenias are caused by reduced granulopoiesis; but, in some patients, the reduced neutrophil counts are caused by increased removal of neutrophils by tissues or by the reticuloendothelial system. Significant shifts of neutrophils from the circulating population to those in the marginal pool attached to the vascular endothelium may also be responsible.

In severe neutropenia there are often painful and intractable infections of the buccal mucosa (Figs. 7.23 & 7.24) and throat, the skin (Fig. 7.25) and in the anal region. Other features of infections associated with severe neutropenia are seen in Chapter 8.

Bone marrow examination is essential in all patients presenting with severe neutropenia. In many there will be evidence of leukaemia or other infiltrations. In those with selective depression of granulopoiesis there is a reduction in granulocyte precursors (Fig. 7.26).

Felty's syndrome

About one percent of patients with rheumatoid arthritis have associated splenomegaly (Fig. 7.27) and neutropenia. Some of these patients also show skin ulceration over the anterior surface of the tibia (Fig. 7.28). The neutropenia in Felty's syndrome is thought to result from neutrophil autoantibodies; the bone marrow characteristically shows increased granulopoiesis. In patients with recurrent infections, splenectomy often results in a return of blood neutrophil numbers to normal.

Causes of Neutropenia
Selective:
Drug-induced: anti-inflammatory: aminopyrine; phenylbutazone
antibacterial: chloramphenicol; co-trimoxazole
anticonvulsants: phenytoin; phenobarbitone
antithyroids: carbimazole
phenothiazines: chlorpromazine; promethazine
miscellaneous: tolbutamide; phenindione
Racial or familial
Cyclical
Infections: viral: particularly parvovirus & hepatitis
bacterial: typhoid; miliary tuberculosis
protozoal: malaria; kala-azar
Autoimmune: idiopathic; Felty's syndrome; systemic lupus erythematosus
Bone marrow failure:
aplastic anaemia; leukaemia; myelofibrosis; marrow infiltrations; megaloblastic anaemia; drugs, chemicals & physical agents, e.g. alkylating agents; antimetabolites
Splenomegaly

Fig. 7.22 Causes of neutropenia.

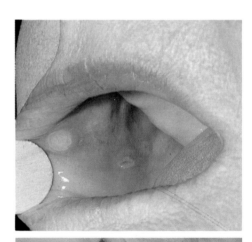

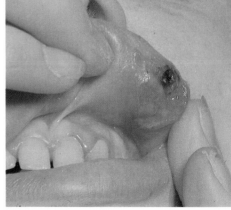

Fig. 7.23 Neutropenia: ulceration of the buccal mucosa (upper) and upper lip (lower) in different patients with severe neutropenia.

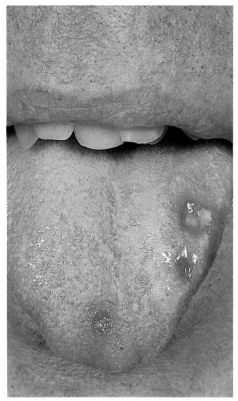 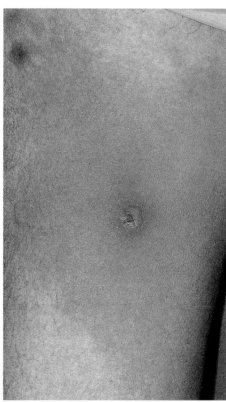 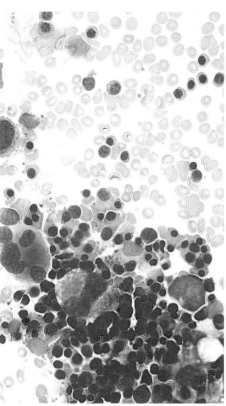

Fig.7.24 Neutropenia: ulceration of the tongue in severe neutropenia.

Fig.7.25 Neutropenia: infected skin lesion with extensive surrounding subcutaneous cellulitis in severe neutropenia. Cultures grew *Staphylococcus aureus* and *Pseudomonas pyocyanea*.

Fig.7.26 Neutropenia: bone marrow aspirate showing an absence of granulopoietic cells. The small fragment and cell trail contain mainly erythroblasts and megakaryocytes.

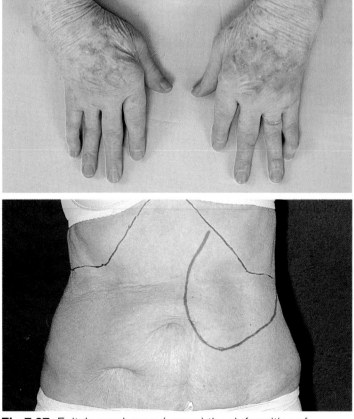 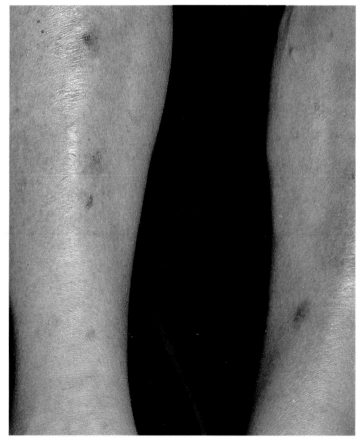

Fig.7.27 Felty's syndrome: (upper) the deformities of rheumatoid arthritis include prominent ulnar styloids, radial deviation of the wrists, swan-neck deformities (best seen in the right fourth finger and left fourth and fifth fingers) and wasting of the intrinsic muscles; (lower) splenic enlargement.

Fig.7.28 Felty's syndrome: skin ulceration on the anterior surfaces of the legs (same patient as in Fig.7.27).

LYMPHOCYTES

Lymphocytes are produced in the bone marrow from the pluripotential stem cell (see Chapter 1) and divide into two main subpopulations: T cells, which are processed in the thymus and form the majority of circulating lymphocytes; and B cells. These populations are indistinguishable morphologically in Romanovsky-stained blood films. The T cells subdivide into two major subsets which are detected by CD8 (T8) and CD4 (T4) monoclonal antibodies to surface membrane antigens. CD8 cells, the major subpopulation of T cells in the marrow, include the suppressor/cytotoxic cells while CD4 (helper) cells predominate in the peripheral blood. T cells form rosettes with sheep erythrocytes. B cells are defined by the presence of surface immuno-globulins (SIgs) which act as antigen receptors. The immunoglobulin may be one of five classes: IgM, IgD, IgG (divided into four subtypes), IgE or IgA (divided into two subtypes), which are determined by which heavy-chain gene (μ, δ, γ, ϵ or α) is expressed. Each molecule also contains a light chain (κ or λ). Both heavy and light chains contain constant and variable regions (see Chapter 1). The heavy-chain genes are situated on chromosome 14 and light-chain genes on chromosomes 2(κ) and 22(λ). The immunoglobulins are expressed in the cytoplasm (in pre-B cells) before they can be detected on the surface (Fig.7.29).

B cells may also express a number of surface antigens, some of which are expressed before SIg, for example, CD10, CD19, CD20 and HLA-DR. The early bone marrow precursors of B cells also express the nuclear enzyme terminal deoxynucleotidyl transferase (TdT). Diversity among different B-cells is produced by differences in the rearrangement of the genes for the variable, diversity and constant regions of the immunoglobulins they secrete (Figs.7.30 & 7.31). This rearrangement from the germ-line configuration takes place first in the heavy chain genes, then in the κ light chain and finally in the λ light chain genes.

The T-cell surface contains an antigen receptor which consists of α and β chains, each with variable and constant portions (Fig.7.32). A γ chain is also present but its function is not yet clear. The genes for these

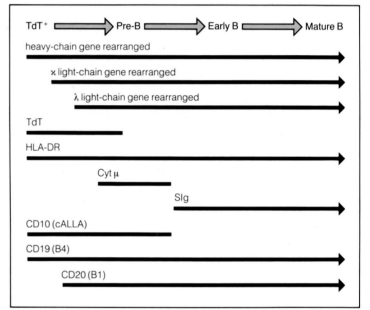

Fig.7.29 The sequence of immunoglobulin gene rearrangements, antigen and immunoglobulin expression during early B-cell development. S = surface; Cyt = cytoplasmic.

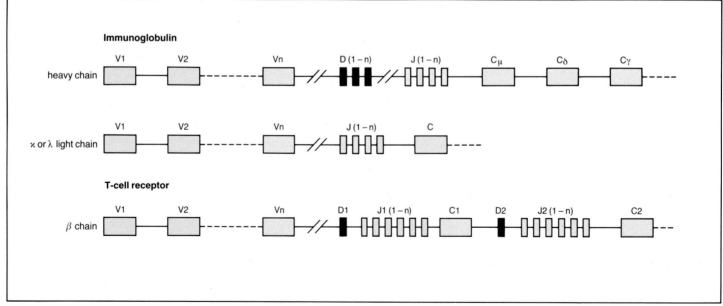

Fig.7.30 Germ-line gene arrangement of Ig molecular chains (retained in all body cells except B cells). Each gene is made up of segments including a number (n) of variable (V), diversity (D), joining (J) and constant (C) genes, the latter for each of the Ig subtypes. Diversity is introduced by the joining of V,D,J and C genes (see Fig.7.31).

polypeptide chains, on chromosomes 14 (α chain) and 7 (β and γ chains), rearrange in T cells in a manner similar to the rearrangement of immunoglobulin genes in B cells, resulting in a wide diversity among T lymphocytes.

The sequence of events in T-cell development appears to be initial expression of nuclear TdT and the surface antigen CD7 followed by CD2. Rearrangement of the T-cell receptor genes occurs in the sequence γ, β and

finally α. The CD5 antigen (which binds sheep red cells) and CD3 antigen (a complex of proteins involved in signal transduction from the T-cell receptor to the cell interior) are expressed on the surface later, although intracytoplasmic CD3 is one of the earliest markers. The CD4 or CD8 antigens are expressed in medullary thymocytes after T-cell receptor gene rearrangement is complete (Fig.7.33).

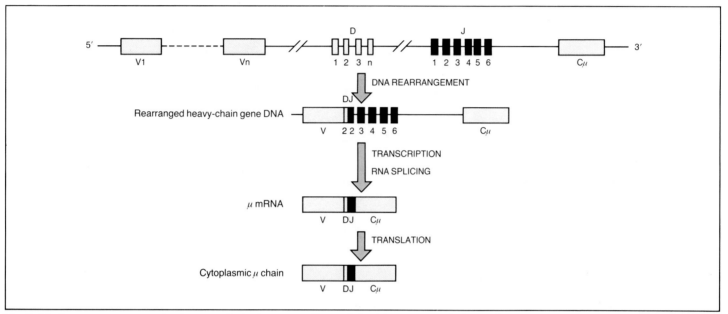

Fig.7.31 Rearrangement of a heavy chain Ig gene. One of the V segments is brought into contact with a D, a J and a C (in this case, Cμ) segment, forming an active transcriptional gene from which the corresponding mRNA is produced. The DJ rearrangement precedes VDJ joining.

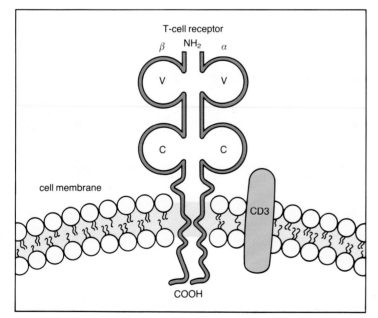

Fig.7.32 The T-cell antigen receptor consists of α and β chains, each of which has a variable (V) and a constant (C) segment. The chains have transmembranous portions but very short intracytoplasmic domains. The associated CD3 complex is involved in signal transduction to the cell interior.

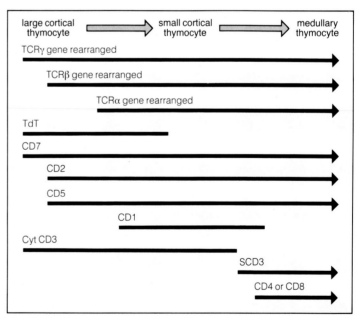

Fig.7.33 The sequence of T-cell receptor gene rearrangements and antigen expression during early T-cell development.

LYMPHOCYTOSIS

The main causes of an increase in the absolute lymphocyte count are listed in Fig.7.34. Greatly raised levels are usually seen in adults with chronic lymphocytic leukaemia. Infants with pertussis and children with acute infectious lymphocytosis, an unusual viral disease, may also have very high lymphocyte counts. Lymphocytoses with large numbers of atypical or 'reactive' cells are most often seen in infectious mononucleosis, in other viral illnesses including infectious hepatitis, and in toxoplasmosis.

Infectious mononucleosis

Infectious mononucleosis (glandular fever) is a disorder characterized by sore throat, fever, lymphadenopathy and atypical lymphocytes in the blood. The disease appears to be the result of infection with Epstein–Barr (EB) virus. In affected patients, heterophil antibodies against sheep red cells are found in the serum at high titres (Paul–Bunnell test).

Most patients present with lethargy, malaise and fever. On examination the majority show significant lymphadenopathy (Fig.7.35). There is usually generalized inflammation of the oral and pharyngeal surfaces with follicular tonsillitis (Fig.7.36), and some patients show palatal petechiae (Fig.7.37). There may be periorbital and facial oedema (Fig.7.38) or a morbilliform rash (Fig.7.39).

Palpable splenomegaly occurs in over half the patients. Occasionally there are subcapsular haematomas of the spleen (Fig.7.40) which have a tendency to rupture. Jaundice due to liver involvement occurs in a minority of patients.

The diagnosis is suspected by finding a moderate lymphocytosis ($10-20 \times 10^9$/l) and large numbers of atypical lymphocytes in the peripheral blood film (Fig.7.41).

Fig.7.34 Causes of lymphocytosis.

Causes of Lymphocytosis
Acute infections:
rubella; pertussis; mumps; infectious mononucleosis; acute infectious lymphocytosis
Chronic infections:
tuberculosis; brucellosis; infective hepatitis; syphilis
Thyrotoxicosis
Chronic lymphocytic leukaemia (see Chapter 9)
Other lymphoid leukaemias & lymphomas (see Chapters 9 & 10)
Chronic T-cell lymphocytosis (see Chapter 9)

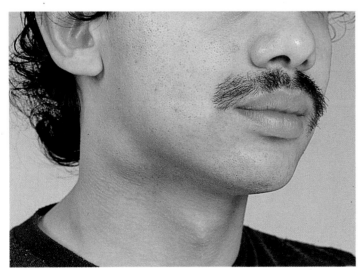

Fig.7.35 Infectious mononucleosis: cervical lymphadenopathy in a 19-year-old man who presented with fever and pharyngitis.

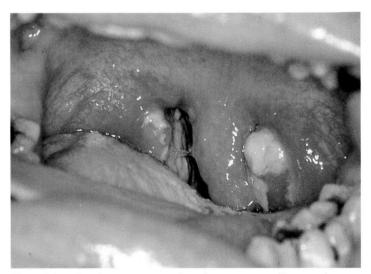

Fig.7.36 Infectious mononucleosis: gross swelling and haemorrhagic erythema of the oropharynx. The tonsils are covered by a purulent exudate.

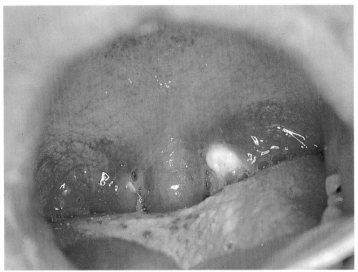

Fig.7.37 Infectious mononucleosis: oropharynx (same case as in Fig.7.36) showing marked swelling of the uvula and tonsils, and palatal petechial haemorrhage.

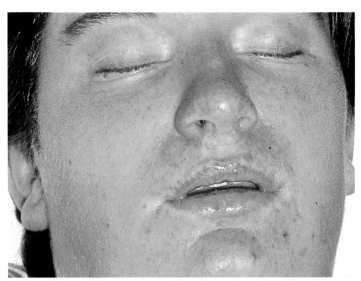

Fig.7.38 Infectious mononucleosis: marked facial and periorbital oedema.

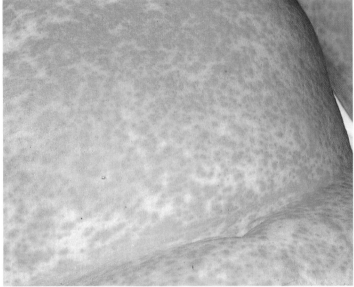

Fig.7.39 Infectious mononucleosis: morbilliform erythematous skin eruption. There was generalized lymphadenopathy and the spleen was enlarged to 3cm below the left costal margin.

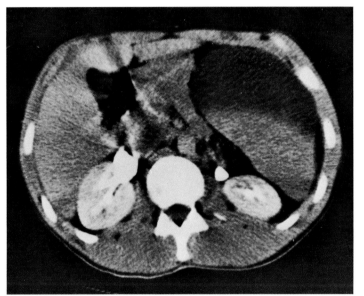

Fig.7.40 Infectious mononucleosis: abdominal CT scan showing massive enlargement of the spleen with a large anterior subcapsular haematoma (area of decreased density).

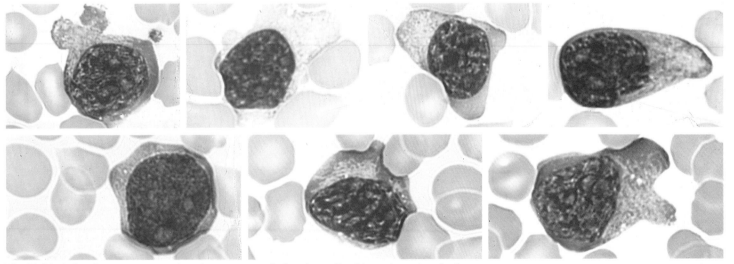

Fig.7.41 Infections mononucleosis: representative 'reactive' lymphocytes in the peripheral blood film of a 21-year-old man. These are T lymphocytes reacting to Epstein-Barr-infected B cells. The cells are large with abundant vacuolated cytoplasm; the nuclei often show a fine blast-like chromatin pattern.

A number of conditions, including acute leukaemia, toxoplasmosis, infectious hepatitis and follicular tonsillitis, are likely to create initial problems of diagnosis. Fine needle aspiration cytology of affected nodes may be helpful. In infectious mononucleosis the cytology is dominated by reactive lymphocyte changes (Fig.7.42) while in toxoplasmosis, characteristic small groups of histiocytes may be found (Fig.7.43).

PRIMARY IMMUNODEFICIENCY DISORDERS

The main types of primary immunodeficiency disease are listed in Fig.7.44. In severe combined immunodeficiency disease, the T- and B-lymphocyte systems fail to develop. There is severe lymphopenia and hypogamma-globulinaemia. Affected infants fail to thrive (Fig.7.45) and die early in life from recurrent infections, such as by

Pneumocystis carinii, cytomegalovirus, other viruses, fungi and bacteria. There is atrophy of the thymus (Fig.7.46); the lymph nodes and spleen are small and devoid of lymphoid cells. The most common cause is deficiency of the enzyme adenosine deaminase (ADA; Fig.7.47). Deficiency of another enzyme, purine nucleoside phosphorylase, causes a more selective lack of T cells. Recently, ADA deficiency has been treated successfully by bone marrow transplantation.

In the very rare syndrome of lymphoreticular dysgenesis, there is failure of development of both the reticuloendothelial and lymphoid systems. Affected infants die soon after birth from overwhelming infection. There is marked lymphopenia, and stigmata of splenic atrophy may be found in the peripheral blood (Fig.7.48).

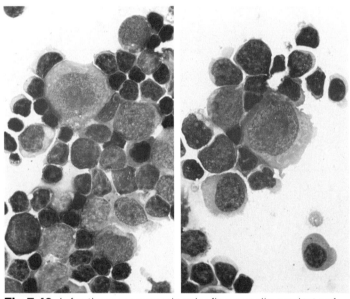

Fig.7.42 Infectious mononucleosis: fine needle aspirate of cervical lymph node showing a pleomorphic lymphoid population including immunoblasts, centroblasts, centrocytes and small lymphocytes.

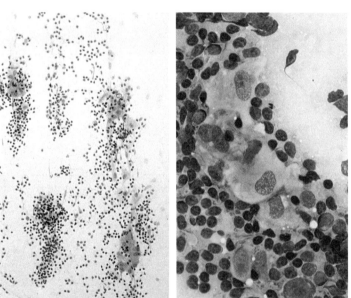

Fig.7.43 Toxoplasmosis: fine needle aspirate of cervical lymph node showing (left) groups of histiocytic cells in the cell trails; (right) at higher magnification these histiocytes are seen to be surrounded by predominantly small lymphocytes. Papanicolaou's stain (left); May-Grünwald/Giemsa stain (right).

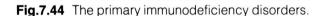

Primary Immunodeficiency Disorders	
X-linked agammaglobulinaemia (Bruton-type immunodeficiency)	Thymoma with immunodeficiency
Thymic hypoplasia (DiGeorge's syndrome)	Selective deficiency of IgA or IgM
Common variable immunodeficiency disease	Miscellaneous: Immunodeficiency associated with: ataxia telangiectasia; Wiskott-Aldrich syndrome; lymphorecticular dysgenesis
Severe combined immunodeficiency disease (SCID or Swiss-type immunodeficiency)	

Fig.7.44 The primary immunodeficiency disorders.

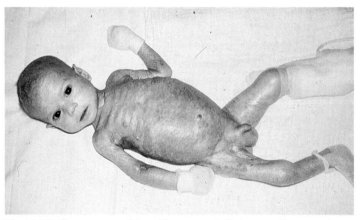

Fig.7.45 Severe combined immunodeficiency disease due to ADA deficiency: severely wasted infant with distended abdomen. There was widespread *Candida* infection of the mouth and chronic diarrhoea. Courtesy of Dr. R.I. Levinsky.

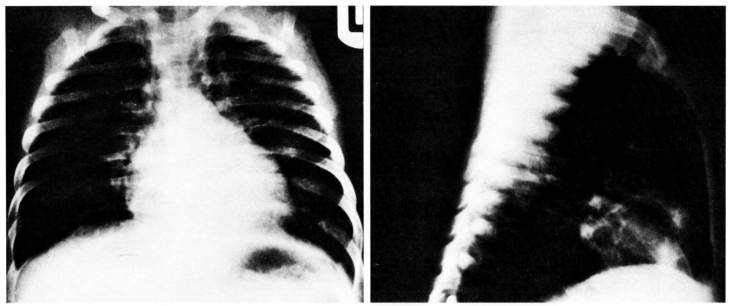

Fig.7.46 Severe combined immunodeficiency disease: chest radiographs of the infant in Fig.7.45. In the PA view (left) there is an absence of thymic shadow in the superior mediastinum; the lateral view (right) confirms the lack of thymus tissue deep to the sternum. Courtesy of Dr. R.I. Levinsky.

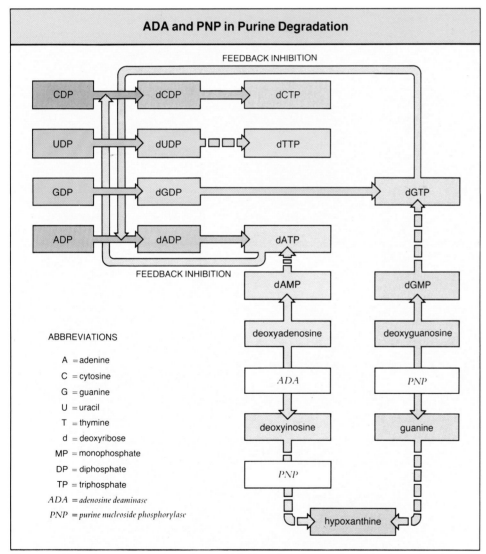

Fig.7.47 Role of adenosine deaminase (ADA) and purine nucleoside phosphorylase (PNP) in purine degradation. ADA deficiency causes death of cortical thymocytes by accumulation of dATP (which inhibits DNA synthesis). PNP deficiency produces toxicity to T cells by accumulation of deoxyguanosine triphosphate (dGTP). ADA and PNP are also involved in adenosine and guanosine degradation respectively. In both deficiencies, other biochemical mechanisms of toxicity to proliferating and non-proliferating lymphoid cells may occur.

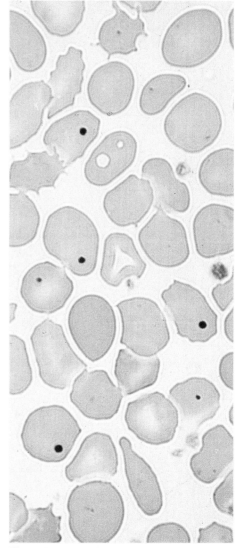

Fig.7.48 Lymphoreticular dysgenesis: peripheral blood film of a one-week-old infant. The large numbers of Howell-Jolly bodies (small granular remnants of DNA) are the result of splenic agenesis. There was a severe lymphopenia. *Absolute lymphocyte count: 0.1x10⁹/l.* 7.15

ACQUIRED IMMUNE DEFICIENCY SYNDROME (AIDS) AND AIDS-RELATED LYMPHADENOPATHY

This increasingly recognized syndrome is particularly common in homosexual men but is also seen in drug users, patients such as haemophiliacs who have undergone transfusion of blood or blood products, and in heterosexual contacts of AIDS cases.

The primary pathology is infection of the lymphoid system with the human immunodeficiency virus (HIV); this is also referred to as HTLV III (human T-lympho-tropic virus)/LAV (lymphadenopathy-associated virus). The patients initially show a prodromal period of non-specific illness with fevers, night sweats, a non-productive cough, intermittent diarrhoea, pruritus and weight loss. During this period, a generalized painful lymphadenopathy is usual (Figs.7.49 & 7.50). There is an alteration in the peripheral blood of T-lymphocyte subsets with a fall from the normal CD4:CD8 (helper:suppressor) ratio of 1.5-2.5:1 to less than 1:1. Dermatitis, alopecia and autoimmune thrombocytopenia occur in some patients.

A wide spectrum of opportunistic infections is seen in AIDS. A proportion of patients develop Kaposi's sarcoma, a vascular skin tumour of endothelial origin (Fig.7.51), and others develop non-Hodgkin's lymphoma.

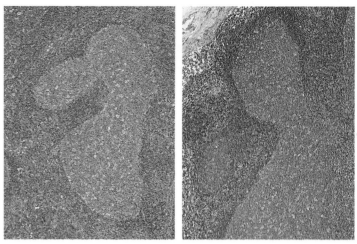

Fig.7.49 Acquired immune deficiency syndrome (AIDS): sections of lymph nodes infected by HIV (HTLV III/LAV) show a spectrum of histological changes. Type I (seen here) includes follicular and paracortical hyperplasia. Mitotically active germinal centres are numerous in the medulla as well as cortex and present a 'geographical outline'. The mantle zones are attenuated and, in places, absent and the follicles appear confluent. The interfollicular tissue shows an increase in small vessels. In the type II pattern, there is loss of germinal centres but diffuse lymphoid hyperplasia; in type III, an end-stage in fatal cases, lymphocyte depletion predominates. Courtesy of Dr. J.E. McLaughlin.

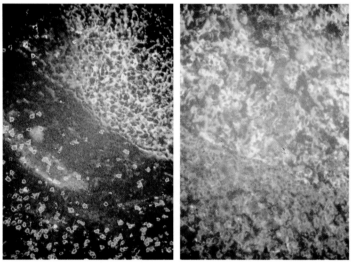

Fig.7.50 Acquired immune deficiency syndrome (AIDS): indirect immunofluorescence of sections of lymph nodes. In the normal nodes (left) the CD8 lymphocytes (orange) are mainly in the paracortex. The germinal centre consists of B lymphocytes and dendritic reticular cells (green). In lymphadenopathy due to HIV infection, the germinal centre is disrupted and invaded by CD8 cells. Courtesy of Prof. G. Janossy.

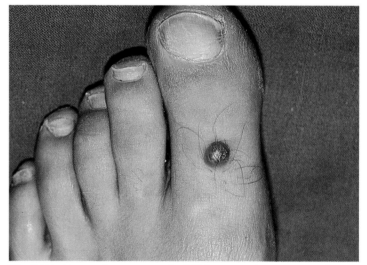

Fig.7.51 Kaposi's sarcoma in AIDS: vascular tumour of endothelial origin on the left big toe in a homosexual male (HIV antigen-positive). Similar tumours of multifocal origin were present elsewhere on the lower limbs and trunk. Courtesy of Dr. L. Fry.

8

ACUTE LEUKAEMIAS

The acute leukaemias are the result of accumulation of early myeloid or lymphoid precursors in the bone marrow, blood and other tissues, and are thought to arise by somatic mutation of a single cell within a minor population of early progenitor cells in the bone marrow or thymus (Fig.8.1). Acute leukaemia may arise *de novo* or be the terminal event in a number of preexisting blood disorders, for instance, polycythaemia rubra vera, chronic granulocytic (myeloid) leukaemia or one of the myelodysplastic syndromes. At presentation at least thirty percent and usually more than eighty percent of the bone marrow cells are 'blasts'.

The diseases are divided into two main subgroups, acute myeloblastic leukaemia (AML) and acute lymphoblastic leukaemia (ALL); these are further subdivided on morphological grounds into various subcategories (Fig.8.2). The French–American–British (FAB) scheme divides acute myeloblastic leukaemia into subtypes M_1 to M_7 and acute lymphoblastic leukaemia

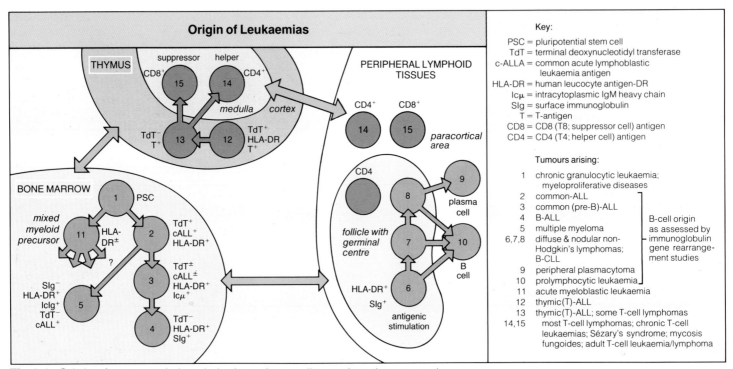

Fig.8.1 Origin of acute and chronic leukaemias, malignant lymphomas and myeloma by clonal expansion of early bone marrow, thymic or peripheral lymphoid cells. Modified from A.V. Hoffbrand & J.E. Pettit (1984) *Essential Haematology, 2nd edition.* Oxford: Blackwell Scientific Publications.

Acute Leukaemia: Morphological Classification*
Myeloid (AML)
M_1: myeloblastic without maturation
M_2: myeloblastic with maturation
M_3: hypergranular promyelocytic
M_4: myelomonocytic
M_5: monocytic
M_6: erythroleukaemia
M_7: megakaryoblastic
Lymphoblastic
L_1: small, monomorphic
L_2: large, heterogeneous
L_3: Burkitt cell-type
*French-American-British (FAB) classification

Fig.8.2 French-American-British (FAB) classification of the acute leukaemias: the myeloblastic leukaemias are divided into 7 types (M_{1-7}) and the lymphoblastic leukaemias into three (L_{1-3}).

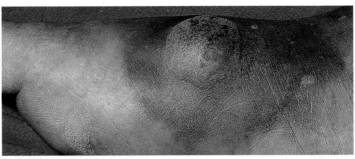
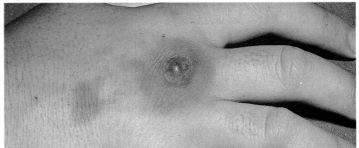

Fig.8.3 Acute myeloblastic leukaemia: (upper) a purplish-black bullous lesion with surrounding erythema caused by infection from *Pseudomonas pyocyanea* on the foot; (right) similar but less-marked infection on the back of the hand.

into subtypes L₁, L₂ and L₃. There are additional unusual types.

CLINICAL FEATURES

Acute leukaemia presents with features of bone marrow failure (anaemia, infections, easy bruising or haemorrhage) and may or may not include features of organ infiltration by leukaemic cells. The organs usually involved are the lymph nodes, spleen and liver, meninges and central nervous system, testes (particularly in acute lymphoblastic leukaemia) and skin (particularly in the M₅ type of acute myeloblastic leukaemia).

Infections are often bacterial in the early stages and particularly affect the skin (Figs.8.3 & 8.4), pharynx, perianal (Fig.8.5) and perineal (Fig.8.6) regions. Fungal infections are particularly common in patients with prolonged periods of neutropenia (Fig.8.7) who have undergone multiple courses of chemotherapy and antibiotic therapy.

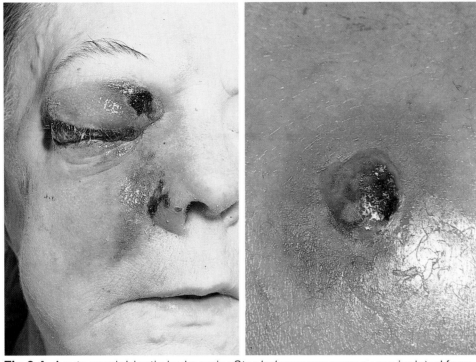

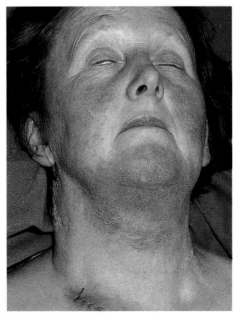

Fig.8.4 Acute myeloblastic leukaemia: *Staphylococcus aureus* was isolated from (left) this infection of the right orbit and surrounding tissue and (right) this necrotic erythematous skin ulcer.

Fig.8.5 Acute myeloblastic leukaemia: this perianal lesion was found to be the result of a mixed infection by *Escherichia coli* and *Streptococcus faecalis*.

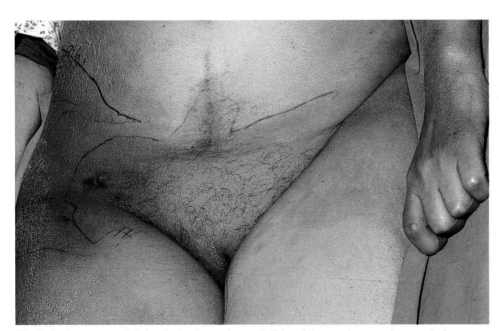

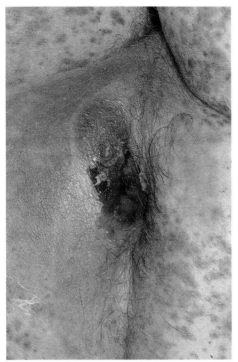

Fig.8.6 Acute myeloblastic leukaemia: cellulitis of the perineum, lower abdomen and upper thighs due to *Pseudomonas pyocyanea*.

Fig.8.7 Acute myeloblastic leukaemia: spreading cellulitis of the neck and chin resulting from mixed streptococcal and *Candida* infection, previous chemotherapy and prolonged periods of neutropenia.

Other viral (especially herpetic), protozoal or fungal infections are frequent, particularly in the mouth (Figs.8.8–8.10). These infections may become generalized and life-threatening. Haemorrhage of the skin or mucous membranes is usually petechial (Figs.8.11 & 8.12).

Infiltration of the skin presenting as a widespread raised, non–itchy, haemorrhagic rash, and swelling of the gums (Fig.8.13) are characteristic of the M_5 type of acute myeloblastic leukaemia; nodular and localized skin infiltrates may also occur (Fig.8.14).

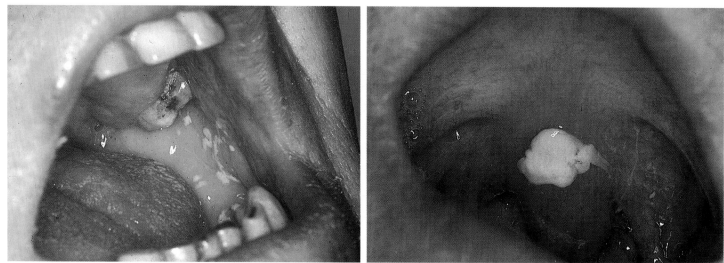

Fig.8.8 Acute myeloblastic leukaemia: plaques of *Candida albicans* (left) in the mouth, with a lesion of herpex simplex on the upper lip and (right) on the soft palate.

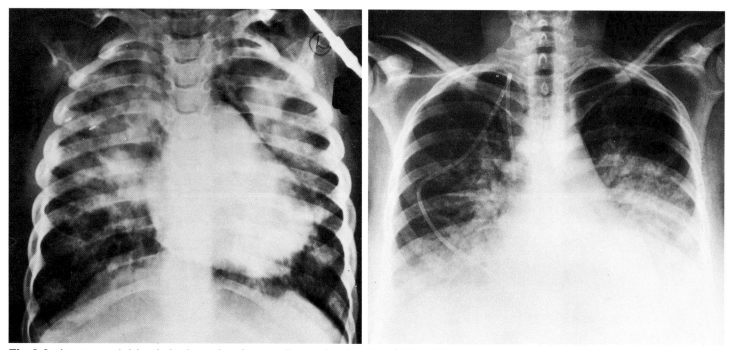

Fig.8.9 Acute myeloblastic leukaemia: chest radiographs showing (left) patchy consolidation bilaterally due to measles infection in a child; (right) interstitial shadowing in lower and mid-zones bilaterally in a 23-year-old female with septicaemia from *Pseudomonas pyocyanea* following chemotherapy. She developed a fatal adult respiratory distress syndrome. Courtesy of Dr. J.M. Chessells (left).

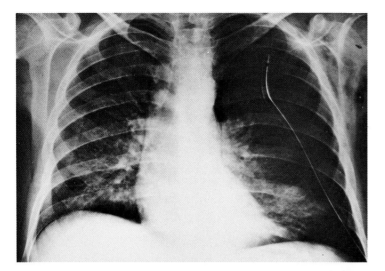

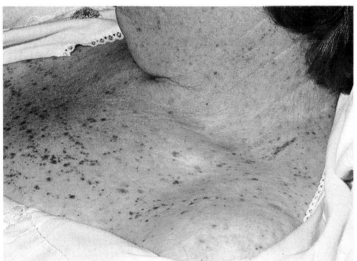

Fig.8.10 Acute lymphoblastic leukaemia: chest radiograph showing consolidation spreading bilaterally from the hilar regions ('bat-wing' shadowing) due to infection by *Pneumocystis carinii*.

Fig.8.11 Acute myeloblastic leukaemia: petechial haemorrhages covering the upper chest and face in severe thrombocytopenia.

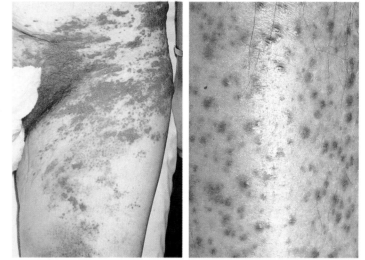

Fig.8.12 Acute myeloblastic leukaemia: (left) marked ecchymoses, petechial haemorrhages and bruises over the groin and thigh; (right) close-up view of petechial haemorrhages over the leg.

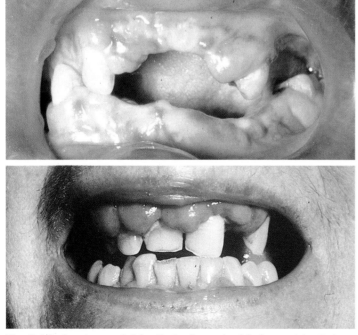

Fig.8.13 Acute myeloblastic leukaemia, M₅ (monoblastic) subtype: leukaemic infiltration of the gums results in their expansion and thickening, and partial covering of the teeth.

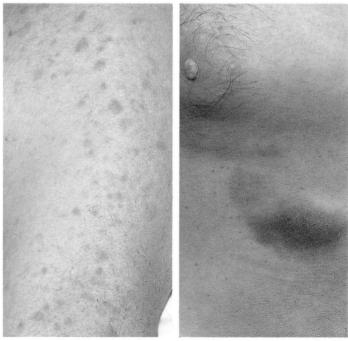

Fig.8.14 Acute myeloblastic leukaemia, M₅ (monoblastic) subtype: (left) multiple, raised, erythematous skin lesions due to leukaemic infiltration; (right) close-up view of nodular skin lesion.

In acute lymphoblastic leukaemia, lymphadenopathy is more common (Fig.8.15). In the T-cell variant (T-ALL), there is often upper mediastinal enlargement due to a thymic mass which responds rapidly to therapy (Fig.8.16). Although meningeal involvement is more frequent in children and younger subjects with acute lymphoblastic leukaemia, it may occur at all ages, presenting with nausea, vomiting, headaches, visual disturbances, photophobia and features of cranial nerve palsies (Fig.8.17). Papilloedema may be found on examination (Fig.8.18) and infiltration may occur at any site (Fig.8.19). Testicular relapse is common although it is only rarely detectable clinically on presentation (Fig.8.20). Bone involvement may produce characteristic radiographic findings (Fig.8.21).

MICROSCOPICAL APPEARANCES
Acute myeloblastic leukaemia
On May-Grünwald/Giemsa staining the M_1 subclass is the least differentiated (Fig.8.22) and often may only be diagnosed with certainty after special staining or electron microscopy. The M_2 subclass shows definite differentiation to promyelocytes (Fig.8.23).

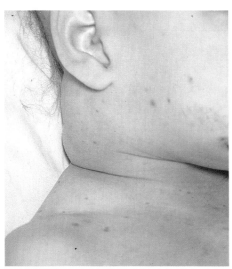

Fig.8.15 Acute lymphoblastic leukaemia: marked cervical lymphadenopathy in a 4-year-old boy. Courtesy of Dr. J.M. Chessells.

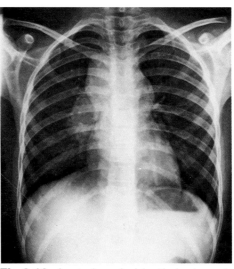

Fig.8.16 Acute lymphoblastic leukaemia, T-ALL subtype: chest radiographs of a 4-year-old boy showing (left) upper mediastinal widening due to thymic enlargement; (right) following one week of therapy with vincristine and prednisolone, the thymic mass has disappeared.

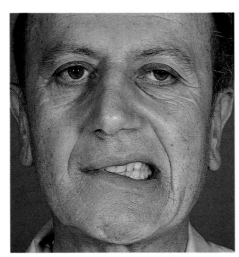

Fig.8.17 Acute lymphoblastic leukaemia: this 59-year-old man has facial asymmetry because of a right lower motor neurone seventh nerve palsy resulting from meningeal leukaemic infiltration. Courtesy of Dr. H.G. Prentice.

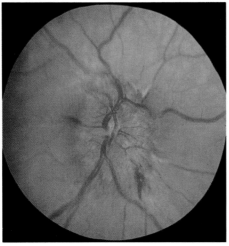

Fig.8.18 Acute lymphoblastic leukaemia: papilloedema due to meningeal disease. There is blurring of the disc margin with venous enlargement and retinal haemorrhages.

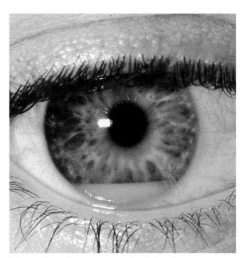

Fig.8.19 Acute lymphoblastic leukaemia: leukaemic infiltration in the anterior chamber of the eye is obscuring the lower rim of the iris.

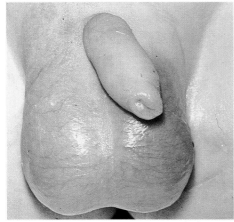

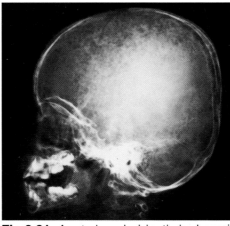

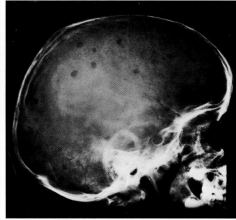

Fig.8.20 Acute lymphoblastic leukaemia: testicular swelling and erythema of the left side of the scrotum due to testicular infiltration. Courtesy of Dr. J.M. Chessells.

Fig.8.21 Acute lymphoblastic leukaemia: radiographs of children's skulls showing (left) a mottled appearance due to widespread leukaemic infiltration of bone and (right) multiple punched-out lesions due to leukaemic deposits. Courtesy of Dr. J.M. Chessells.

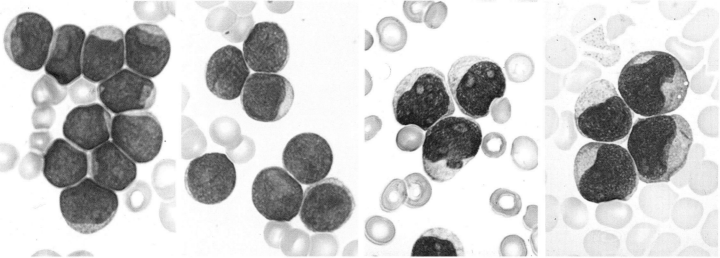

Fig.8.22 Acute myeloblastic leukaemia, M$_1$ (myeloblastic without maturation) subtype: bone marrow aspirates showing blasts with large, often irregular, nuclei with one or more nucleoli, and with varying amounts of eccentrically placed cytoplasm. There is either no definite granulation or a few azurophilic granules and occasional Auer rods. At least 3% of cells stain by Sudan black or myeloperoxidase.

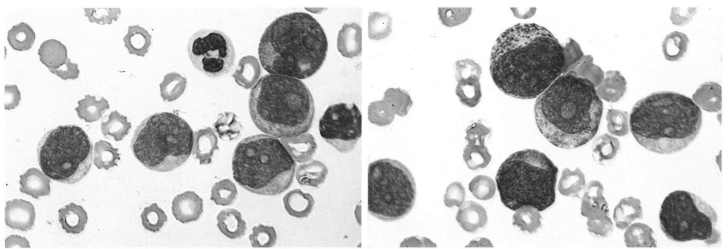

Fig.8.23 Acute myeloblastic leukaemia, M$_2$ (myeloblastic with maturation) subtype: bone marrow aspirates showing (left) blasts similar to those in Fig.8.22 but promyelocytes with azurophilic granules are also present; (right) blast cells with folded nuclei, one or two nucleoli, varying numbers of azurophilic granules and occasional Auer rods.

The typical form of M₃ (acute promyelocytic leukaemia) shows bundles of rod-like structures ('faggots' or Sultan bodies) which are aggregates of granules and can be seen with special stains (Fig.8.24). These cells contain procoagulant material which, when released into the circulation, causes disseminated intravascular coagulation (DIC); this type also has a microvariant (Fig.8.25).

M₄ (myelomonocytic leukaemia) shows a mixture of blasts with promyelocytic and monocytic differentiation, the latter consisting of less than twenty percent of the total (Fig.8.26). In one subtype, there are abnormal eosinophils and inversion (inv) of chromosome 16 (Fig.8.26, right).

M₅ or acute monoblastic or monocytic leukaemia (Fig.8.27) shows over twenty percent monoblasts or differentiated 'promonocytes' or monocytic cells. Serum and urinary lysozyme are high.

In subclass M̄₆ (erythroleukaemia) over fifty percent of cells are erythroid precursors with bizarre dyserythropoietic forms (Figs.8.28 & 8.29). Features of myelodysplasia are also present in other cell lines.

Acute megakaryoblastic leukaemia (M₇) is rare. It is often associated with fibrosis of the marrow and recognized by the appearance of the blasts, special staining for platelet peroxidase, electron microscopy and monoclonal antibodies to cell surface antigens (Fig.8.30).

Acute lymphoblastic leukaemia
Lymphoblasts show little evidence of differentiation. Cases with smaller, more uniform, cells with scanty cytoplasm are classified as L₁ (Fig.8.31) whereas cases with blasts differing widely in size, with prominent nucleoli and great amounts of cytoplasm, are classified as L₂ (Fig.8.32). L₂ tends to include more of the adult cases and also most of those immunologically typed as T-ALL.

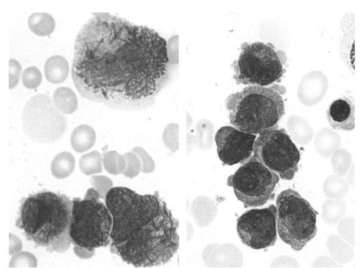

Fig.8.24 Acute myeloblastic leukaemia, M₃ (hypergranular promyelocytic) subtype: promyelocytes containing coarse azurophilic granules and Sultan bodies which stain similarly to those of the granules. The nuclei contain one or two nucleoli. The subtype is associated with the 15:17 chromosome translocation (see Fig.8.60).

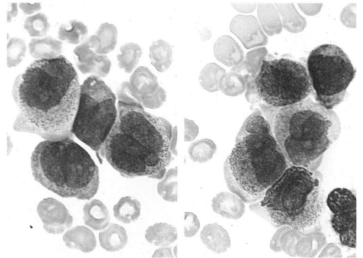

Fig.8.25 Acute myeloblastic leukaemia, M₃ (promyelocytic) subtype: microgranular variant. The usually bilobed cells contain numerous small azurophilic granules.

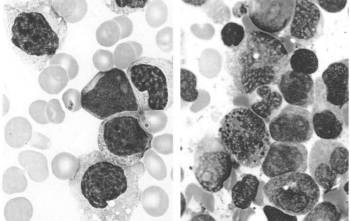

Fig.8.26 Acute myeloblastic leukaemia, M₄ (myelomonocytic) subtype: blast cells contain cytoplasmic granules (myeloblasts and promyelocytes) or pale cytoplasm with occasional vacuoles and granules, and folded or rounded nuclei (monoblasts); (right) eosinophil with basophilic granules. Courtesy of Dr. M. Bilter & Prof. J. Rowley (right).

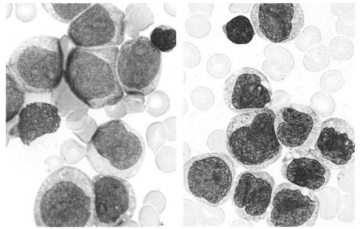

Fig.8.27 Acute myeloblastic leukaemia, M₅ (monoblastic) subtype: blast cells with pale cytoplasm or perinuclear 'halos' and cytoplasmic vacuoles but only occasional granules. Their usually centrally placed nuclei are folded, rounded or kidney-shaped.

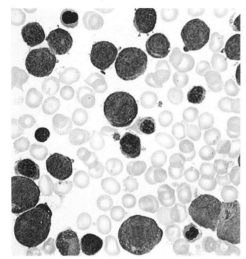

Fig.8.28 Acute myeloblastic leukaemia, M_6 (erythroleukaemia) subtype: there is a preponderance of erythroid cells at all stages of development.

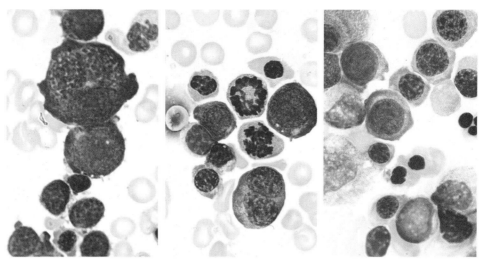

Fig.8.29 Acute myeloblastic leukaemia, M_6 (erythroleukaemia) subtype: high power views of bone marrow aspirate showing erythroid predominance with many dyserythropoietic features, such as multinucleated cells, vacuolated cytoplasm, abnormal mitoses and megaloblastic nuclei.

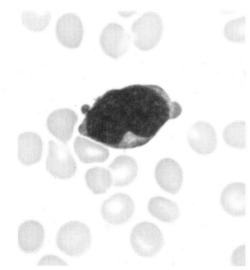

Fig.8.30 Acute myeloblastic leukaemia, M_7 (megakaryoblastic): a cell with scanty cytoplasm and pseudopodoid margins, an appearance associated with but not confined to this.

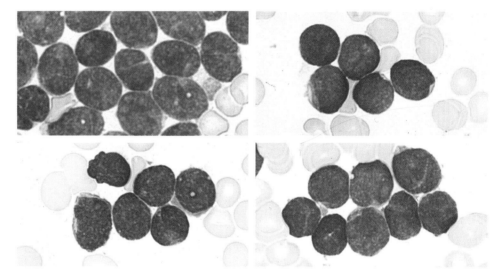

Fig.8.31 Acute lymphoblastic leukaemia, L_1 subtype: rather small, uniform blast cells with scanty cytoplasm, and rounded or cleft nuclei with usually only one nucleolus.

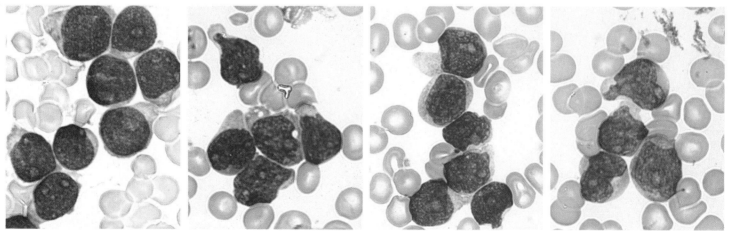

Fig.8.32 Acute lymphoblastic leukaemia, L_2 subtype: blast cells which vary considerably in size and amount of cytoplasm; the nuclear/cytoplasmic ratio is rarely as high as in L_1. The nuclei are variable in shape and often contain many nucleoli.

The L_3 variant shows multiple small vacuoles throughout a basophilic cell cytoplasm and often overlying the nucleus (Fig.8.33). This appearance corresponds usually to the rare B-cell or Burkitt type. The bone marrow in all variants is hypercellular with leukaemic blasts comprising eighty percent or more of the marrow cell total (Fig.8.34). In acute lymphoblastic leukaemia, blasts are often seen in the cerebrospinal fluid (Fig.8.35) or testes (Fig.8.36).

CYTOCHEMISTRY

In acute myeloblastic leukaemia, special stains such as myeloperoxidase or Sudan black are used to confirm the presence of granules in the myeloid cells (Fig.8.37). Monocytic differentiation is demonstrated by non-specific esterase staining which may be combined with chloracetate staining to distinguish monoblasts and myeloblasts in the same case (Fig.8.38). The periodic acid–Schiff reagent may show block positivity in the M_6

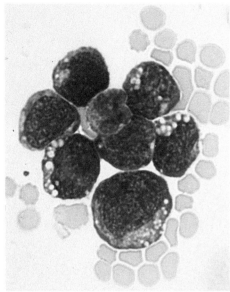

Fig.8.33 Acute lymphoblastic leukaemia, L_3 subtype: blast cells with deeply staining blue cytoplasm containing numerous small perinuclear vacuoles. This appearance is usually associated with the B-cell type (B-ALL).

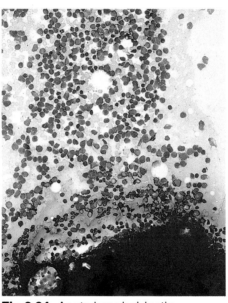

Fig.8.34 Acute lymphoblastic leukaemia: low power view of bone marrow fragment showing hypercellularity of cellular trails which are over eighty percent blast cells.

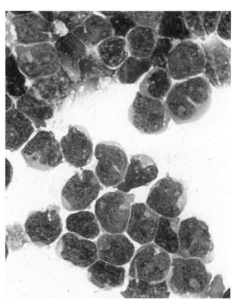

Fig.8.35 Acute lymphoblastic leukaemia: high power view of cytospin of cerebrospinal fluid showing a deposit of blast cells of varying morphology. The patient presented with the features of meningeal leukaemia.

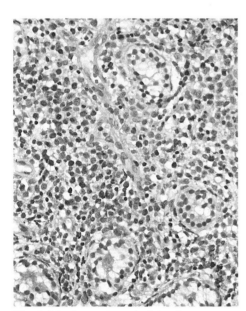

Fig.8.36 Acute lymphoblastic leukaemia: low power view of testicular infiltrate showing leukaemic blast cells in the interstitial tissues and in the seminiferous tubular epithelium.

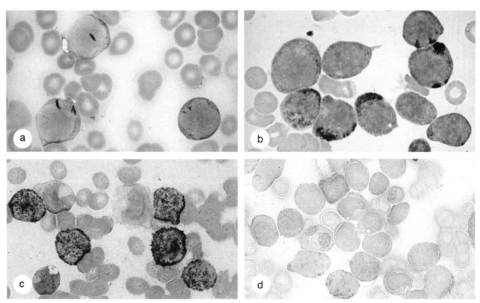

Fig.8.37 Acute myeloblastic leukaemia: bone marrow aspirates of (a & b) M_2 subtypes show black-staining cytoplasmic granules and Auer rods; (c) M_4 subtype shows myeloblasts with black cytoplasmic granules. The monoblasts show only background staining; (d) M_2 subtype shows multiple blue-staining cytoplasmic granules. Sudan black (a-c) and myeloperoxidase (d) stains.

variant (Fig.8.39). The presence of monoblasts may also be shown by measuring serum lysozyme or demonstrating microscopically lysozyme secretion by the monoblasts (Fig.8.40).

In acute lymphoblastic leukaemia, the special stains of value are: periodic acid-Schiff which shows block positiv-ity in non-B, non-T-ALL usually showing the c-ALL antigen (c-ALLA; Fig.8.41); acid phosphatase which shows eccentric, Golgi-body staining in T-ALL (Fig.8.42); and oil red-O which stains lipid material (Fig.8.43) which appears as vacuoles on conventional May-Grünwald/Giemsa staining.

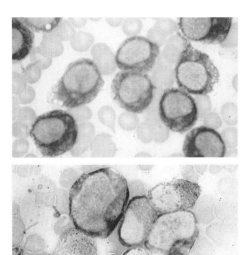

Fig.8.38 Acute myeloblastic leukaemia: bone marrow aspirates of (upper) M_5 subtype shows deep orange staining by non-specific esterase; (lower) M_4 subtype shows deep orange staining of the monoblast cytoplasm by non-specific esterase and blue staining of myeloblast cytoplasm by chloracetate.

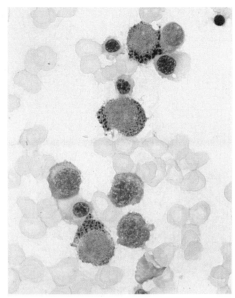

Fig.8.39 Acute myeloblastic leukaemia, M_6 subtype: bone marrow aspirate in which the cytoplasm of some of the erythroblasts shows block positive red staining by periodic acid-Schiff.

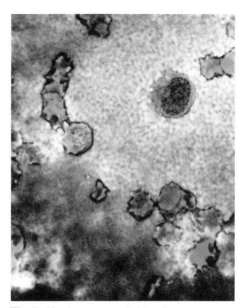

Fig.8.40 Acute myeloblastic leukaemia, M_5 subtype: the bone marrow aspirate plate has been layered with the organism *Micrococcus lysodeikticus*. There is clearing of the organism around a monoblast because of secretion of lysozyme (muramidase) by the cell. Courtesy of Dr. D. Catovsky.

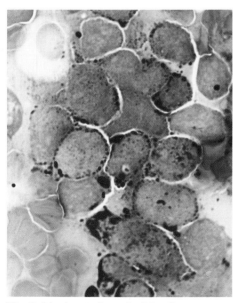

Fig.8.41 Acute lymphoblastic leukaemia, non-B non-T c-ALL: bone marrow aspirate showing cells with one or more coarse granules in the cytoplasm. Periodic acid-Schiff stain.

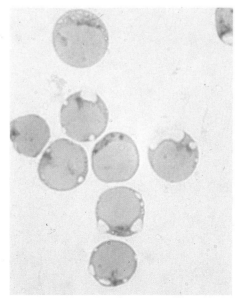

Fig.8.42 Acute lymphoblastic leukaemia, T-ALL subtype: bone marrow aspirate shows red cytoplasmic staining with marked coloration of the Golgi zone adjacent to or indented into the nucleus. Acid-phosphatase stain.

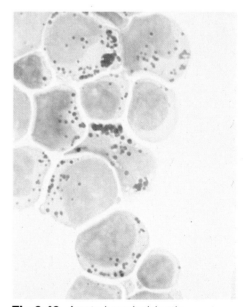

Fig.8.43 Acute lymphoblastic leukaemia, L_3 subtype: bone marrow aspirate stained with oil red-O shows prominent cytoplasmic lipid collections corresponding to some of the vacuoles shown by Romanowsky staining (see Fig.8.33).

IMMUNOLOGICAL MARKERS

Immunological testing by immunofluorescence, peroxidase or alkaline phosphatase-antialkaline phosphate (AP-AAP) techniques is particularly useful in acute leukaemia. A typical panel of (monoclonal) antibodies used includes:

a) Precursor associated:3C5 or MY10; TdT; HLA-DR
b) Myeloid: MY9; MY7; MSC2
c) Monocytic: Mo2; UCHM1
d) Erythroid: anti-glycophorin
e) Megakaryoblastic: J15
f) Common ALL & B: CD19(B or Leu 12); CD10(J5 or RF-AL3); CD26(B1); anti-IgM
g) T-associated: CD7(3A1, RFT2); CD2(T11); CD5(T1); CD3(OKT3 or Leu 4).

The sequence of expression of these antigens is given in

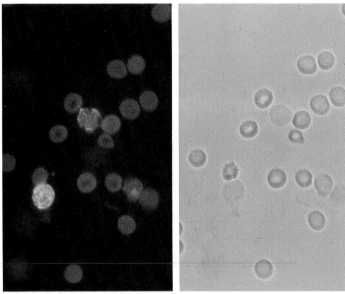

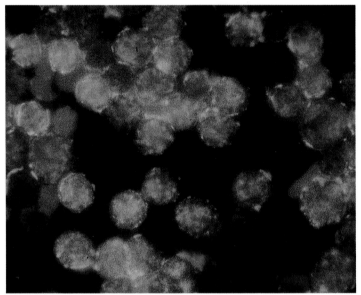

Fig.8.44 Acute lymphoblastic leukaemia, common-ALL subtype: bone marrow aspirates (left) seen by indirect immunofluorescent staining for the nuclear enzyme terminal deoxynucleotidyl transferase (TdT) using fluorescein labelling (green), and the common-ALL antigen (c-ALLA) using avidin labelling (orange). One of the cells is double-stained; (right) the same cells seen by phase. Courtesy of Prof. G. Janossy.

Fig.8.45 Acute lymphoblastic leukaemia, common-ALL subtype: bone marrow aspirate seen by indirect immunofluorescence shows nuclear TdT (green) and membrane HLA-DR antigen (orange). Most cells are double-stained but some cells show only one or the other antigen. Courtesy of Prof. G. Janossy.

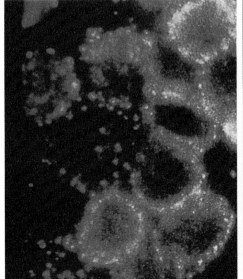
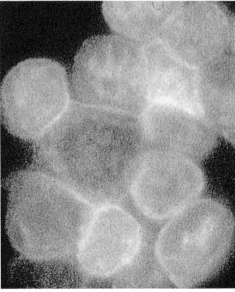
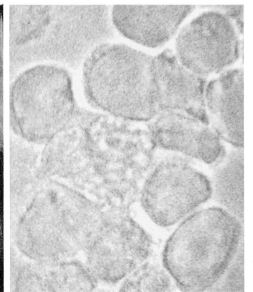

Fig.8.46 Acute lymphoblastic leukaemia, T-ALL subtype: bone marrow aspirates seen by indirect immunofluorescence shows (left) red cell membrane T antigen and (middle) green-staining nuclear TdT; (right) the same cells seen by phase. Courtesy of Prof. G. Janossy.

Figs.7.29 and 7.33. The blasts are usually positive for the nuclear enzyme terminal deoxynucleotidyl transferase (TdT). Tests for this may be combined with membrane staining for HLA-DR (Ia) or for the common acute lymphoblastic leukaemia antigen (c-ALLA) which are both usually positive in c-ALL, or for the T-cell antigens which are positive in T-ALL (Figs.8.44–8.46). TdT testing is particularly valuable for detecting blasts at extramedullary sites, since no TdT-positive cells occur normally outside the marrow or thymus (Figs.8.47 & 8.48), and for detecting populations of lymphoblasts in cases of mixed ALL/AML arising *de novo* or during transformation of chronic granulocytic leukaemia (Figs.8.49 & 8.50).

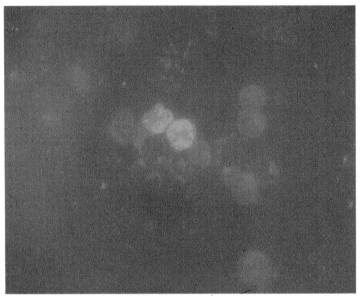

Fig.8.47 Acute lymphoblastic leukaemia: cerebrospinal fluid seen by indirect immunofluorescent staining for TdT. These few cells, difficult to recognize morphologically, show nuclear TdT staining typical of lymphoblasts. Courtesy of Dr. K.F. Bradstock.

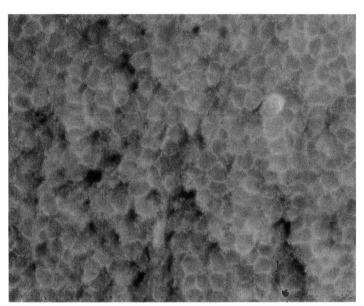

Fig.8.48 Acute lymphoblastic leukaemia, common-ALL subtype: testicular infiltrate seen by indirect immunofluorescence shows nuclear TdT as green and membrane HLA-DR (Ia) antigen as orange. Courtesy of Prof. G. Janossy.

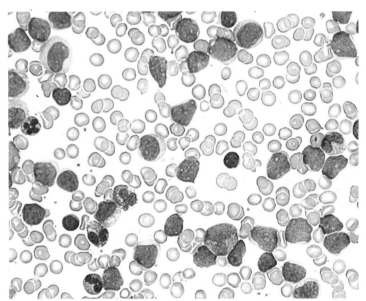

Fig.8.49 Acute leukaemias, mixed cell (myeloblastic/lymphoblastic) type: bone marrow aspirate showing blasts of varying size and morphology. Some show scanty cytoplasm without granules while others, usually larger, show eccentric nuclei, substantial cytoplasm and granules.

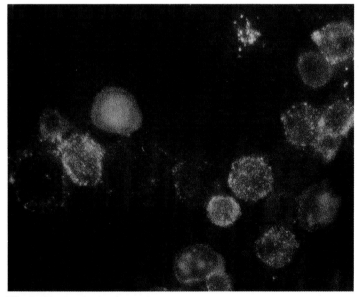

Fig.8.50 Acute leukaemia, mixed cell type: bone marrow aspirate seen by indirect immunofluorescence shows one population of cells (lymphoblastic) to have nuclear TdT (green) while another population (myeloblastic) has myeloid surface antigen (yellow/orange). Courtesy of Prof. G. Janossy.

In so-called pre-B-ALL, intracytoplasmic immunoglobulin is expressed and may be detected by indirect immunofluorescence (Fig.8.51). In B-ALL, surface immunoglobulin is present but TdT is invariably negative (Fig.8.52). Characteristic antigens may also be demonstrated by enzyme-linked cytochemistry instead of immunofluorescence (Fig.8.53). Immunoglobulin gene probes show that the cell in c-ALL, pre-B-ALL and B-ALL show clonal rearrangements of their immunoglobulin genes, thus confirming their B-cell origin. This is also the case for B-cell chronic lymphocytic leukaemia, B-cell non-Hodgkin's lymphoma, myeloma and hairy cell leukaemia (Fig.8.54). The T-cell receptor genes (γ, β and α) may show clonal rearrangement in the T-cell tumours, for example, T-ALL, T-CLL, T-cell lymphoma and Sézary's disease.

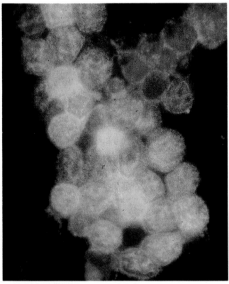

Fig.8.51 Acute lymphoblastic leukaemia, pre-B subtype: bone marrow aspirate seen by indirect immunofluorescence. The blast cells show nuclear TdT as green and intracytoplasmic immunoglobulin (IgM) as orange. Courtesy of Prof. G. Janossy.

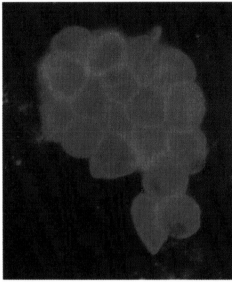
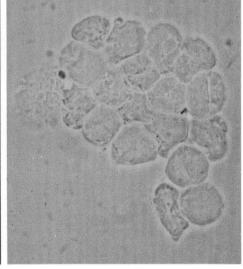

Fig.8.52 Acute lymphoblastic leukaemia, B subtype: bone marrow aspirate seen by indirect immunofluorescence. The cells (left) are invariably negative for nuclear TdT but show the presence of surface immunoglobulin (SIg); (right) as seen by phase. Courtesy of Prof. G. Janossy.

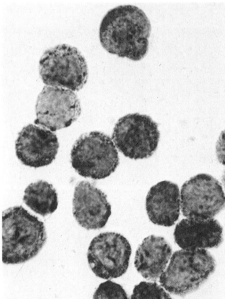

Fig.8.53 Acute lymphoblastic leukaemia: bone marrow aspirate stained by the alkaline phosphatase-antialkaline phosphatase (AP-AAP) technique to demonstrate the presence of the HLA-DR (Ia) antigen. Courtesy of Dr. D. Campana.

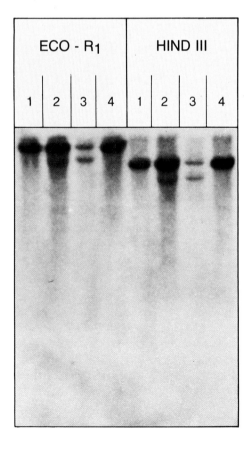

Fig.8.54 Autoradiograph of Southern blot DNA analysis in ALL: DNA extracted from the peripheral blood of a patient with c-ALL has been digested by restriction enzymes ECO-R_1 and HIND III. Track 1 is of normal leucocytes; tracks 2 and 3 are of leukaemic blasts; and track 4 is of the promyelocytic cell line HL60. In all tracks except 2 the cells have been concentrated before DNA extraction. The DNA digests have been subjected to electrophoresis in agarose and transferred to nitrocellulose. A ^{32}P-labelled genomic DNA probe to the JH region of the IgM heavy-chain gene has been added to hybridize with complementary DNA in the DNA digests.

All the tracks show a band of similar molecular weight corresponding to the JH region in the germline configuration. Tracks 2 and 3 show an additional band of lower molecular weight due to clonal rearrangement of the heavy-chain gene in the c-ALL DNA. Courtesy of Dr. R. Taheri and Dr. J. D. Norton.

CONGENITAL ACUTE LEUKAEMIA

Fig.8.55 illustrates a rare type of acute leukaemia, congenital acute leukaemia. This is usually myeloblastic and characterized by extensive extramedullary infiltration, including of the skin.

CYTOGENETICS

Cytogenetic analysis of acute leukaemia cells may help to confirm the diagnosis and indicate the subtype in which characteristic abnormalities may occur (see Appendix). The presence of a translocation, particularly if no normal karyotypes are present, usually implies a poor prognosis. The cytogenetic abnormalities hypodiploidy (Fig.8.56) or hyperdiploidy (Fig.8.57) are more common in ALL than AML. Some of the more common translocations include t(4;11)(q21;q23) in ALL (Fig.8.58), t(8;21)(q22;q22) in AML, M₂ (Fig.8.59) and t(15;17)(q22;q12) in AML, M₃ (Fig.8.60).

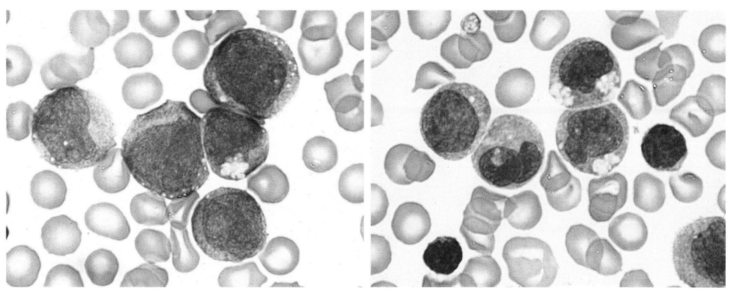

Fig.8.55 Congenital acute myeloblastic leukaemia: peripheral blood films of a male infant who presented at birth with anaemia, hepatosplenomegaly and skin lesions. There are large numbers of myeloblasts with prominent cytoplasmic vacuolation. *Hb:10.1g/dl; WBC:92x10⁹/l; blasts:85%; platelets:15x10⁹/l.* Courtesy of Dr. J.M. Chessells.

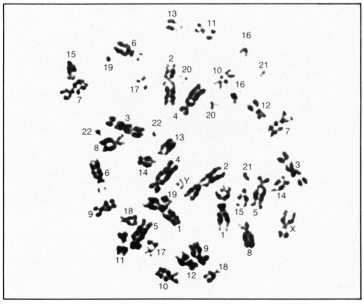
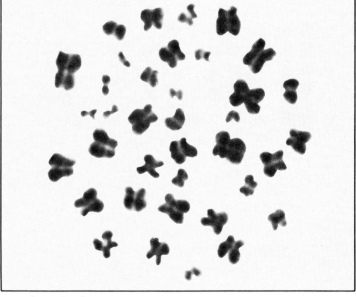

Fig.8.56 Chromosomes (adult male): (left) normal 46 chromosomes in metaphase from a G-banded marrow cell; (right) only 37 chromosomes in hypodiploid metaphase from a marrow cell. The contracted, poorly banded, chromosomes are characteristic of those from a leukaemic clone. Courtesy of Dr. L.M. Secker-Walker.

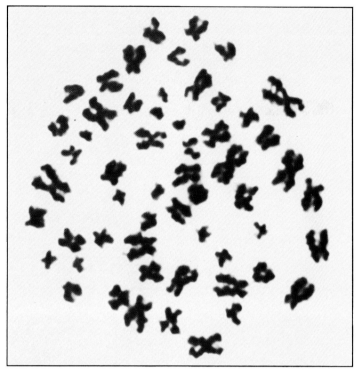

Fig.8.57 Acute lymphoblastic leukaemia, L₁ subtype: 56 chromosomes in hyperdiploid metaphase from a marrow cell. The contracted, poorly banded, chromosomes are characteristic of leukaemic tissue. Courtesy of Dr. L.M. Secker-Walker.

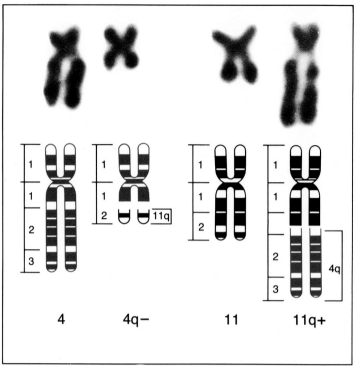

Fig.8.58 Acute lymphoblastic leukaemia, L₁ subtype: (upper) partial karyotypes of G-banded chromosomes 4 and 11 from a patient with blasts of null phenotype (TdT⁺, c-ALL⁻). The translocated chromosomes are on the right in each pair; (lower) diagrammatic systematized description of the structural aberration. Courtesy of Dr. L.M. Secker-Walker.

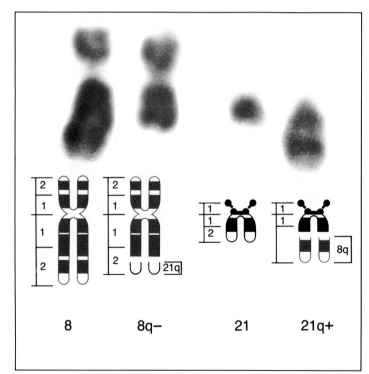

Fig.8.59 Acute myeloblastic leukaemia, M₂ subtype: (upper) partial karyotypes of G-banded chromosomes 8 and 21. The translocated chromosomes are on the right in each pair; (lower) diagrammatic systematized description of the structural aberration. Courtesy of Dr. L.M. Secker-Walker.

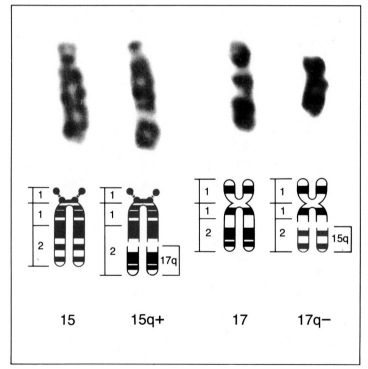

Fig.8.60 Acute myeloblastic leukaemia, M₃ subtype (acute promyelocytic leukaemia; APL): (upper) partial karyotypes of G-banded chromosomes 15 and 17. The translocated chromosomes are on the right in each pair; (lower) diagrammatic systematized description of the structural aberration. Courtesy of Dr. L.M. Secker-Walker.

9

CHRONIC LEUKAEMIA AND MYELODYSPLASIA

CHRONIC LYMPHOCYTIC LEUKAEMIA (CLL)

Chronic lymphocytic (lymphatic) leukaemia, predominantly a disease of the elderly, is characterized by large numbers of lymphocytes which accumulate in the blood, spleen, liver and lymph nodes. In the majority of cases, the cells are a monoclonal population of immature B-lymphocytes showing low-density surface immunoglobulin. Prolymphocytes (see Fig.9.18) are also seen in variable proportions in the peripheral blood, the proportion increasing in more advanced disease in some cases.

Symmetrical enlargement of superficial lymph nodes is found in most patients (Figs.9.1-9.3) and, rarely, there is tonsillar involvement (Fig.9.4). In advanced disease there is splenomegaly and hepatomegaly, and patients with thrombocytopenia may show bruising and extensive skin purpura (Fig.9.5). Infections are frequent due to immunoglobulin deficiency, neutropenia and lymphoid dysfunction. In many patients there may be associated herpes zoster (Figs.9.6 & 9.7) or herpes simplex (Fig.9.8) infections, and oral candidiasis and other infections are also a frequent occurrence (Fig.9.9).

The blood count in chronic lymphocytic leukaemia reveals an absolute lymphocytosis (between 20-200x10⁹/l is usual), and the peripheral blood has a characteristic lymphoid morphology (Figs.9.10 & 9.11). In advanced disease there is often a normochromic anaemia and thrombocytopenia. About ten percent of patients develop a secondary warm-type autoimmune haemolytic anaemia (Fig.9.12) and, in a smaller number of cases, an autoimmune thrombocytopenia occurs. Approximately twenty percent of patients with chronic lymphocytic leukaemia are asymptomatic and the diagnosis is made only when a routine blood test is performed.

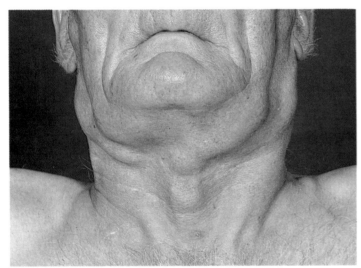

Fig.9.1 Chronic lymphocytic leukaemia: bilateral cervical lymphadenopathy in a 65-year-old man. *Hb:12.5g/dl; WBC:150x10⁹/l (lymphocytes:140x10⁹/l); platelets:120x10⁹/l.*

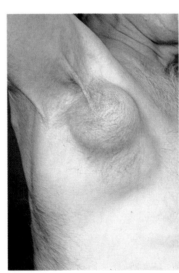
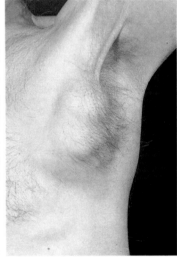

Fig.9.2 Chronic lymphocytic leukaemia: bilateral axillary lymphadenopathy (same patient as in Fig.9.1).

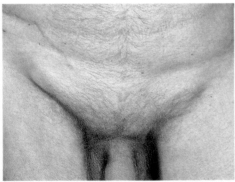
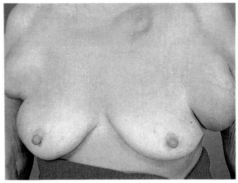
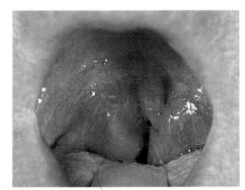

Fig.9.3 Chronic lymphocytic leukaemia: (upper) bilateral inguinal lymphadenopathy (same patient as in Fig.9.1); (lower) gross enlargement of the lymph nodes in both axillary regions in a 69-year-old female.

Fig.9.4 Chronic lymphocytic leukaemia: massive enlargement of the pharyngeal tonsils (same patient as in Fig.9.1).

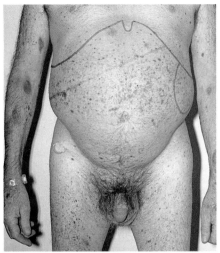

Fig.9.5 Chronic lymphocytic leukaemia: purpuric haemorrhage and abdominal swelling in a 54-year-old man. The extent of liver and splenic enlargement is indicated. *Hb:10.9g/dl;WBC:250x10⁹/l (lymphocytes: 245x10⁹/l); platelets:35x10⁹/l.*

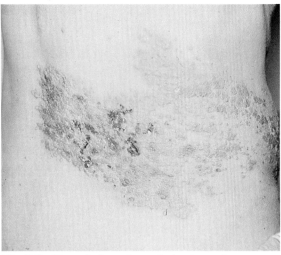

Fig.9.6 Chronic lymphocytic leukaemia: herpes zoster infection in a 68-year-old female.

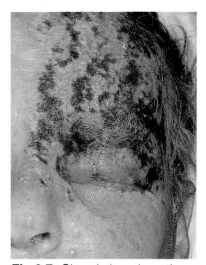

Fig.9.7 Chronic lymphocytic leukaemia: herpes zoster infection in the territory of the ophthalmic division of the fifth cranial nerve.

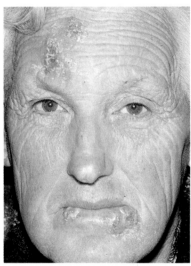

Fig.9.8 Chronic lymphocytic leukaemia: herpes simplex eruptions of the lower lip and skin of the forehead.

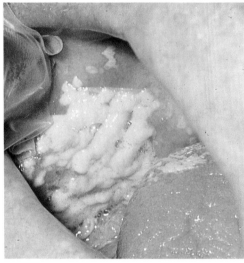

Fig.9.9 Chronic lymphocytic leukaemia: extensive *Candida albicans* infection of the buccal mucosa of a 73-year-old female.

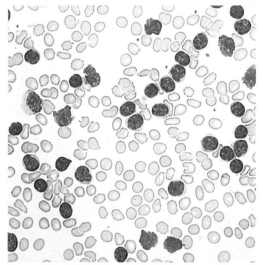

Fig.9.10 Chronic lymphocytic leukaemia: peripheral blood film showing the increased numbers of lymphocytes and occasional 'smear' cells characteristic of this condition. *Hb:9.0g/dl; WBC:190x10⁹/l; platelets:70x10⁹/l.*

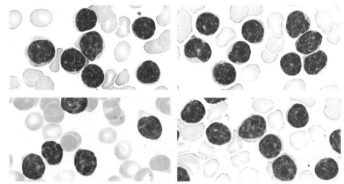

Fig.9.11 Chronic lymphocytic leukaemia: lymphocytes in the peripheral blood of four different patients show a thin rim of cytoplasm, condensed coarse chromatin and only rare nucleoli.

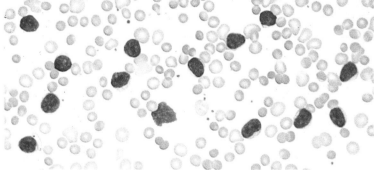

Fig.9.12 Chronic lymphocytic leukaemia with autoimmune haemolytic anaemia: peripheral blood film shows increased numbers of lymphocytes, red cell spherocytosis and polychromasia. The direct Coombs test was strongly positive with IgG on the surface of the cells. *Hb:8.3g/dl; reticulocytes:150x10⁹/l; WBC:110x10⁹/l (lymphocytes:107x10⁹/l); platelets:90x10⁹/l.*

Bone marrow examination shows extensive replacement of normal marrow elements by lymphocytes, reaching thirty to ninety-five percent of the marrow cell total. Trephine biopsies (Figs.9.13 & 9.14) show either nodular or diffuse collections of abnormal cells. Patients with nodular histology have a better prognosis. In patients with autoimmune haemolytic anaemia or thrombocytopenia the spleen is sometimes removed and shows a characteristic histology (Fig.9.15).

Although marker studies (Fig.9.16) indicate that the majority of patients with chronic lymphocytic leukaemia have B-cell disease, occasional patients are found to have a T-cell form of the disease (Fig.9.17).

PROLYMPHOCYTIC LEUKAEMIA

This variant of chronic lymphocytic leukaemia usually occurs in the elderly and is associated with marked splenomegaly, absolute lymphocytosis usually over 100×10^9/l and minimal lymph node enlargement. The blood film shows larger lymphocytes than are found in classical CLL (Fig.9.18). In the majority of patients, surface marker studies indicate a B-cell origin of

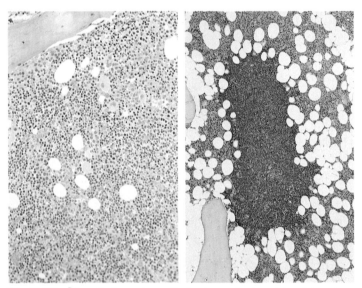

Fig.9.13 Chronic lymphocytic leukaemia: trephine biopsies showing (left) a marked diffuse increase in marrow lymphocytes (closely packed cells with small dense nuclei); (right) a nodular pattern of lymphocyte accumulation (in a different patient).

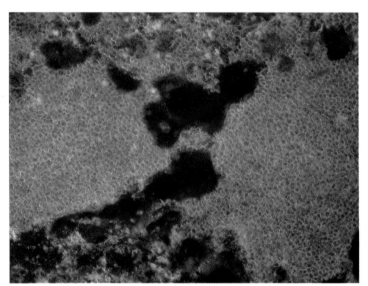

Fig.9.14 Chronic lymphocytic leukaemia: trephine biopsy with two neoplastic lymphoid nodules containing predominantly B-cells with positive reaction for IgM (green fluorescein staining). Numerous reactive T-cells are identified by a monoclonal antibody to the CD$_5$ antigen (red rhodamine staining). Courtesy of Dr. G. Pizzolo and Dr. M. Chilosi.

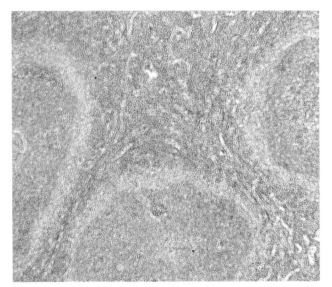

Fig.9.15 Chronic lymphocytic leukaemia: histological section of spleen in a patient with secondary autoimmune haemolytic anaemia. There is expansion of lymphoid tissue in the periarterial sheaths of the white pulp and obvious red cell entrapment in the reticuloendothelial cords and splenic sinuses.

	B-CLL	B-PLL	HCL	T-CLL, T-PLL
Surface Ig	±(IgM±IgD)	++(IgM±IgD)	+(IgM or IgG (or IgA)	−
MRBC rosettes	++	±	±	−
SRBC rosettes	−	−	−	+
Surface antigens				
HLA-DR	+	+	+	−
CD19 (B4)	+	+	+	−
CD20 (B1)	+	+	+	−
CD5 (T1)	+	−	−	−
CD2 (T11)	−	−	−	+
CD3 (T3)	−	−	−	+
FMC7	−	+	±	−
Gene rearrangement				
IgH	+	+	+	−
TCRβ	−	−	−	+

Fig.9.16 The immunological markers and immunoglobin (Ig) heavy chain (H) and T-cell receptor (TCR) β-chain rearrangement in B-cell CLL, PLL and HCL, and in T-cell CLL and PLL. M = mouse; S = sheep.

prolymphocytes, but occasional patients are seen with a T-cell variant of this disease (Fig.9.19) and have a prognosis which is less predictable.

CHRONIC T-CELL LYMPHOCYTOSIS (LARGE GRANULAR LYMPHOCYTE LEUKAEMIA)

In this recently recognized syndrome, patients with chronic neutropenia and/or anaemia show an increase in peripheral blood lymphocytes which may be large and with a granular appearance (Fig.9.20). A proportion of the patients show seropositive rheumatoid arthritis and splenomegaly as a subgroup of Felty's syndrome. The cells are of CD8 (T8) phenotype and suppressor function, and show the antigen characteristic of natural killer (NK) cells detected by the monoclonal antibody HNK-1. The cells, in most cases, are a monoclonal population of T-lymphocytes shown by rearrangement of the genes for the β-chain of the T-cell antigen receptor. Nevertheless, the disease usually runs a chronic benign course.

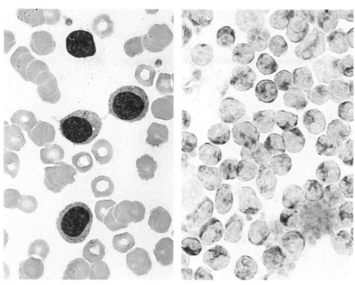

Fig.9.17 Chronic lymphocytic leukaemia: peripheral blood films in a T-cell variant showing (left) abnormal lymphocytes and (right) characteristic 'clump' positivity in the Golgi zone using acid phosphatase staining.

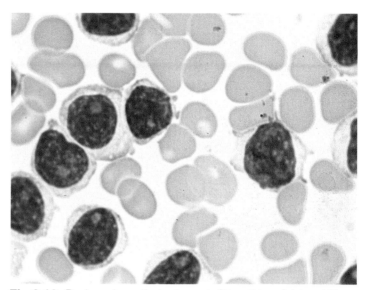

Fig.9.18 Prolymphocytic leukaemia(B-cell type): blood film showing prolymphocytes which have prominent central nucleoli and an abundance of pale cytoplasm. A high density of surface immunoglobulin confirmed their B-cell nature. *Hb:9g/dl; WBC:350x10⁹/l (lymphocytes:317x10⁹/l); platelets:75x10⁹/l.* Courtesy of Dr. D. Catovsky.

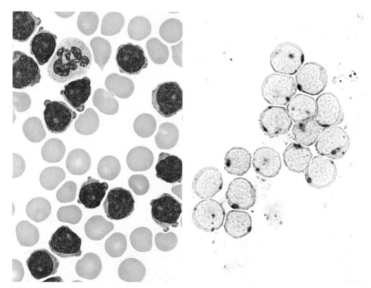

Fig.9.19 Prolymphocytic leukaemia(T-cell type): blood films showing (left) prolymphocytes and a single neutrophil. Cell marker studies showed positive reactions with anti-T-cell antisera and an absence of surface immunoglobulin; (right) 'clump' positivity of these cells using acid phosphatase staining. *Hb:10.5g/dl; WBC:240x10⁹/l; platelets:60x10⁹/l.* Courtesy of Dr. D. Catovsky.

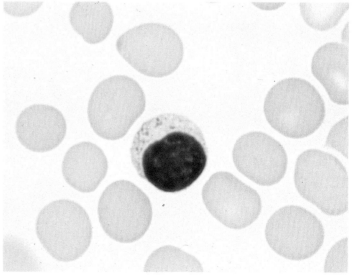

Fig.9.20 Chronic T-cell lymphocytosis: peripheral blood film showing a large lymphocyte with multiple coarse azurophilic, cytoplasmic granules. Immunological marker studies showed the cells to be CD8⁺ (T8⁺), CD3⁺ (T3⁺) and HNK-1⁺. The patient had rheumatoid arthritis, splenomegaly, chronic neutropenia and lymphocytosis. *Absolute lymphocyte count:8.6x10⁹/l.*

9.5

HAIRY CELL LEUKAEMIA (LEUKAEMIC RETICULOENDOTHELIOSIS)

Patients with hairy cell leukaemia usually present with pancytopenia and splenomegaly without lymphadenopathy. The characteristic cells of B-lymphocyte origin are seen in the peripheral blood (Fig.9.21) and may also be found in large numbers in marrow aspirates or from splenic imprints in patients

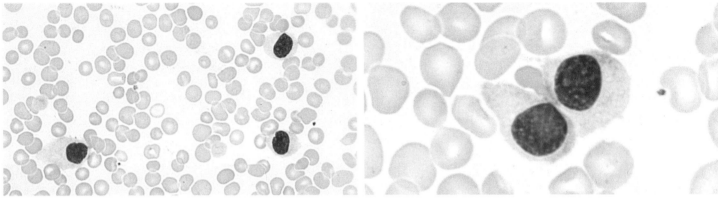

Fig.9.21 Hairy cell leukaemia: peripheral blood films showing (left) typical 'hairy' cells which have round or oval nuclei and a moderate amount of finely mottled, pale grey cytoplasm with irregular serrated ('hairy') edges. The chromatin pattern has less density than typical small lymphocytes; (right) at higher magnification the nucleoli are clearly visible. *Hb:9.4g/dl; WBC:5.5x10^9/l (hairy cells:4.3x10^9/l); platelets:90x10^9/l.*

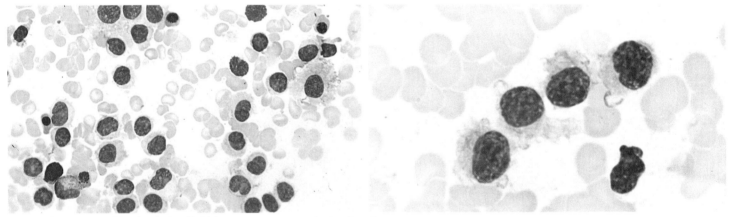

Fig.9.22 Hairy cell leukaemia: (left) bone marrow aspirate showing a predominance of hairy cells in the cell trail; (right) splenic imprints showing typical nuclear and cytoplasmic features of the abnormal hairy cells.

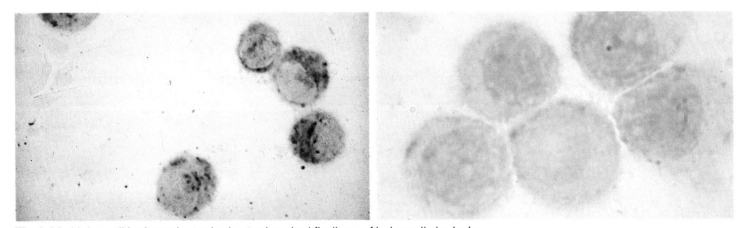

Fig.9.23 Hairy cell leukaemia: typical cytochemical findings of hairy cells include (left) a strongly positive reaction to tartaric acid-resistant acid phosphatase and (right) a fine granular positivity with crescentic accumulation at one side of the nucleus following alpha-naphthyl butyrate esterase staining.

who have had a splenectomy (Fig.9.22). Hairy cells also show characteristic cytochemical reactions (Fig.9.23).

In many patients the marrow is difficult to aspirate and trephine biopsy is necessary for diagnosis. In these cases, diffuse infiltration by hairy cells (Fig.9.24) and a dense reticulin fibre pattern (Fig.9.25) are seen.

Histological sections of the spleen (Figs.9.26 & 9.27) and liver (Figs.9.28 & 9.29) may demonstrate unusual vascular 'lakes' caused by hairy cell infiltration of these organs.

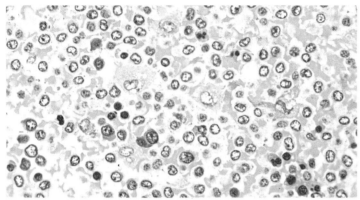

Fig.9.24 Hairy cell leukaemia: trephine biopsy showing extensive replacement of normal haemopoietic tissue by discrete mononuclear hairy cells. The nuclei are typically surrounded by a clear zone of cytoplasm. Methacrylate section.

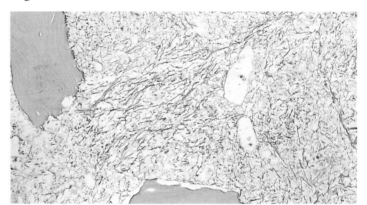

Fig.9.25 Hairy cell leukaemia: trephine biopsy showing increased fibre density and thickness in the reticulin fibre pattern. Silver impregnation technique.

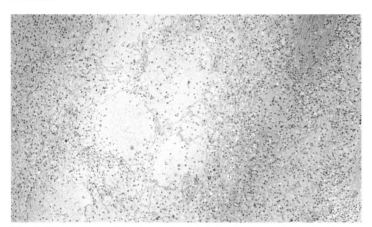

Fig.9.26 Hairy cell leukaemia: histological section of spleen shows hairy cell infiltration of reticuloendothelial cords and sinuses. Numerous blood 'lakes' are seen in the centre of the field.

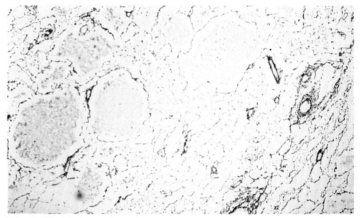

Fig.9.27 Hairy cell leukaemia: histological section of spleen (same case as in Fig.9.26) shows more clearly the reticulin fibre pattern outlining the abnormal venous 'lakes'. The presence of these structures may explain the extensive splenic red cell pooling that occurs in this disease. Silver impregnation technique.

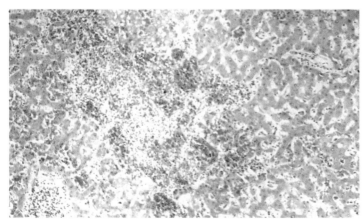

Fig.9.28 Hairy cell leukaemia: histological section of liver shows hairy cell infiltration of sinusoids and portal tracts. There is sinusoidal ectasia and pseudoangiomatous transformation of hepatic blood vessels.

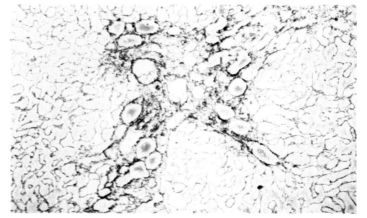

Fig.9.29 Hairy cell leukaemia: histological section of liver (same case as in Fig.9.28) shows the reticulin fibre pattern clearly, confirming the gross distortion of hepatic vascular architecture. It is thought that attachment of large numbers of hairy cells to the sinusoidal lining cells causes cell damage which results in these characteristic vascular abnormalities in the liver and spleen. Silver impregnation technique.

CHRONIC GRANULOCYTIC LEUKAEMIA (CGL)

Chronic granulocytic (myeloid) leukaemia is most frequently seen in the middle-aged. In most patients there is a replacement of normal marrow by cells with an abnormal G-group chromosome, the Philadelphia or Ph[1] chromosome (Fig.9.30). This abnormality is a result of reciprocal translocation involving chromosome 9 band q34 and chromosome 22 band q11. The cellular oncogene c-abl, which codes for a tyrosine protein kinase, is translocated to a specific breakpoint cluster region (bcr) of chromosome 22. Part of the bcr gene (the 5' end) remains on chromosome 22, the 3' end moving to chromosome 9 together with the oncogene c-sis (which codes for a protein with close homology to one of the two subunits of platelet-derived growth factor). As a result of the translocation onto chromosome 22, a chimeric bcr/c-abl messenger RNA (mRNA) is produced (Fig.9.31), suggesting that an abnormal chimeric protein may be important in the excess haemopoietic cell

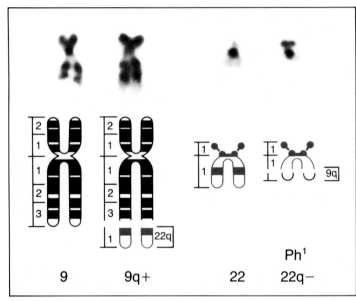

Fig.9.30 Chronic granulocytic leukaemia: (upper) partial karyotypes of G-banded chromosomes 9 and 22. The translocated chromosomes are on the right in each pair. Ph[1] is the Philadelphia chromosome; (lower) diagrammatic systematized description of the structural aberration. Courtesy of Dr. L. M. Secker-Walker.

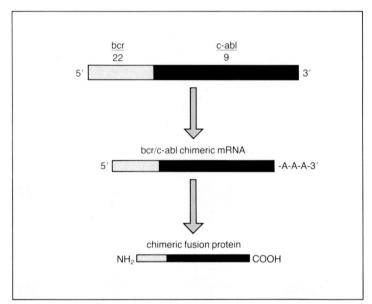

Fig.9.31 Chronic granulocytic leukaemia: chimeric bcr/c-abl mRNA encoded for partly by the bcr (breakpoint cluster region) of chromosome 22 and partly by the c-abl oncogene translocated from chromosome 9 to 22.

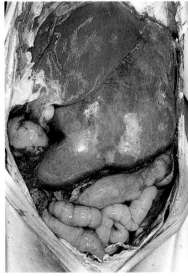

Fig.9.32 Chronic granulocytic leukaemia: abdominal contents at autopsy of a 54-year-old man. The grossly enlarged spleen extends towards the right iliac fossa. The central pale area covered by fibrinous exudate overlay an extensive splenic infarct. The liver is moderately enlarged.

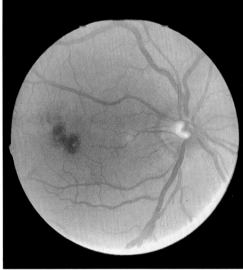

Fig.9.33 Chronic granulocytic leukaemia: ocular fundus in the hyperviscosity syndrome shows distended retinal veins and deep retinal haemorrhages at the macula. *Hb:14g/dl; WBC:590x10⁹/l; platelets:1050x10⁹/l.*

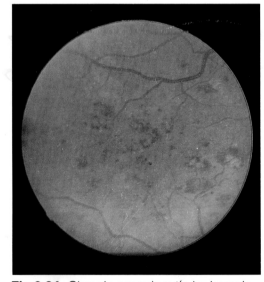

Fig.9.34 Chronic granulocytic leukaemia: ocular fundus (same case as in Fig.9.33) showing prominent leukaemic infiltrates fringed by areas of retinal haemorrhage.

proliferation. A clonal proliferation of these abnormal cells leads to a progressive expansion of the total body granulocyte mass.

The symptoms are related to hypermetabolism and include anorexia, lassitude, weight loss and night sweats. Splenomegaly is usual and frequently massive (Fig.9.32). There may also be features of anaemia, a bleeding disorder, visual disturbance due to retinal disease (Figs.9.33 & 9.34), neurological symptoms and occasionally gout (Fig.9.35). As in chronic lymphocytic leukaemia, this condition is only discovered in some patients during routine blood counting. The white cell count is usually between 50-500x10^9/l and a complete spectrum of granulocytic cells are seen in the blood film (Figs.9.36-9.38). Basophils are often prominent and the level of myelocytes, metamyelocytes and neutrophils exceeds that of the more primitive blast cells and promyelocytes. The bone marrow is hypercellular with a granulocytic predominance.

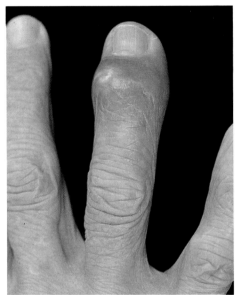

Fig.9.35 Chronic granulocytic leukaemia: acute inflammation and swelling of the fourth finger due to uric acid deposition. *Hb:8.6g/dl; WBC:540x10^9/l; platelets:850x10^9/l; serum uric acid:0.85mmol/l.*

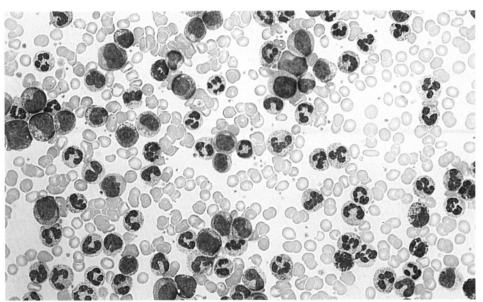

Fig.9.36 Chronic granulocytic leukaemia: peripheral blood film showing cells of all stages in granulopoietic development. *Hb:16.8g/dl; WBC:260x10^9/l; platelets:140x10^9/l.*

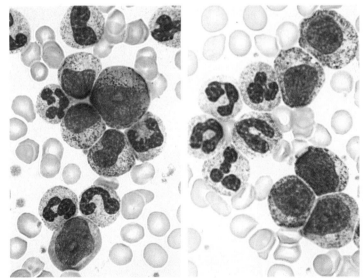

Fig.9.37 Chronic granulocytic leukaemia: peripheral blood films showing a myeloblast, promyelocytes, myelocytes, metamyelocytes, and band and segmented neutrophils.

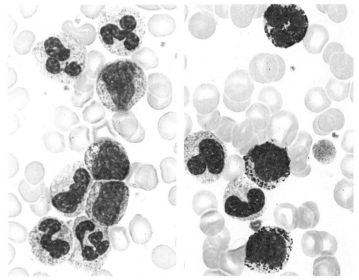

Fig.9.38 Chronic granulocytic leukaemia: peripheral blood films showing (left) myelocytes, a metamyelocyte, and band and segmented neutrophils and (right) basophils.

In about seventy percent of patients there is a terminal metamorphosis to an acute malignant form of leukaemia (Figs.9.39 & 9.40) which is associated with a rapid deterioration of the patient and progressive bone marrow failure. There may be infiltration of the skin (Figs.9.41 & 9.42) and other non-haemopoietic tissues. The transformation may be myeloblastic, lymphoblastic or mixed.

Philadelphia-negative chronic granulocytic leukaemia

Occasional patients have a variant of chronic granulocytic leukaemia which is associated with fewer myelocytes, more monocytoid cells and atypical neutrophils in the peripheral blood. Severe anaemia and thrombocytopenia are more frequent than in classical CGL. The Philadelphia chromosome is not found in these patients but the chimeric bcr/c-abl mRNA is produced.

A juvenile form of Philadelphia-negative CGL occurs in children, often with marked lymphadenopathy and eczematoid rashes (Fig.9.43). As in the adult form, there are morphological differences from classical chronic granulocytic leukaemia (Figs.9.44 & 9.45).

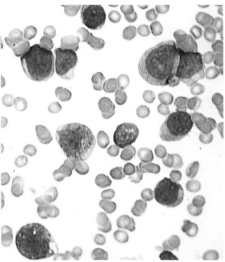

Fig.9.39 Chronic granulocytic leukaemia: peripheral blood film showing blast cell transformation. Over half the white cells seen are primitive blast forms. *Hb:8.5g/dl; WBC:110x10⁹/l (blasts:65x10⁹/l); platelets:45x10⁹/l.*

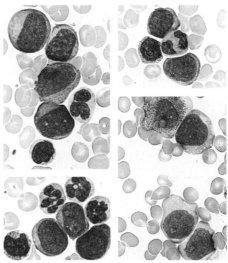

Fig.9.40 Chronic granulocytic leukaemia: peripheral blood films at high magnification showing blast cell transformation. There are numerous myeloblasts, atypical neutrophils and an abnormal promyelocyte (lower right).

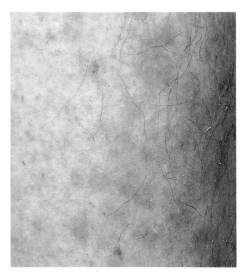

Fig.9.41 Chronic granulocytic leukaemia: nodular leukaemic infiltrates in the skin over the anterior surface of the tibia in a 48-year-old woman with blast cell transformation.

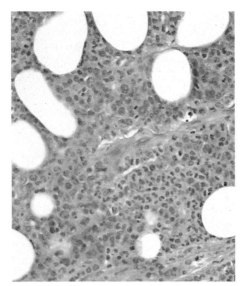

Fig.9.42 Chronic granulocytic leukaemia: histological section of skin lesion in Fig.9.41 shows extensive perivascular infiltration with mononuclear cells and polymorphs in the deeper layers of the dermis.

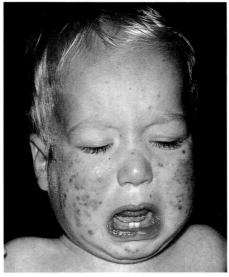

Fig.9.43 Juvenile chronic granulocytic leukaemia: eczematoid facial rash and lip bleeding in an 8-month-old infant. There was moderate splenomegaly. Cytogenetic studies failed to demonstrate the presence of the Philadelphia chromosome. *Hb:10.5g/dl; WBC: 120x10⁹/l; platelets:85x10⁹/l.* Courtesy of Dr. J.M. Chessells.

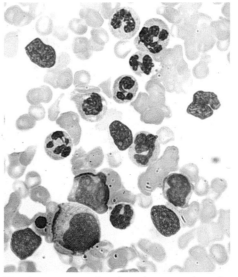

Fig.9.44 Juvenile chronic granulocytic leukaemia: peripheral blood film from the infant in Fig.9.43 shows a predominance of myelomonocytoid cells.

MYELODYSPLASTIC SYNDROMES (MDS)

The myelodysplastic syndromes usually occur in elderly subjects presenting with an anaemia which proves refractory to treatment by haematinics, with persistent neutropenia and thrombocytopenia or various combinations of these. Typically there is no enlargement of the liver, spleen and lymph nodes.

Within this group of patients, some present with an absolute monocytosis of greater than $1.0 \times 10^9/l$ with or without splenomegaly. This has been referred to as 'chronic myelomonocytic leukaemia'. Gum hypertrophy and skin deposits do not usually occur.

The myelodysplastic syndromes have been classified into five subgroups (Fig.9.46). Clinically these patients have symptoms related to bone marrow failure with frequent infective episodes (Figs.9.47 & 9.48) and bleeding abnormalities (Fig.9.49). Many patients die as a consequence of these complications of severe neutropenia or thrombocytopenia but, in others, the disease progresses to frank acute myeloblastic leukaemia. In the past these syndromes, particularly those with normal numbers of blasts (<5%) in the marrow, have been referred to as 'preleukaemia'.

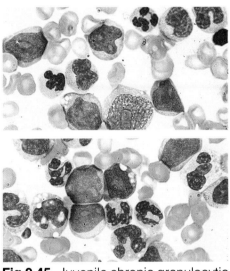

Fig.9.45 Juvenile chronic granulocytic leukaemia: peripheral blood films at higher magnification showing occasional blast forms, myelomonocytic cells, and atypical agranular band and segmented neutrophils.

FAB Classification of the Myelodysplastic Syndromes

1 Refractory anaemia (RA)

2 RA with ring sideroblasts
   (ring sideroblasts > 15%)

3 RA with excess blasts (RAEB; blasts 5-20%)

4 Chronic myelomonocytic leukaemia (CMML)

5 RAEB 'in transformation' (blasts 20-30%)

Fig.9.46 The myelodysplastic syndromes: the French-American-British (FAB) classification.

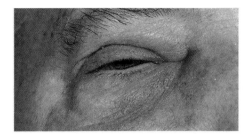
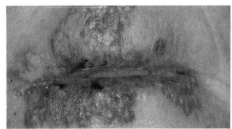

Fig.9.47 Myelodysplastic syndrome: (upper) skin infection spreading from the eyelids; (lower) extensive herpes simplex eruptions spreading from the lip margins to adjacent skin. Both patients had Type III disease (refractory anaemia with excess blasts).

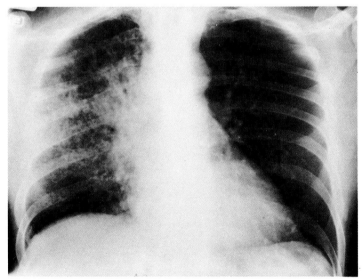

Fig.9.48 Myelodysplastic syndrome: chest radiograph (portable film) of a 62-year-old male with Legionnaire's disease. There is widespread patchy consolidation throughout the right lung.

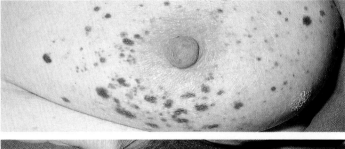
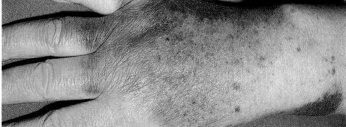

Fig.9.49 Myelodysplastic syndrome: (upper) extensive purpura of the skin of the breast in a 35-year-old woman with refractory anaemia (Type I); (lower) extensive ecchymoses and purpura of the skin over the back of the hand (same patient). *Hb:8g/dl; WBC:4x10^9/l; platelets:20x10^9/l.*

The blood film abnormalities in each subgroup are highly variable. General features include macrocytic red cells, qualitative granulocytic and monocytic changes (see below), and giant platelets. In patients with Type I, there may be no gross morphological changes (Fig.9.50). In Type II, there is frequently a dimorphic red cell population (Fig.9.51). Patients with Type III often show leucoerythroblastic changes. The greatest number of blast cells is seen in Type V (see Fig.9.62), and abnormal myelomonocytic cells and monocytosis (Figs.9.52 & 9.53) are characteristic of Type IV.

The bone marrow in the myelodysplastic syndromes is typically hypercellular and shows morphological abnormalities, often in all three series of haemopoietic cells. Cytogenetic abnormalities are common, particularly in secondary MDS (see Chapter 1). There is usually evidence of dyserythropoiesis with nuclear atypia, some megaloblastosis and ring sideroblasts (Figs.9.54–9.59). In some cases, there is an increase in reticulin while occasional cases are hypocellular.

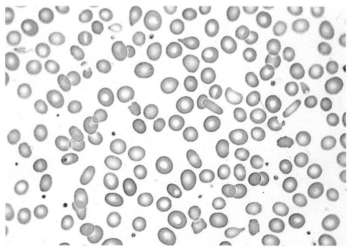

Fig.9.50 Myelodysplastic syndrome: peripheral blood film in refractory anaemia (Type I) shows marked anisocytosis and poikilocytosis. *Hb:7.9g/dl; WBC:5.4x10⁹/l (neutrophils: 1.8x10⁹/l); platelets:120x10⁹/l.*

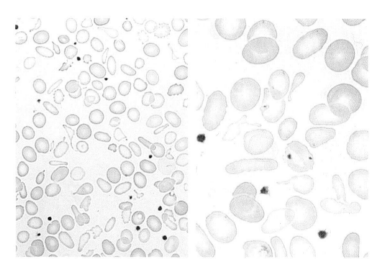

Fig.9.51 Myelodysplastic syndrome: peripheral blood films in acquired sideroblastic anaemia (Type II) showing (left) marked red cell anisocytosis and poikilocytosis. Although the majority of cells are markedly hypochromic, there is a second population of normochromic cells; (right) at higher magnification the central red cell shows two small basophilic inclusions (Pappenheimer bodies). Perls' staining demonstrated that similar inclusions were Prussian blue-positive (siderotic granules).These granules are far more numerous after splenectomy.

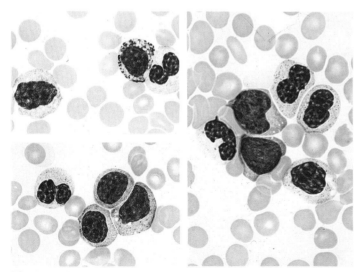

Fig.9.52 Myelodysplastic syndrome: peripheral blood films showing white cells in chronic myelomonocytic leukaemia (Type IV). There are many atypical myelomonocytic cells and pseudo-Pelger neutrophils, some of which are agranular.

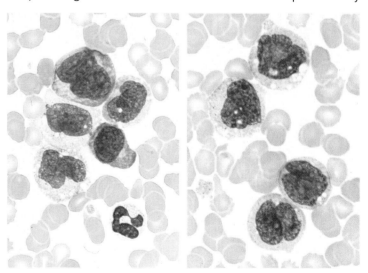

Fig.9.53 Myelodysplastic syndrome: peripheral blood films showing white cells in chronic myelomonocytic leukaemia (Type IV). The majority of cells are more monocytoid than those in Fig.9.52 and the neutrophil shown is agranular.

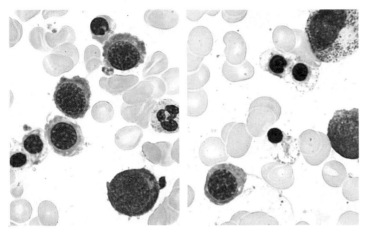

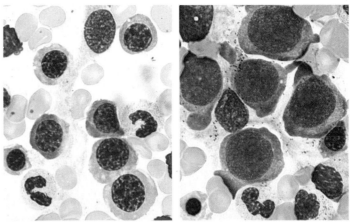

Fig.9.54 Myelodysplastic syndrome: bone marrow cell trails in acquired sideroblastic anaemia (Type II) showing marked defective haemoglobinization and vacuolation in later stage polychromatic and pyknotic erythroblasts.

Fig.9.55 Myelodysplastic syndrome: bone marrow cell trails in Type II showing erythroblasts with (left) vacuolation of cytoplasm in later cells, mild megaloblastic features and (right) a prominent group of proerythroblasts.

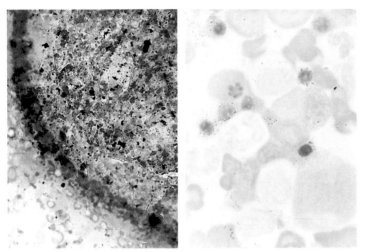

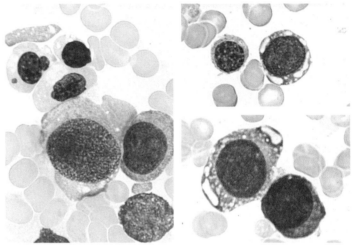

Fig.9.56 Myelodysplastic syndrome: bone marrow fragment in Type II showing (left) increased iron stores and (right) pathological ring sideroblasts at higher magnification. Perls' stains.

Fig.9.57 Myelodysplastic syndrome: bone marrow aspirates in Type III showing (left) abnormal proerythroblasts and megaloblast-like changes and (right) prominent cytoplasmic vacuolation in the basophilic erythroblasts, evidence of dyserythropoiesis.

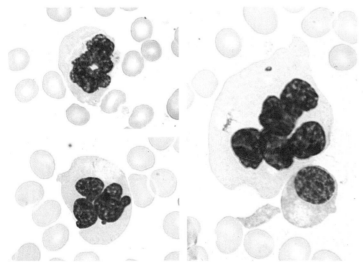

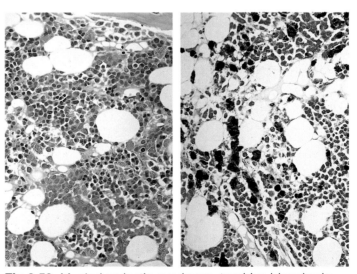

Fig.9.58 Myelodysplastic syndrome: bone marrow aspirates in Type III showing three examples of polyploid multinucleated polychromatic erythroblasts, further evidence of gross dyserythropoiesis.

Fig.9.59 Myelodysplastic syndrome: trephine biopsies in Type III showing (left) clusters of blast forms and prominent haemosiderin-laden macrophages; (right) the gross increase in reticuloendothelial iron stores confirmed by Perls' staining.

Granulocytic abnormalities include hypogranular or agranular myelocytes, metamyelocytes and neutrophils, pseudo–Pelger cells and hypersegmented or polyploid neutrophils (Fig.9.60). Megakaryocyte abnormalities include small mononuclear or binuclear forms (Fig.9.61) or large megakaryocytes with multiple round nuclei and large granules in the cytoplasm.

In the more advanced myelodysplastic syndromes, there is also an increase in the blast cell population but, by definition, these cells remain less than thirty percent of the marrow cell total (Fig.9.62). When the level of blast cells exceeds this figure, it is assumed that an evolution to acute myeloblastic leukaemia has occurred.

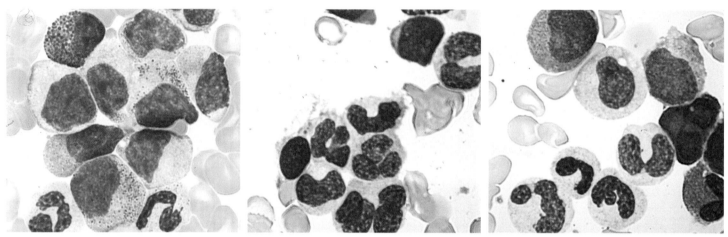

Fig.9.60 Myelodysplastic syndrome: bone marrow aspirates in Type III showing disturbed granulopoiesis with (left) agranular promyelocytes and (middle & right) agranular neutrophils and abnormal myelomonocytic cells; some cells ('paramyeloid' cells) are difficult to classify as monocytic or granulocytic.

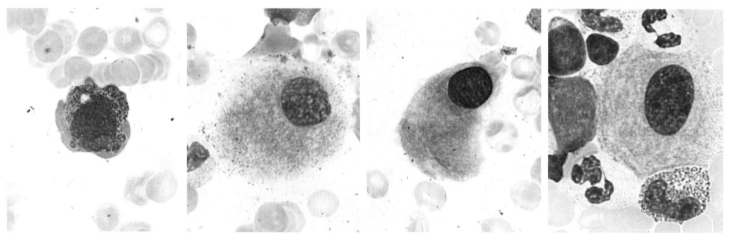

Fig.9.61 Myelodysplastic syndrome: bone marrow aspirates showing an atypical megakaryoblast and three atypical mononuclear megakaryocytes, all of which show evidence of cytoplasmic maturation and granulation.

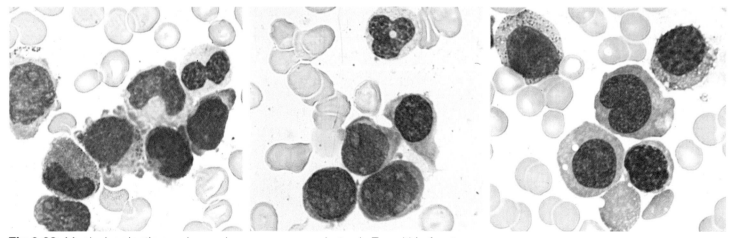

Fig.9.62 Myelodysplastic syndrome: bone marrow aspirates in Type V (refractory anaemia with excess blasts in transformation) showing increased numbers of blast cells, some of which have atypical features. The blast cells comprised 23% of the marrow cell total. Agranular neutrophils and myelomonocytic cells are also evident.

MALIGNANT LYMPHOMAS

The term 'malignant lymphoma' embraces a variable group of proliferative diseases that originate in the lymph nodes or extranodal lymphatic tissues, the most well-defined being Hodgkin's disease. The remainder, known collectively as the non-Hodgkin's lymphomas, vary from highly proliferative and rapidly fatal disorders to malignancies which are very well tolerated for ten to twenty years or more.

In all of these diseases, there is replacement of normal lymphoid structure by abnormal cells. The presence of Reed-Sternberg cells is diagnostic in Hodgkin's disease; in the others, there are diffuse or follicular (nodular) collections of cells which closely resemble normal B- or T-lymphoid cells at different stages of development. Rarely, these tumours may be composed of cells derived from histiocytes of the monocyte/phagocyte system. The clonal nature of the non-Hodgkin's lymphomas of B- or T-cell origin can be shown by using: cytogenetic markers; intracytoplasmic or surface immunoglobulin of single light-chain type; recombinant DNA techniques to detect immunoglobulin or T-cell receptor gene rearrangements, supported by a variety of mono- or polyclonal antibodies to cellular surface antigens.

HODGKIN'S DISEASE
This is the most common malignant tumour of lymphoid tissue and is closely related to the other malignant lymphomas. The aetiology is unknown. In many patients the disease at presentation is localized to a single peripheral lymph node region and studies of its natural history indicate that its subsequent progression is initially by direct contiguity within the lymphatic system.

With advanced disease there is dissemination to involve non-lymphatic tissue. The disease may affect all age groups but is particularly common in young and middle-aged adults. Most patients present with a painless, asymmetrical, firm

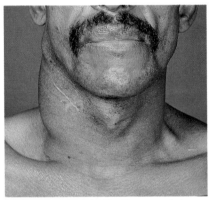

Fig. 10.1 Hodgkin's disease: right-sided cervical lymphadenopathy. The scar of a previous biopsy incision is well healed.

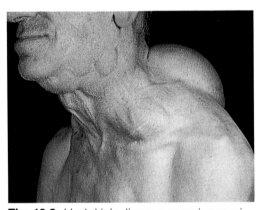

Fig. 10.2 Hodgkin's disease: massive cervical lymphadenopathy in a 73-year-old man who presented with extensive disease.

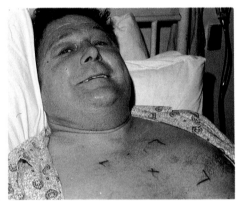

Fig. 10.3 Hodgkin's disease: cyanosis and oedema of the face, neck and upper trunk due to superior vena cava obstruction caused by mediastinal node involvement. The skin markings over the anterior chest indicate the field of radiotherapy.

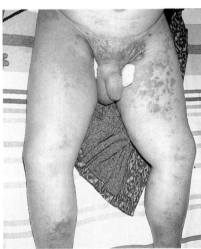

Fig. 10.4 Hodgkin's disease: gross oedema of the legs, genitals and lower abdominal wall with umbilical herniation due to lymphatic obstruction resulting from extensive involvement of the inguinal and pelvic lymph nodes. There is a staphylococcal infection in the skin folds of the groins. The CT scan of this case is shown in Fig. 10.26

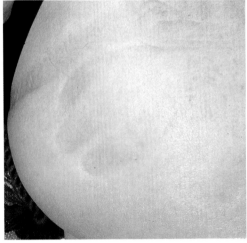
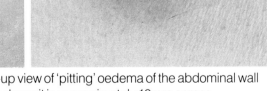

Fig. 10.5 Hodgkin's disease: (left) close-up view of 'pitting' oedema of the abdominal wall (same case as in Fig. 10.4); (right) this skin deposit is approximately 10mm across.

and discrete enlargement of the superficial lymph nodes (Figs. 10.1 & 10.2). Mediastinal disease, occasionally accompanied by an obstructed superior vena cava (Fig. 10.3), and involvement of retroperitoneal lymph nodes may be detected during staging procedures. Clinical splenomegaly occurs during the course of the disease in fifty percent of patients. Rarely, patients may present with lymphatic obstruction (Fig. 10.4).

The disease may involve the liver, skin (Fig. 10.5) and other organs, for example, the gastrointestinal tract or brain and, in rare patients, the retina (Fig. 10.6). There is also depressed cell-mediated immunity which is associated with an increased incidence of infections, particularly herpes zoster (Fig. 10.7), fungal diseases and tuberculosis.

The diagnosis is usually made from histological examination of excised lymph nodes. The affected nodes are enlarged and show pale translucent cut surfaces (Fig. 10.8). Initially the nodes remain discrete but, later in the disease, they become matted together and there may be invasion of surrounding tissues. Hodgkin's tissue in other organs has a similar pale, flesh-like, appearance (Fig. 10.9).

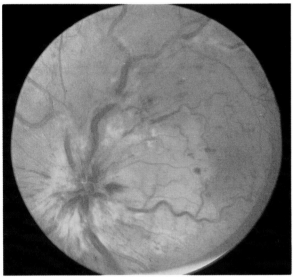

Fig. 10.6 Hodgkin's disease: extensive infiltration of the optic disc and surrounding retina.

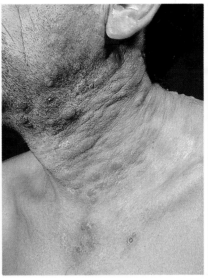
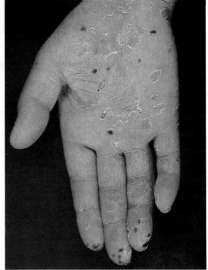

Fig. 10.7 Hodgkin's disease: (left) vesicular cutaneous eruption of the neck due to herpes zoster; (right) atypical herpetic eruption of the palmar surface of the hand.

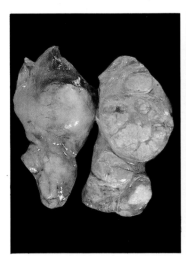
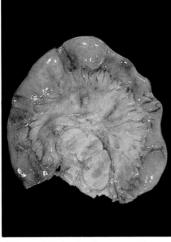

Fig. 10.8 Hodgkin's disease: (left) matted block of resected involved cervical nodes showing in cross-section the pale translucent, fleshy, tumour tissue with areas of fibrosis and necrosis; (right) para-aortic lymph nodes removed at necropsy showing in cross-section the typical moist 'fish-flesh' appearance of this tumour.

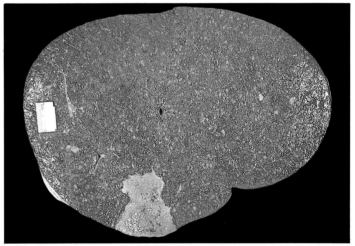

Fig. 10.9 Hodgkin's disease: cross-section of a spleen removed at laparotomy shows a single large Hodgkin's deposit adjacent to the capsule. There are also numerous focal greyish-yellow areas up to 4mm in diameter scattered throughout the tissue.

Microscopically the presence of polypoid Reed–Sternberg cells is characteristic (Fig. 10.10). Associated inflammatory cells include lymphocytes, histiocytes, neutrophils, eosinophils and plasma cells. There is a variable fibrous reaction.

The histological classification includes four subtypes (Fig. 10.11), each of which implies a different prognosis. Patients with lymphocyte-predominant disease have the most favourable prognosis, possibly because they have a

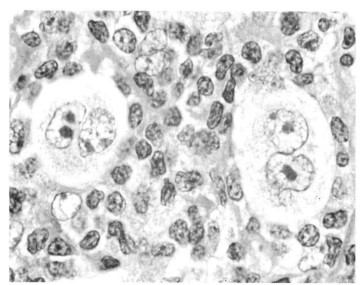

Fig. 10.10 Hodgkin's disease: high power view of lymph node biopsy showing two typical multinucleated Reed-Sternberg cells surrounded by lymphocytes.

Histological Classification of Hodgkin's Disease	
Type	**Features**
Lymphocyte-predominant	Lymphocyte proliferation dominates; Few Reed-Sternberg cells seen; Nodular & diffuse patterns
Nodular sclerosis	Tumour nodules surrounded by collagen bands extending from nodal capsule; Characteristic 'lacunar cell' variant of Reed-Sternberg cell often seen; Infiltrate may be lymphocyte-predominant, mixed cellular or lymphocyte-depleted type
Mixed cellularity	Numerous Reed-Sternberg cells seen; Intermediate numbers of lymphocytes
Lymphocyte-depleted	'Reticular' pattern with predominant Reed-Sternberg cells & sparse lymphocytes or 'diffuse fibrosis' with disordered connective tissue, few lymphocytes and infrequent Reed-Sternberg cells

Fig. 10.11 Hodgkin's disease: histological classification.

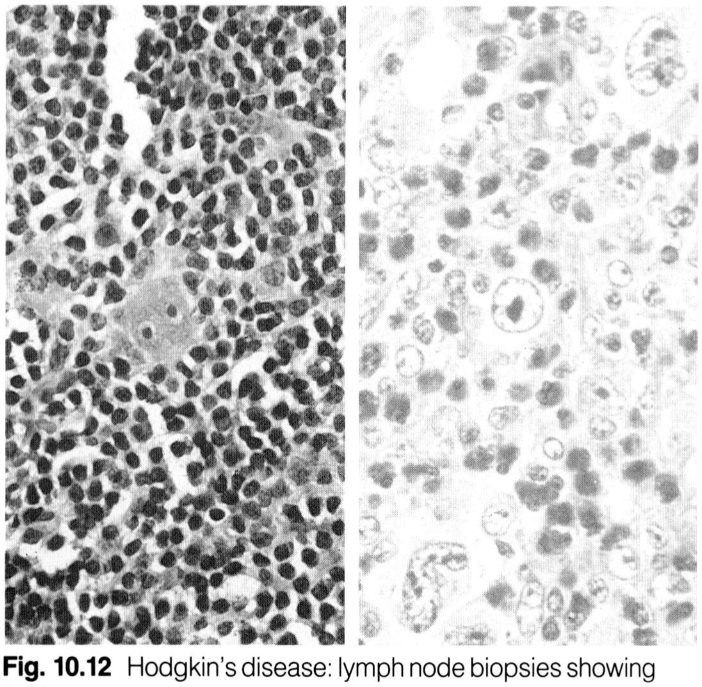

Fig. 10.12 Hodgkin's disease: lymph node biopsies showing (left) a single Reed-Sternberg cell surrounded by lymphocytes and other mononuclear cells in lymphocyte-predominant disease; (right) large numbers of Reed-Sternberg cells and atypical mononuclear cells, prominent eosinophils but only small numbers of lymphocytes. This appearance is typical of lymphocyte-depleted disease.

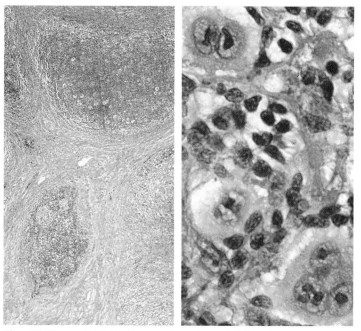

Fig. 10.13 Hodgkin's disease: lymph node biopsies showing (left) abundant bands of collagenous connective tissue separating areas of abnormal Hodgkin's tissue in the nodular sclerosis type of disease; (right) high power view of mixed cellular disease showing Reed-Sternberg cells surrounded by lymphocytes.

more effective cellular immune response than patients with lymphocyte-depleted disease, which has a relatively poor prognosis. The histopathology and cytology of Hodgkin's disease is illustrated in Figs. 10.12 to 10.15. A number of monoclonal antibodies have been described recently which react, although not specifically, with antigens on the Reed-Sternberg cell and may help in diagnosis (Fig. 10.16). The exact nature of this cell remains obscure.

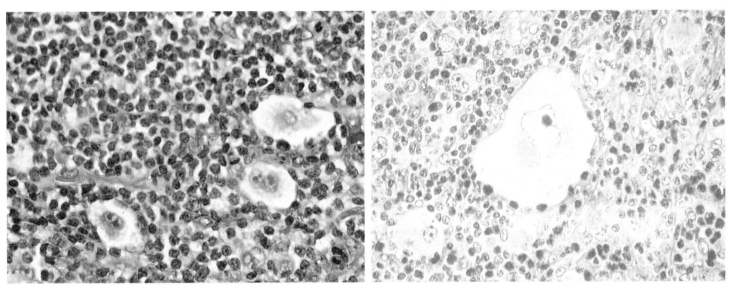

Fig. 10.14 Hodgkin's disease: high power views of 'lacunar' variants of Reed-Sternberg cells.

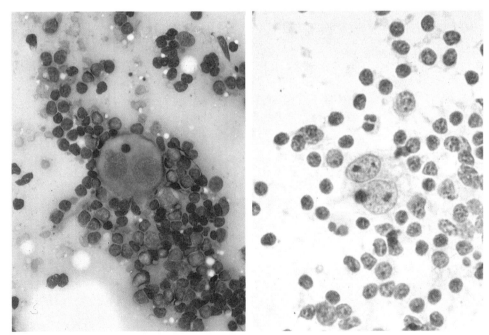

Fig. 10.15 Hodgkin's disease: fine needle aspirates of involved lymph nodes showing Reed-Sternberg cells stained by May-Grünwald/Giemsa (left) and Papanicolaou (right) techniques.

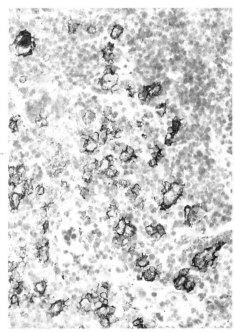

Fig. 10.16 Hodgkin's disease: lymph node biopsy showing a positive reaction of the monoclonal antibody Ki 1 with Reed-Sternberg cells. This antibody reacts particularly, but not exclusively, with Reed-Sternberg cells. Alkaline phosphatase-anti-alkaline phosphatase (AP-AAP) technique. Courtesy of Prof. H. Stein.

Staging techniques

The prognosis and selection of the best possible treatment depends on accurate staging of the disease (Fig. 10.17). After thorough clinical examination, a number of laboratory and radiological procedures are employed in the initial assessment. Many patients have a normochromic normocytic anaemia with a leucocytosis and/or eosinophilia, and bone marrow aspirates and trephine biopsies may provide diagnostic material (Figs. 10.18–10.20). Mediastinal, hilar node or lung involvement may be detected by chest radiography (Figs. 10.21 & 10.22), liver involvement by percutaneous biopsy, and para-aortic or pelvic lymph node involvement by abdominal radiography (Fig. 10.23) and lymphangiography (Figs. 10.24 & 10.25). Computerized tomographic (CT) scanning is now used extensively in the search for thoracic and abdominal lymph node and organ involvement (Fig. 10.26).

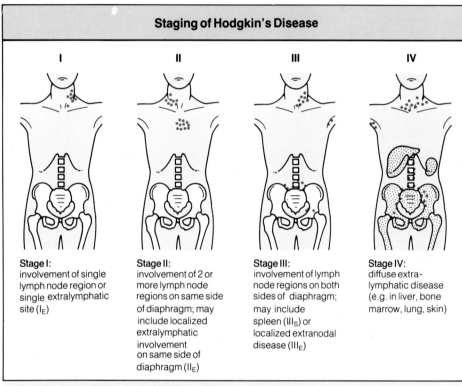

Staging of Hodgkin's Disease

I	II	III	IV

Stage I: involvement of single lymph node region or single extralymphatic site (I_E)

Stage II: involvement of 2 or more lymph node regions on same side of diaphragm; may include localized extralymphatic involvement on same side of diaphragm (II_E)

Stage III: involvement of lymph node regions on both sides of diaphragm; may include spleen (III_S) or localized extranodal disease (III_E)

Stage IV: diffuse extralymphatic disease (e.g. in liver, bone marrow, lung, skin)

NB: if unexplained weight loss of >10% body weight in preceding 6 months and/or fevers of >38°C and night sweats, classified as 'B'; if absent, 'A'.

Fig. 10.17 Hodgkin's disease: clinical staging. Stage I: node involvement in one area; Stage II: two or more areas confined to one side of diaphragm; Stage III*: areas above and below diaphragm; Stage IV: extranodal areas including bone marrow and liver. The stage number is followed by either 'A' (absence) or 'B' (presence) referring to: unexplained fever above 38°C; night sweats; loss of more than 10% of body weight within 6 months. A subscript 'E' indicates localized extranodal extension from a nodal mass, for example, I_E describes mediastinal disease with contiguous spread to the lung or spinal theca. Modified from A.V. Hoffbrand and J.E. Pettit, *Essential Haematology, second edition,* Oxford: Blackwell Scientific Publications.

*Splenic involvement is included in this classification because it is often a prelude to widespread haematogenous spread.

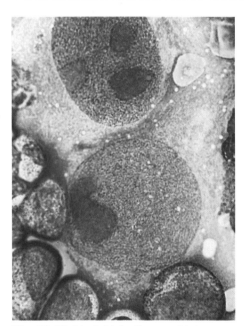

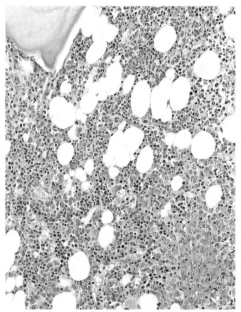

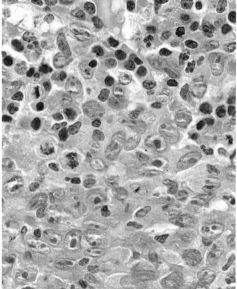

Fig. 10.18 Hodgkin's disease: high power view of bone marrow aspirate showing a Reed-Sternberg call.

Fig. 10.19 Hodgkin's disease: trephine biopsy showing (left) Hodgkin's tissue replacing normal haemopoietic elements in the lower right field; (right) higher power view shows extensive replacement of haemopoietic tissue by lymphocyte-depleted Hodgkin's tissue comprising Reed-Sternberg cells and other atypical mononuclear cells in the centre and lower fields.

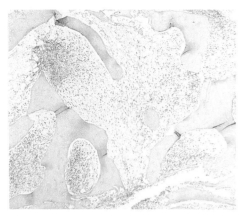

Fig. 10.20 Hodgkin's disease: trephine biopsy in the fibrotic variant of lymphocyte-depleted disease showing almost complete replacement of haemopoietic tissue by Hodgkin's deposits accompanied by abundant fibrous tissue in the intertrabecular space.

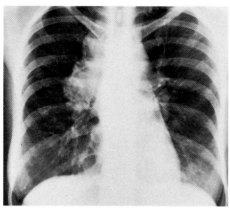

Fig. 10.21 Hodgkin's disease: chest radiograph showing prominent right paratracheal and hilar lymph node enlargement. There is less marked enlargement of the anterior mediastinal, subcarinal and left hilar nodes, and significant narrowing of the proximal regions of both major bronchi. Contrast material in the apical lymph node on the left is from a previous lymphangiogram.

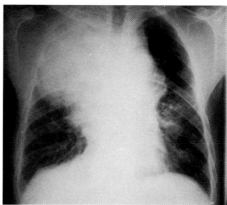

Fig. 10.22 Hodgkin's disease: chest radiograph showing widespread enlargement of hilar and mediastinal lymph nodes with associated collapse of the right upper lobe, and infiltration or possibly pneumonic changes in the mid-zone of the left lung.

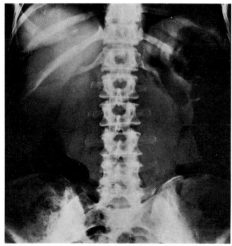

Fig. 10.23 Hodgkin's disease: plain abdominal radiograph showing bilateral massive para-aortic lymph node enlargement. Courtesy of Dr. D. Nag.

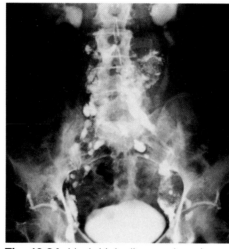

Fig. 10.24 Hodgkin's disease: lymphangiogram with IVP shows enlarged para-aortic lymph nodes (particularly on the left and lower left pelvis) with displacement of the ureter.

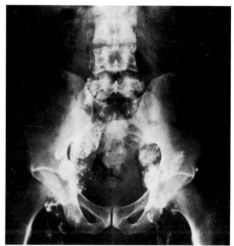

Fig. 10.25 Hodgkin's disease: lymphangiogram showing bilateral external iliac and lower para-aortic lymph node enlargement and filling defects.

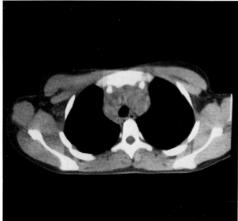
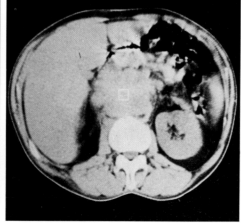
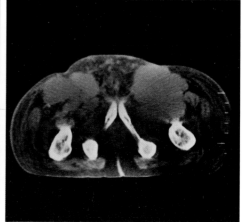

Fig. 10.26 Hodgkin's disease: computerized tomographic (CT) scans of (left) chest showing paratracheal and anterior mediastinal lymph node enlargement; (middle) abdomen showing massive para-aortic lymph node enlargement displacing the pancreas forwards; (right) pelvis showing massive bilateral inguinal and pelvic lymphadenopathy with marked oedema of the lower abdominal wall (see also Fig. 10.4).

As staging procedures are not always reliable, laparotomy may be performed, combined with abdominal node and liver biopsies, and splenectomy in cases considered to be stage I or II after clinical examination and the initial staging procedures. Involvement of the gastrointestinal tract may be revealed by barium studies (Fig. 10.27) and compression of the spinal cord by paravertebral deposits using myelography (Fig. 10.28).

NON-HODGKIN'S LYMPHOMAS
Although the clinical presentation of these lymphomas has many similarities with that of Hodgkin's disease, the natural history is more variable, the pattern of spread is not as regular and a greater proportion of patients present with disease in organs other than lymph nodes or with leukaemic manifestations.

Patients usually present with asymmetric painless enlargement of lymph nodes in one or more peripheral lymph node regions (Figs. 10.29 & 10.30). As well as retroperitoneal involvement, the mesenteric nodes are frequently affected,

and the liver and spleen are often enlarged (Fig. 10.31).

Of the extranodal sites, the bone marrow shows focal involvement in about twenty percent of patients. After the marrow, liver and spleen, the gastrointestinal tract is most frequently involved and patients may present with acute abdominal symptoms. The skin is not infrequently affected (Fig. 10.32), and is primarily involved in two unusual, closely related, T-lymphocytic lymphomas, mycosis fungoides and Sézary syndrome (see below).

The gross pathology of non-Hodgkin's lymphoma is similar to that of Hodgkin's disease (Figs. 10.33 & 10.34). The differential diagnosis is therefore made by histological examination of excised lymph nodes or extranodal tumours. In recent years, this has been one of the most difficult areas of diagnostic histopathology, but recognition that the majority of these tumours arise from follicular centre cells (FCC) and that the architecture is either follicular or diffuse was a major conceptual advance in understanding and classifying these diseases (Fig. 10.35).

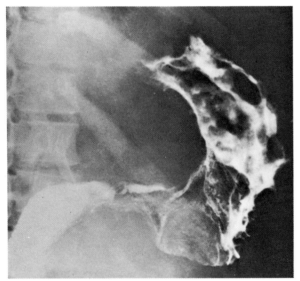

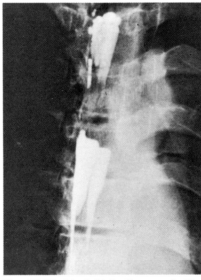

Fig. 10.27 Hodgkin's disease: barium meal demonstrating extensive mucosal and gastric wall involvement of the body and pylorus of the stomach. Courtesy of Dr. D. Nag.

Fig. 10.28 Hodgkin's disease: (left) cisternogram showing partial block of contrast at the level of T4 and a complete block at the lower part of T6; (right) sagittal section post-mortem shows extradural extension of tumour from the body of T4 (uppermost) and more extensive cordal involvement at T7 and T9. There is patchy involvement of other vertebral bodies and spinous processes. Extensive paravertebral tumour is seen anteriorly below the level of T5.

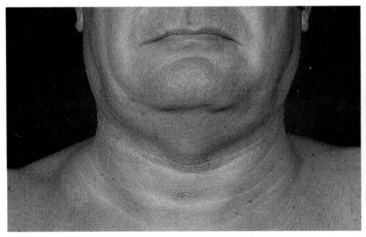

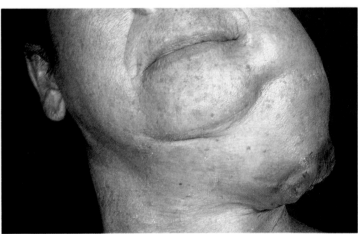

Fig. 10.29 Non-Hodgkin's lymphoma: (left) bilateral cervical lymphadenopathy in a patient with diffuse lymphocytic lymphoma; (right) massive enlargement of lymph nodes in the left submandibular area with extensive ulceration of the overlying skin in a patient with immunoblastic lymphoma.

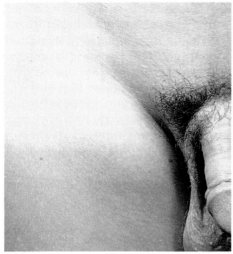

Fig. 10.30 Non-Hodgkin's lymphoma: inguinal lymphadenopathy in a 13-year-old patient with lymphoblastic lymphoma.

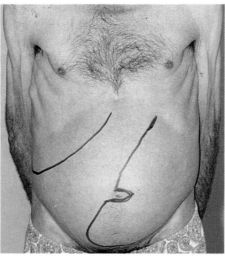

Fig. 10.31 Non-Hodgkin's lymphoma: massive enlargement of the spleen and hepatomegaly in diffuse lymphocytic lymphoma. *Hb:9.5g/dl; WBC:6.0×10⁹/l; lymphocytes:2.7×10⁹/l; platelets:80×10⁹/l.*

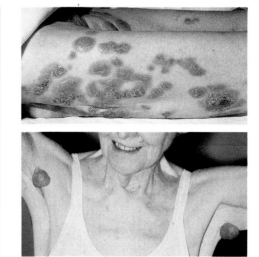

Fig. 10.32 Non-Hodgkin's lymphoma: (upper) extensive skin deposits in advanced centroblastic lymphoma; (lower) pedunculated skin deposits in centrocytic/centroblastic lymphoma.

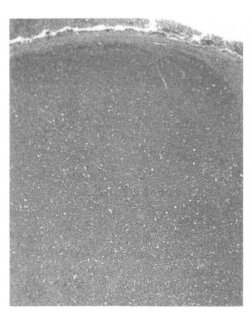

Fig. 10.33 Non-Hodgkin's lymphoma: enlarged lymph nodes of the porta hepatis seen post-mortem from a patient with immunoblastic lymphoma.

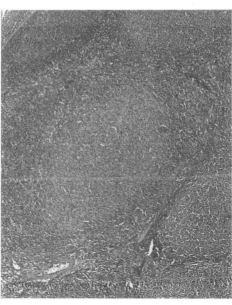

Fig. 10.34 Non-Hodgkin's lymphoma: section of spleen removed at laparotomy from a patient with immunoblastic lymphoma showing widespread replacement of splenic tissue by pale tumour with extensive areas of necrosis.

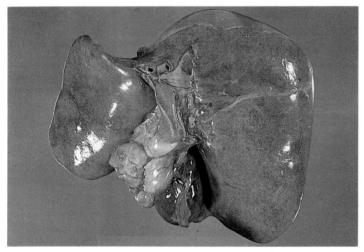
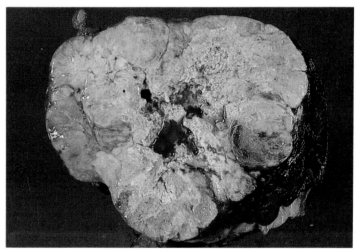

Fig. 10.35 Non-Hodgkin's lymphoma: histological sections of lymph nodes showing (left) diffuse pattern of involvement in lymphocytic lymphoma. The normal architecture has been totally replaced by a uniform population of neoplastic lymphocytes; (right) follicular pattern in centrocytic lymphoma. The 'follicles' or 'nodules' of neoplastic cells are surrounded by small, darkly staining, lymphocytes.

The four important classifications of non-Hodgkin's lymphomas in current use are the Kiel, Rappaport, Lukes-Collins and the National Cancer Institute (NCI) Working Formulation (Fig.10.36). These all depend on the cytological appearance of the tumour cell and whether the tumour is arranged in a follicular (nodular) or diffuse pattern. The Kiel and Lukes-Collins classifications also include the immunological phenotype of the lymphoma cells. The account given here is the Kiel classification.

The malignant lymphomas are named according to the normal counterpart of the predominant tumour cell type. It is assumed that the tumour consists of a clone of cells in which maturation is fixed at a particular stage of development with an inability to proceed beyond it (see Fig.8.1). Patients with centrocytic and centroblastic lymphomas (Fig.10.37) with a follicular pattern and those with relatively small lymphoid cells (lymphocytes and lymphoplasmacytoid cells; Fig.10.38) have a more favourable natural history and survival. The high-grade malignancy group of tumours with a poor prognosis are characterized by larger 'blast' forms.

Nearly all follicular and most diffuse lymphomas are derived from B lymphocytes. Less than one-tenth carry membrane features of T cells and a similar proportion have neither B- nor T-cell markers and are designated as 'null' cell

Classifications of Non-Hodgkin's Lymphomas

Kiel (Lennert)	Lukes-Collins	Rappaport (modified)	National Cancer Institute Working Formulation

Low-grade malignancy
  lymphocytic (including CLL,
    hairy cells & others)
  lymphoplasmacytoid
  centrocytic
  centrocytic/centroblastic
    follicular
    follicular & diffuse
    diffuse
  cutaneous T-cell group
  T-zone lymphoma
 	
High-grade malignancy
  centroblastic
  lymphoblastic [B, T
    (convoluted) or Burkitt types]
  immunoblastic (B or T)
 	
True histiocytic tumours
	Undefined
	
	B-cell
	  small lymphocytic
	  plasmacytoid (lymphocytic)
	  follicular centre cell (FCC)
	    types (nodular or diffuse):
	    small cleaved
	    large cleaved
	    large non-cleaved
	    immunoblastic sarcoma
	
	T-cell
	  small lymphocytic
	  convoluted lymphocytic
	  cerebriform (cutaneous)
	  lymphoepithelioid
	  immunoblastic sarcoma
	
	Histiocytic
		Nodular and/or diffuse
		  poorly differentiated lymphocytic
		  mixed
		  Burkitt's
		  undifferentiated non-Burkitt's
		  'histiocytic'
		
		Diffuse
		  well differentiated lymphocytic (WDL)
		  WDL with plasmacytoid differentiation
		  intermediate lymphocytic
		  immunoblastic
		  lymphoblastic
		  'Lennert' type
		  mycosis fungoides
		  plasmacytoma
		  unclassifiable
		  composite
		  malignant histiocytosis
			Low-grade malignancy
			  A. small lymphocytic with or without plasmacytoid
			    differentiation
			  B. follicular, small cleaved
			  C. follicular, mixed small cleaved & large cell
			
			Intermediate grade malignancy
			  D. follicular, large cell
			  E. diffuse, small cleaved
			  F. diffuse, mixed small & large cell
			  G. diffuse, large cell
			
			High-grade malignancy
			  H. large cell immunoblastic
			  I. lymphoblastic (convoluted or non-convoluted)
			  J. small non-cleaved cell (Burkitt & non-Burkitt
			    types)
			
			Miscellaneous
			  composite
			  histiocytic
			  mycosis fungoides
			  hairy cell
			  unclassifiable
			  others

Fig. 10.36 Non-Hodgkin's lymphoma: histological classification.

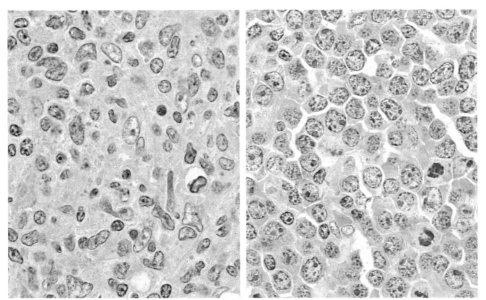

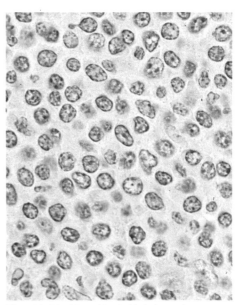

Fig. 10.37 Non-Hodgkin's lymphoma: (left) centrocytic lymphoma shows large cells with considerable nuclear pleomorphism and pale indistinct cytoplasm. The deformed nuclei have a light chromatin pattern and may contain nucleoli; (right) centroblastic lymphoma shows neoplastic cells which are much larger than lymphocytes and have a round nucleus with prominent nucleoli, many of which are adjacent to the nuclear membrane. A number of mitotic figures are seen.

Fig. 10.38 Non-Hodgkin's lymphoma: lymphocytic lymphoma shows predominating small lymphocytes with round nuclei containing densely clumped heterochromatin.

tumours. Gene rearrangement studies show that many of these are indeed of B-cell origin. True histiocytic lymphomas are rare (see below).

The lymphocytic lymphomas (Fig. 10.38) are closely related to chronic lymphocytic leukaemia; many regard the tumours with diffuse histology as a tissue phase of this disease. The characteristic small mature-appearing lymphocyte is, after the lymphoblast, probably the least differentiated lymphoid cell, the so-called 'virgin' B cell which has not been stimulated by antigen to react and divide. Many patients with this condition are elderly with a slowly progressive disease. Some lymphoplasmacytoid lymphomas may be associated with the production of monoclonal paraproteins. If there are significant amounts of IgM, the condition is known as Waldenström's macroglobulinaemia (see Chapter 11).

Patients with follicular tumours are more likely to be middle-aged than those with diffuse lymphomas, and their disease often follows a benign course for many years. However, sudden transformation may occur into aggressive blast cell and diffuse tumours which are sometimes associated with a leukaemic phase.

The blastic or high-grade malignancy group of lymphomas are associated with a fast rate of cellular proliferation. Histologically, in immunoblastic types (Fig. 10.39) there is widespread destruction of nodal architecture, often with extension through the capsule into surrounding perinodal tissues. Progressive infiltration may affect the gastrointestinal tract, the brain or spinal cord, the kidneys or other organs.

The lymphoblastic lymphomas (Fig. 10.40) occur mainly in children and young adults and merge clinically and morphologically with acute lymphoblastic leukaemia of the poor prognosis type. Young patients presenting with mediastinal masses may be diagnosed as T-cell lymphoblastic lymphoma or T-cell lymphoblastic leukaemia (T-ALL).

Immunological and cytological studies provide additional diagnostic information in patients with malignant lymphoma (Figs. 10.41–10.45). Attempts are made to stage the extent of the disease as in Hodgkin's disease.

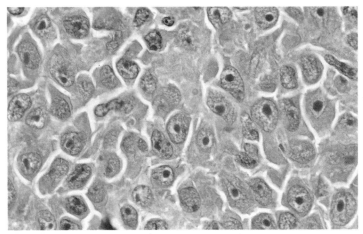

Fig. 10.39 Non-Hodgkin's lymphoma: immunoblastic lymphoma shows large neoplastic cells with a single prominent central nucleolus and abundant, darkly staining, cytoplasm.

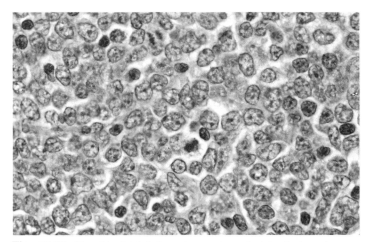

Fig. 10.40 Non-Hodgkin's lymphoma: lymphoblastic lymphoma. The lymphoblasts have round or oval nuclei with delicate, evenly dispersed, chromatin patterns and one to three nucleoli, and only a scanty rim of cytoplasm. The darker cells are small lymphocytes.

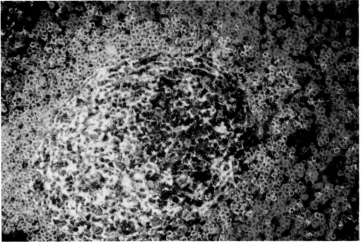 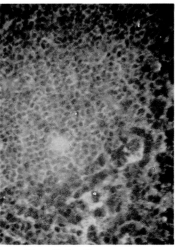 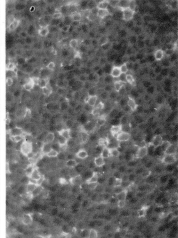

Fig. 10.41 Reactive lymph node: indirect immunofluorescence for T- and B-cell distribution shows that (left) T cells (red rhodamine labelling) occupy the paracortical area surrounding the mainly B-lymphocyte corona expressing IgM (green fluorescein labelling). A number of T cells are scattered within the germinal centre where immune complexes are also stained strongly by the IgM antisera; (middle) T cells within the paracortical area are a mixture of CD4 (T4;helper phenotype)-positive (red) and CD8 (T8;suppressor/cytotoxic phenotype)-positive (green) cells; (right) at the edge of a germinal centre is a mixture of B lymphocytes expressing ϰ (red) or λ (green) light chains. Courtesy of Dr. M. Chilosi, Prof. G. Janossy and Dr. G. Pizzolo.

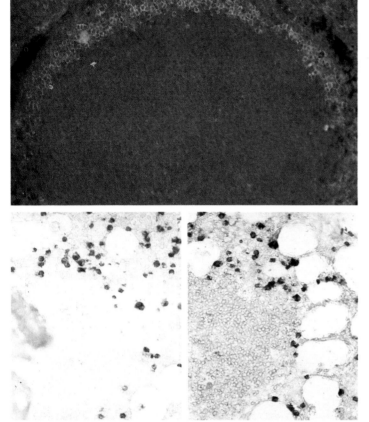

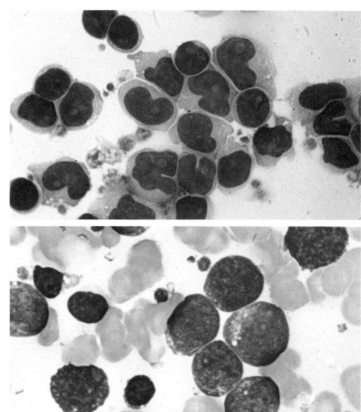

Fig. 10.42 Non-Hodgkin's lymphoma: (upper) lymph node seen by indirect immunofluorescence to demonstrate monoclonality of malignant cells in follicular or non-follicular lymphomas shows ϰ light chain exclusively (red) and no reaction for λ chain (green). Around the edge of the follicle, the residual normal lymphocyte corona is a mixture of B cells with ϰ and λ light chains. Trephine biopsy stained by immunoperoxidase shows (lower left) brown ring staining for ϰ in the malignant lymphoid nodule and (lower right) no labelling for λ, confirming the monoclonal origin of the lymphoma. The strong brown staining around the edges of some of the cells is unblocked endogenous peroxidase within eosinophils. Courtesy of Prof. G. Janossy and Dr. G. Pizzolo.

Fig. 10.43 Non-Hodgkin's lymphoma: fine needle aspirates showing (upper) centrocytic and (lower) centroblastic lymphoma. May-Grünwald/Giemsa stain.

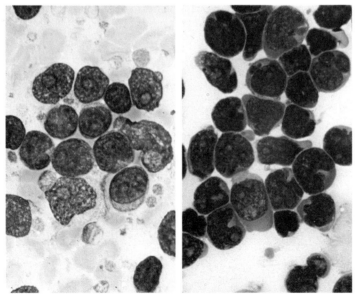

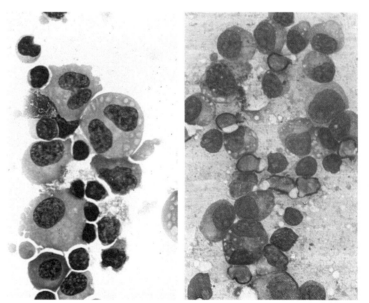

Fig. 10.44 Non-Hodgkin's lymphoma: fine needle aspirates showing (left) immunoblastic and (right) lymphoblastic lymphoma. May-Grünwald/Giemsa stain.

Fig. 10.45 Non-Hodgkin's lymphoma: fine needle aspirates showing (left) plasmacytic lymphoma and (right) immunoblastic lymphoma with plasmacytic differentiation. May-Grünwald/Giemsa stain.

Bone marrow involvement is assessed using aspirates and trephine biopsies (Figs. 10.46–10.48) and, in some cases, lymphoma cells are found in peripheral blood (Fig. 10.49). Chest radiography may detect thoracic involvement (Figs. 10.50–10.52); liver biopsy, lymphangiography and computerized tomography (Fig. 10.53) are employed in the search for occult abdominal disease. There is less support for exploratory laparotomy and splenectomy in non-Hodgkin's lymphoma than in Hodgkin's disease, but these procedures are sometimes required to make the initial diagnosis in patients with primary disease in the abdomen.

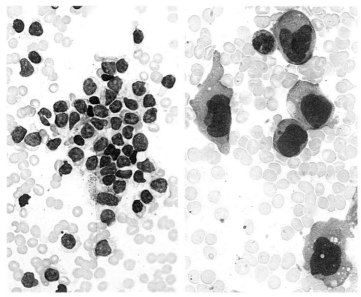

Fig. 10.46 Non-Hodgkin's lymphoma: bone marrow aspirates showing (left) a dominance of neoplastic lymphocytes in the cell trail in lymphocytic lymphoma; (right) higher power view of large neoplastic immunoblasts in immunoblastic lymphoma. The smaller cell is a monocyte.

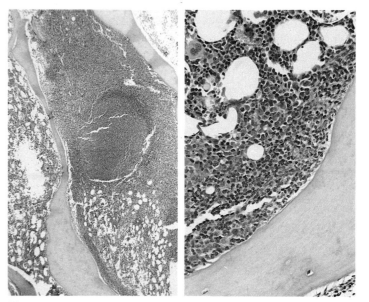

Fig. 10.47 Non-Hodgkin's lymphoma: trephine biopsy in centrocytic/centroblastic lymphoma showing (left) almost complete replacement of normal haemopoietic tissue in the upper field and a paratrabecular collection of neoplastic lymphoid cells below; (right) higher power shows the demarcation between the paratrabecular centrocytes and centroblasts and the normal haemopoietic cells and fat.

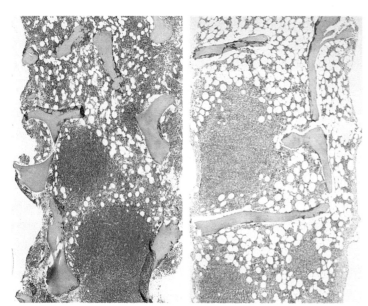

Fig. 10.48 Non-Hodgkin's lymphoma: trephine biopsies from two different patients showing extensive focal deposits of lymphoma cells.

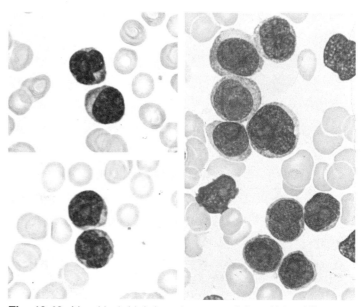

Fig. 10.49 Non-Hodgkin's lymphoma: peripheral blood films showing (left) nucleolated lymphoid cells, two of which show prominent nuclear clefts, in a patient with follicular lymphoma; (right) abnormal large 'blast' forms or 'lymphosarcoma' cells in a patient with widely disseminated and terminal centroblastic lymphoma.

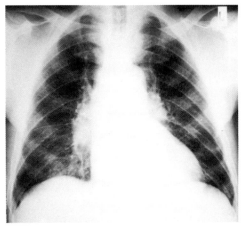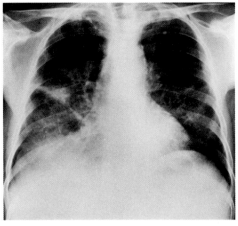

Fig. 10.50 Non-Hodgkin's lymphocytic lymphoma: chest radiographs showing (left) bilateral hilar lymph node enlargement and (right) interstitial and confluent shadowing, particularly in the lower and mid-zones, which biopsy showed to be due to lymphomatous infiltration.

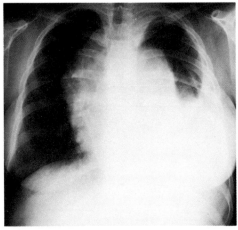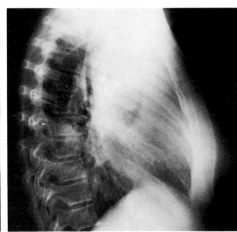

Fig. 10.51 Non-Hodgkin's T-lymphoblastic lymphoma: chest radiographs showing (left) gross enlargement of the mediastinal lymph nodes and a pleural effusion on the left; (right) the lateral view confirms anterior mediastinal disease with posterior displacement of the trachea.

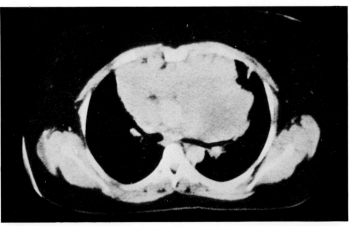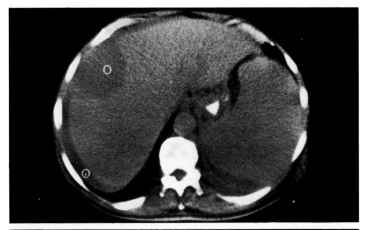

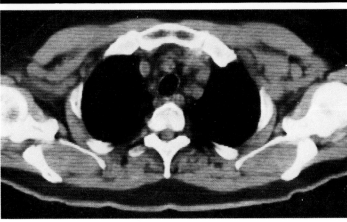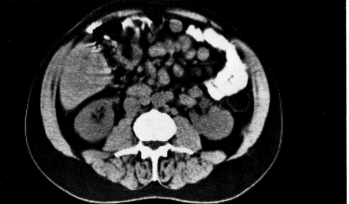

Fig. 10.52 Non-Hodgkin's lymphoma: computerized tomographic scans through the mid-thorax show (upper) gross enlargement of anterior mediastinal, paratracheal and hilar nodes in T-lymphoblastic lymphoma; (lower) anterior mediastinal and paratracheal lymph node enlargement in centrocytic/centroblastic lymphoma.

Fig. 10.53 Non-Hodgkin's lymphoma: computerized tomographic scans through the abdomen show (upper) hepatic and splenic enlargement and a prominent radiolucent focus in the right lobe of the liver. Ascitic fluid is present and there is contrast medium in the gut; (lower) mesenteric and some para-aortic lymph node enlargement.

Ten to fifteen percent of patients with non-Hodgkin's lymphoma present with extranodal disease involving the gastrointestinal tract (Fig. 10.54), thyroid (Fig. 10.55), the lungs (Fig. 10.56) or other organs, such as the skin (Fig. 10.57) or brain (Fig. 10.58).

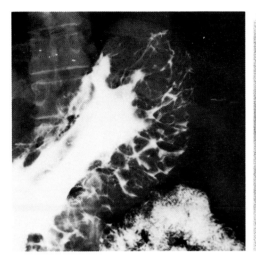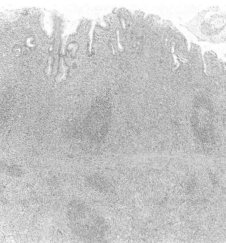

Fig. 10.54 Non-Hodgkin's lymphoma: (left) barium study shows mucosal and mural involvement of the fundus and body of the stomach; (right) histological section of a primary centrocytic/centroblastic lymphoma of the stomach showing invasion of the gastric glands, lamina propria and deeper areas by sheets of tumour cells. Courtesy of Dr. D. Nag (left).

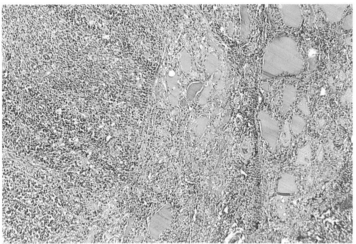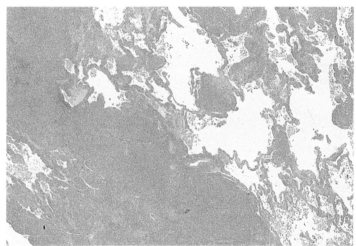

Fig. 10.55 Non-Hodgkin's lymphoma: histological section of thyroid with primary centroblastic lymphoma shows sheets of neoplastic centroblasts (on the left) and remaining colloid-filled acini (on the right). Immunoperoxidase staining for light chains confirmed the monoclonality of the tumour cells.

Fig. 10.56 Non-Hodgkin's lymphoma: lower power view of histological section of lung with primary lymphocytic lymphoma shows sheets of neoplastic lymphocytes at the edge of the tumour infiltrating the surrounding lung along bronchovascular bundles and alveolar septae.

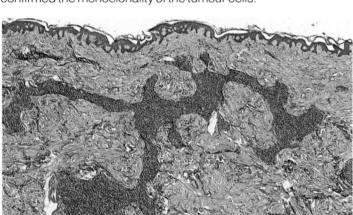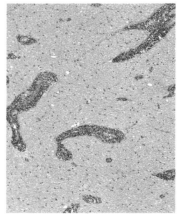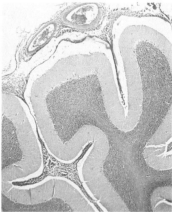

Fig. 10.57 Non-Hodgkin's lymphoma: histological section of skin with centrocytic/centroblastic lymphoma shows sheets of tumour cells in the reticular dermis. Immunoperoxidase staining of the tumour demonstrated monoclonal B-cell characteristics.

Fig. 10.58 Non-Hodgkin's lymphoma: sections of brain in CNS relapse in lymphoblastic lymphoma showing (left) nodular invasion along perivascular spaces and (right) extensive involvement of the meninges. A similar pattern of involvement occurs in primary lymphoma of the brain. In the past, these primary tumours have been categorized as microgliomas. Courtesy of Dr. B.B. Berkeley.

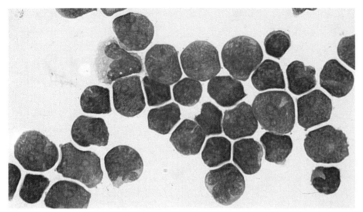

Fig. 10.59 Non-Hodgkin's lymphoma: high power view of cytospin preparation of cerebrospinal fluid in CNS relapse in lymphoblastic lymphoma showing typical lymphoblasts.

In patients with disease of the central nervous system, examination of the cerebrospinal fluid usually shows lymphoma cells (Fig. 10.59). Extradural deposits may produce compression of the spinal cord (Fig. 10.60).

Burkitt's (African) lymphoma

This unusual B-lymphoblastic lymphoma is found in young African children. The Epstein–Barr virus has been identified in Burkitt-cell cultures and the tumour may result from an inability of the immune response to deal effectively with this virus. There is an unusual predilection for massive jaw lesions (Fig. 10.61), extranodal abdominal involvement and, in females, ovarian tumours (Fig. 10.62). Sections of involved tissue show the characteristic 'starry sky' appearance of B-lymphoblastic lymphomas with histiocytic reticular cells scattered among the neoplastic lymphoblasts (Fig. 10.63). A characteristic cytogenetic abnormality of the tumour cells is

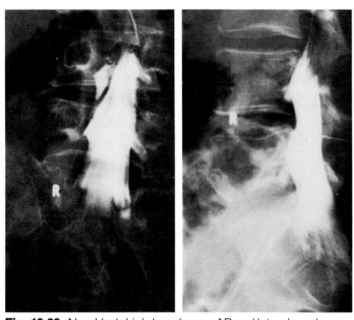

Fig. 10.60 Non-Hodgkin's lymphoma: AP and lateral myelograms demonstrating an extradural deposit in the anterior lumbar canal commencing at L4. Courtesy of Dr. D. Nag.

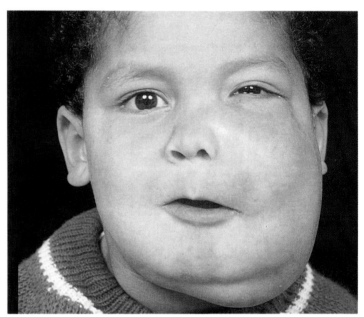

Fig. 10.61 Burkitt's lymphoma: characteristic facial swelling due to extensive tumour involvement of the mandible and surrounding soft tissues. Courtesy of Dr. J.M. Chessells.

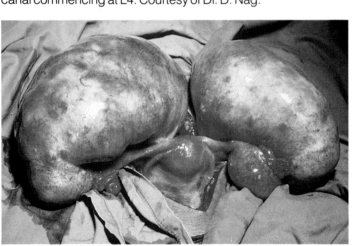

Fig. 10.62 Burkitt's lymphoma: gross bilateral involvement of the ovaries.

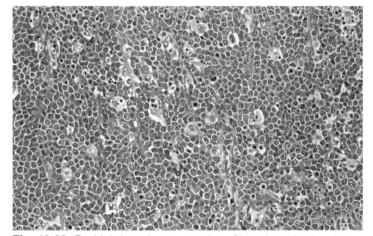

Fig. 10.63 Burkitt's lymphoma: section of lymph node showing sheets of lymphoblasts with prominent nuclear membranes and 'starry sky' tingible-body macrophages.

found in many patients (Fig. 10.64). A non-endemic form of the disease occurs elsewhere in older subjects and involves lymphoid tissue especially of the ileocaecal or cervical regions.

Mycosis fungoides and Sézary syndrome

Mycosis fungoides, a chronic lymphoma of the skin, usually evolves through three stages: a premycotic stage with lesions similar to eczema or psoriasis (Fig. 10.65); an infiltrative or plaque stage (Fig. 10.66), sometimes with generalized exfoliative erythroderma (Figs. 10.67 & 10.68) and invasion of the blood by typical convoluted neoplastic lymphoid cells (Fig. 10.69; the so-called Sézary syndrome); and a nodular or tumour stage associated with deeper invasion by the tumour (Fig. 10.70) and infiltration of lymph nodes and other organs. The Sézary cells in the blood and in the cells of the skin lesion have surface markers of T cells usually of CD4 subtype.

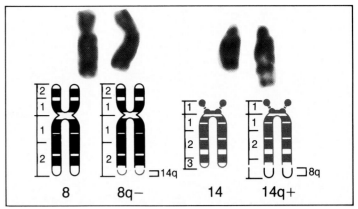

Fig. 10.64 Burkitt's lymphoma: (upper) partial karyotypes of G-banded chromosomes 8 and 14 from a child. The translocated chromosomes are on the right in each pair. The cellular oncogene c-myc moves with the translocated portion of chromosome 8; (lower) diagrammatic systematized description of the structural aberration. Other cases show translocations t(8;22) or t(2;8). Courtesy of Dr. L.M. Secker-Walker.

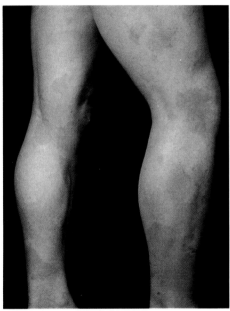

Fig. 10.65 Mycosis fungoides: typical eczematoid lesions at presentation.

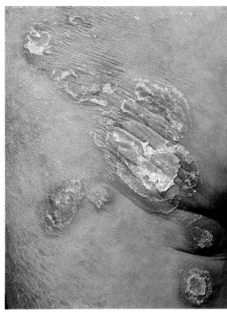

Fig. 10.66 Mycosis fungoides: these psoriasiform plaques appeared six months later (same patient as in Fig. 10.65).

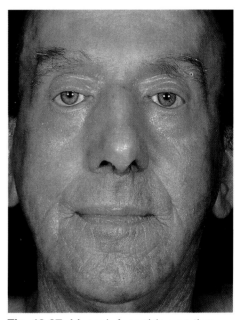

Fig. 10.67 Mycosis fungoides: erythroderma in advanced disease.

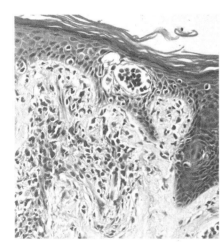

Fig. 10.68 Mycosis fungoides: typical histology shows a focal intraepidermal collection of abnormal lymphoid cells (Pautrier's abscess) and similar groups of tumour cells in the papillary dermis.

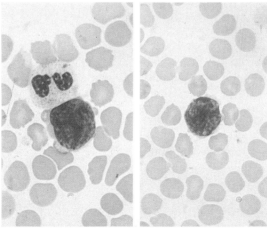

Fig. 10.69 Mycosis fungoides: the characteristic atypical large lymphoid cells have cerebriform nuclei with fine chromatin patterns and scanty cytoplasm.

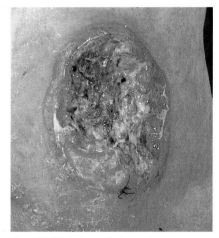

Fig. 10.70 Mycosis fungoides: extensive ulceration of the abdominal skin indicative of the invasive tumour stage.

Adult T-cell lymphoma-leukaemia (ATLL)

This unusual lymphoproliferative malignancy occurs predominantly in Japan and in blacks of the West Indies and Caribbean countries, and USA. Typically the lymphoma evolves rapidly with early involvement of the lymph nodes, skin (Fig. 10.71), blood and bone marrow. The cells are $CD4^+$, $CD3^+$, TdT^-.

The neoplastic lymphoid cells vary in size and have an irregular nucleus, often with marked convolutions (Figs. 10.72 & 10.73). Associated hypercalcaemia may lead to death in coma. The disease is caused by a C-type RNA retrovirus now designated as human T-cell lymphoma-leukaemia virus I (HTLV I).

T-zone lymphoma

In this rare aggressive disease, the T-dependent paracortical areas of lymph nodes are expanded by pleomorphic T lymphocytes with irregular and/or convoluted nuclei. Plasma and eosinophilic cells and epithelioid venules may also be present (Fig. 10.74).

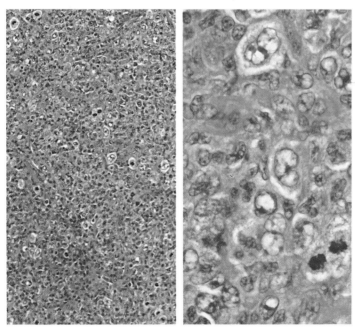

Fig. 10.71 Adult T-cell lymphoma-leukaemia syndrome: extensive involvement of the skin. Courtesy of Dr. J.W. Clark.

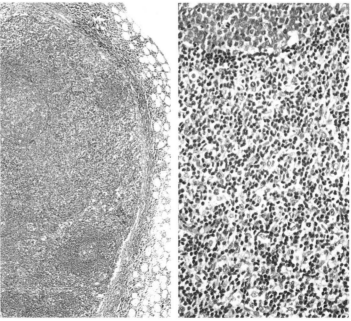

Fig. 10.72 Adult T-cell lymphoma-leukaemia syndrome: peripheral blood films showing the characteristic abnormal lymphocytes with convoluted nuclei. Courtesy of Dr. D. Catovsky.

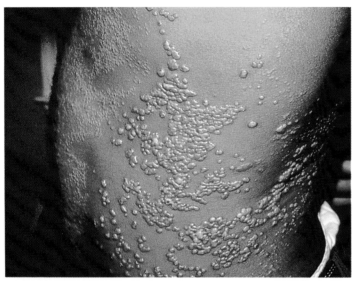

Fig. 10.73 Adult T-cell lymphoma-leukaemia syndrome: histological sections of lymph node showing (left) replacement of normal architecture by pleomorphic lymphoid cells; (right) occasional bizarre polylobulated giant cells and prominent mitotic figures at high magnification.

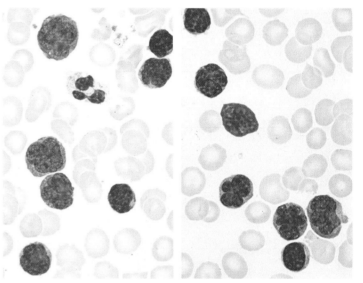

Fig. 10.74 T-zone lymphoma: (left) expansion of paracortical region with wide separation of germinal follicles; (right) high power shows many T-lymphocytes with clear cytoplasm, eosinophils and prominent venules. Courtesy of Dr. J.E. McLaughlin.

Lymphoepithelioid (Lennert's) lymphoma

This disease shows some similarities histologically to Hodgkin's disease. The lesion involves numerous epithelioid cell granulomata and a mixture of small and large T lymphocytes, the larger including multinucleated cells which may resemble Reed–Sternberg cells (Fig. 10.75).

Angioimmunoblastic lymphadenopathy

This premalignant lymphoproliferative disorder is characterized by the replacement of normal lymph node architecture by a mixed population of immunoblasts, lymphocytes, plasma cells, histiocytic cells and granulocytes, as well as a marked vascular proliferation (Fig. 10.76). Trephine biopsies may show bone marrow involvement (Fig. 10.77) and skin rashes are frequent (Fig. 10.78).

The condition is associated with polyclonal increases in serum immunoglobulin and an increased susceptibility to infection. The aetiology is unknown but an uncontrolled response to antigen would appear to be important in its pathogenesis. In many patients, an evolution to an immunoblastic lymphoma occurs. Gene rearrangement studies show a T-cell origin in most cases.

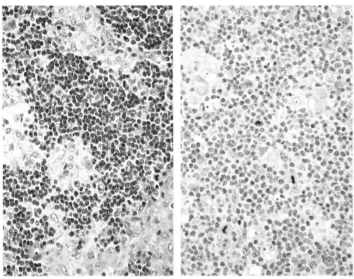

Fig. 10.75 Lymphoepithelioid (Lennert's) lymphoma: clumps of epithelioid cells interspersed with a mixed population of small and large (T) lymphocytes with occasional mitoses and large atypical cells resembling Reed–Sternberg cells. The small cells show irregular angular nuclei. The tumour T-cells are thought to produce lymphokines which cause epithelioid cell formation from histiocytes. Courtesy of Dr. J.E. McLaughlin.

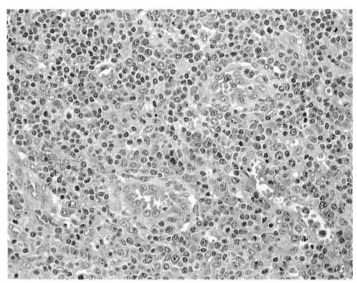

Fig. 10.76 Angioimmunoblastic lymphadenopathy: histological section of lymph node showing replacement of normal architecture by a pleomorphic infiltrate of immunoblasts, plasma cells and lymphocytes. Numerous small blood vessels lined with plump endothelial cells are seen.

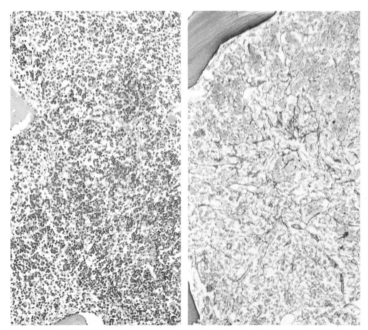

Fig. 10.77 Angioimmunoblastic lymphadenopathy: bone marrow trephine biopsy (same case as in Fig. 10.76) shows (left) extensive replacement of haemopoietic cells by abnormal lymphoid tissue; (right) silver impregnation staining outlines the characteristic arborizing vascular pattern of the condition.

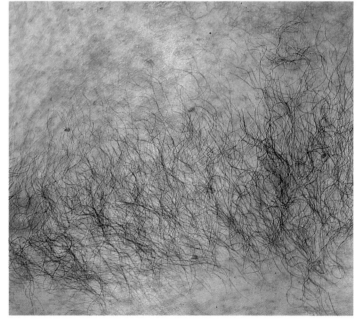

Fig. 10.78 Angioimmunoblastic lymphadenopathy: skin appearances of a 65-year-old man who presented with fever, an erythematous rash and lymphadenopathy, and subsequently died of an overt lymphoma.

TRUE HISTIOCYTIC LYMPHOMAS AND OTHER HISTIOCYTIC PROLIFERATIONS

In the Rappaport classification, histiocytic lymphoma is a major class and includes lymphomas of large cells with moderate or abundant cytoplasm and oval or round nuclei. Phenotypic studies have shown that the majority of these tumours are B cell in type (principally immunoblastic or centroblastic tumours) while some are T-cell immunoblastic tumours.

True histiocytic (monocyte/phagocyte system) cell tumours of lymph nodes (Figs. 10.79-10.81) are rare. Other tumours derived from true histiocytes are also uncommon. These include monocytic leukaemia (M_5 variant of acute myeloblastic leukaemia) with secondary involvement of the liver, spleen and lymph nodes (see Chapter 8), disseminated malignant histiocytosis (including histiocytic medullary reticulosis and childhood Letterer-Siwe disease) and histiocytosis confined to bone. Other unusual histiocytic proliferations are even more rare, such as virus-associated haemophagocytic syndrome, familial haemophagocytic reticulosis and sinus histiocytosis with massive lymphadenopathy.

The disseminated malignant histiocytosis of early childhood (Letterer-Siwe disease) usually affects children within the first three years of life. There is usually hepatosplenomegaly, lymphadenopathy and eczematoid skin eruptions (Fig. 10.82). Localized lesions occur frequently in the skull (Figs. 10.83 & 10.84), ribs and long bones, and the bone marrow is sometimes involved (Fig. 10.85).

Variants of malignant histiocytosis have been described as 'histiocytosis X' and include Hand-Schüller-Christian disease and eosinophilic granuloma of bone (Fig. 10.86). Patients with histiocytosis confined to bone have a more favourable prognosis than patients with disseminated malignant histiocytosis.

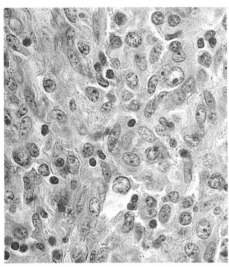

Fig. 10.79 Histiocytic lymphoma: histological section of lymph node showing replacement of normal architecture by sheets of abnormal histiocytic cells with abundant cytoplasm.

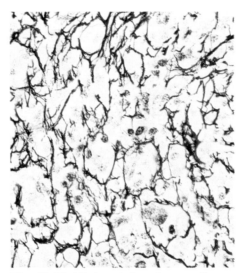

Fig. 10.80 Histiocytic lymphoma: silver impregnation staining of the same case as in Fig. 10.79 shows a prominent dense reticulin fibre network surrounding individual tumour cells.

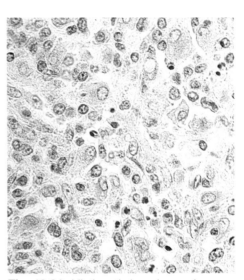

Fig. 10.81 Histiocytic lymphoma: immunoperoxidase staining for lysozyme (muramidase) of the same case as in Fig. 10.79 shows a high proportion of positive cells, indicating their monocytic origin. The cells were also positive for α-1-antitrypsin.

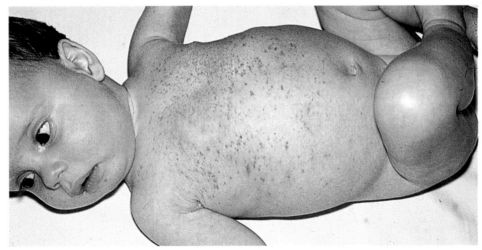

Fig. 10.82 Disseminated malignant histiocytosis: typical haemorrhagic eczematoid rash in a 10-month-old child with Letterer-Siwe disease. Courtesy of Dr. M.D. Holdaway.

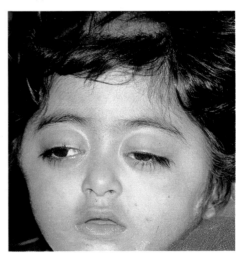

Fig. 10.83 Disseminated malignant histiocytosis: prominent bossing of the frontal bone and proptosis in a child with multiple skull deposits (Hand-Schüller-Christian disease). Courtesy of Dr. U. O'Callaghan.

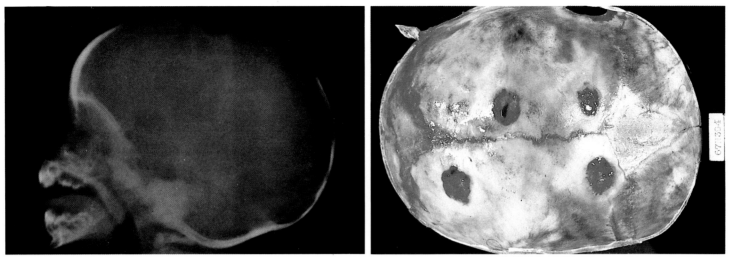

Fig. 10.84 Disseminated malignant histiocytosis: skull of an infant with Letterer-Siwe disease seen (left) radiographically and (right) at necropsy showing the typical osteolytic deposits in the vault.

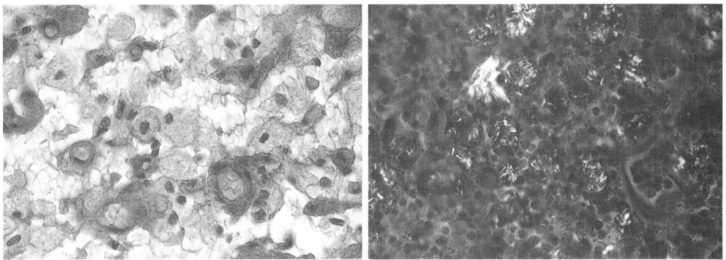

Fig. 10.85 Disseminated malignant histiocytosis: frozen sections of a skeletal lesion stained using the Sudan IV technique and viewed under (left) normal and (right) polarized light. The staining reaction indicates accumulation of neutral fat and cholesterol in the cytoplasm.

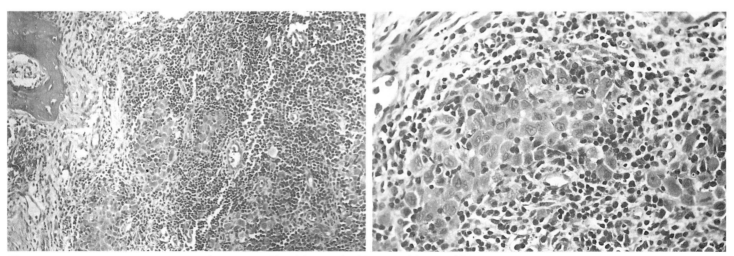

Fig. 10.86 Eosinophilic granuloma of bone: trephine biopsy of a 28-year-old man with skeletal lesions shows (left) replacement of normal haemopoietic tissue by sheets of histiocytes and eosinophils; (right) higher power view of the abnormal histiocytes and eosinophils.

10.21

Disseminated malignant histiocytosis in adults is associated with extensive marrow, liver and splenic involvement by the malignant histiocytes (Figs. 10.87–10.90). In the variant known as histiocytic medullary reticulosis, the cells phagocytose red cells, actively causing a haemolytic anaemia with prominent jaundice (Figs. 10.91 & 10.92).

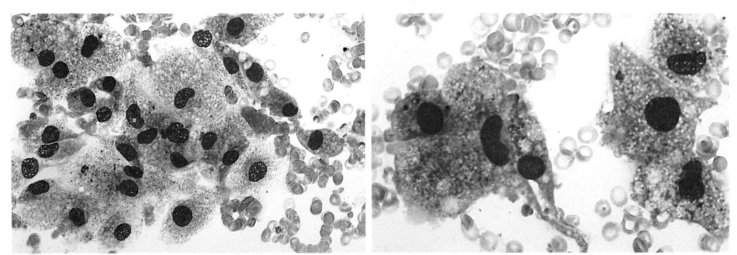

Fig. 10.87 Malignant histiocytosis: bone marrow aspirate showing (left) abnormal histiocytes in a 64-year-old patient who presented with pancytopenia, hepatomegaly and splenomegaly; (right) higher power view showing the considerable nuclear pleomorphism and abundant vacuolated cytoplasm of the malignant cells.

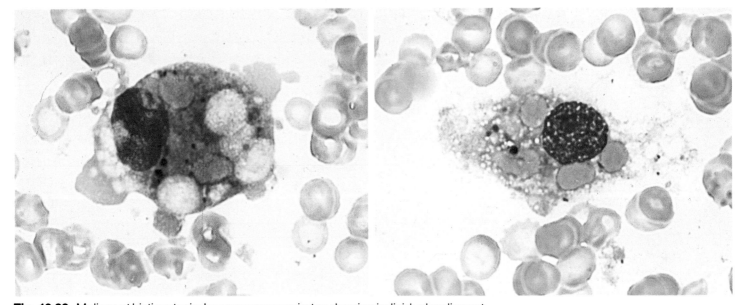

Fig. 10.88 Malignant histiocytosis: bone marrow aspirates showing individual malignant histiocytes and prominent phagocytosis of red cells.

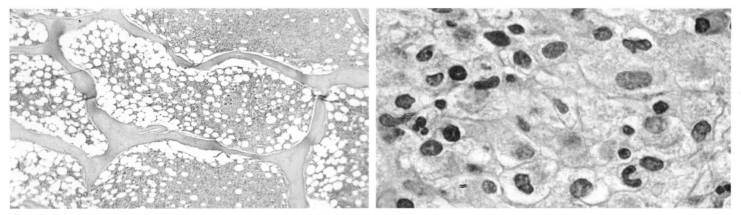

Fig. 10.89 Malignant histiocytosis: trephine biopsy showing (left) extensive replacement of normal intratrabecular haemopoietic tissue by sheets of abnormal histiocytes; (right) at higher magnification the tumour cells show pleomorphic and hyperchromatic nuclei and abundant vacuolated cytoplasm.

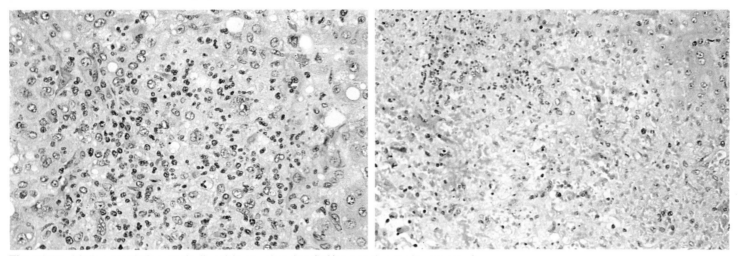

Fig. 10.90 Malignant histiocytosis: liver biopsy showing (left) extensive replacement of liver parenchymal cells by sheets of neoplastic histiocytes and (right) associated areas of liver cell necrosis.

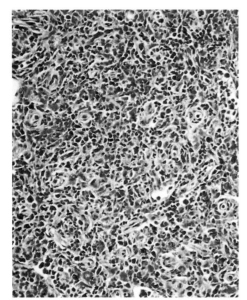

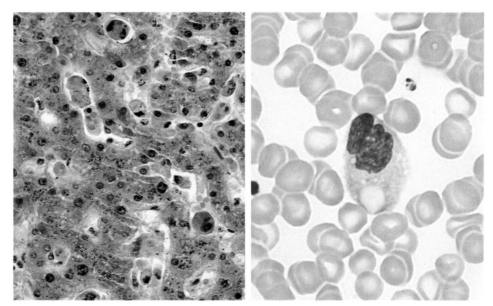

Fig. 10.91 Histiocytic medullary reticulosis: extensive histiocytic infiltration of the hepatic sinusoids. Many of the abnormal cells show erythrophagocytosis. The 61-year-old patient presented with jaundice, lymphadenopathy, hepatomegaly, splenomegaly and pancytopenia. Courtesy of Dr. J.E. McLaughlin.

Fig. 10.92 Histiocytic medullary reticulosis: (left) liver biopsy showing Kupffer cell erythrophagocytosis; (right) peripheral blood film showing a phagocytosed red cell in the cytoplasm of a monocyte.

10.23

In the virus-associated haemophagocytic syndrome, histiocytic proliferation has been associated with infection by herpes or other viruses. Affected patients have high fever, hepatosplenomegaly, lymphadenopathy and peripheral blood cytopenias. Bone marrow aspirates and histological preparations from involved tissues show histiocytic hyperplasia with prominent haemophagocytosis (Fig. 10.93).

Familial haemophagocytic reticulosis is a rare disorder with a recessive inheritance pattern affecting infants and young children. Usually, there is a high fever, hepatosplenomegaly, pancytopenia, rapid deterioration and death from haemorrhage, sepsis, liver dysfunction and central nervous system involvement (Fig. 10.94).

Sinus histiocytosis with massive lymphadenopathy is a rare condition seen most frequently in young blacks and is characterized by lymphadenopathy, fever, leucocytosis and hypergammaglobulinaemia. It is thought to be due to an abnormal reaction to viral infection. The cervical nodes are usually involved (Fig. 10.95). Histologically the nodes show marked sinusoidal dilatation by macrophages with foamy cytoplasm (Fig. 10.96) and plasma cells. Although the disease may follow a protracted course, there is usually a spontaneous and total recovery.

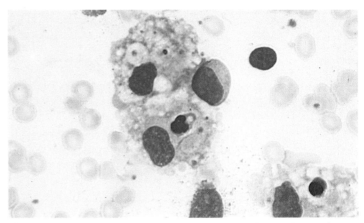

Fig. 10.93 Virus-associated haemophagocytic syndrome: bone marrow aspirate showing a group of histiocytes which have engulfed red cells and erythroblasts. This reactive condition associated with viral infection may be confused with malignant histiocytosis. Courtesy of Dr. S. Knowles.

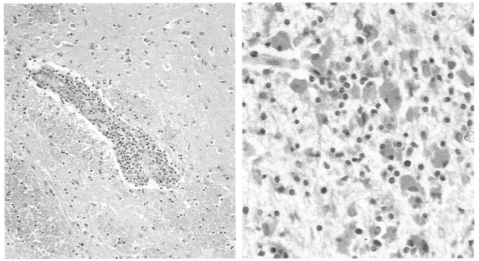

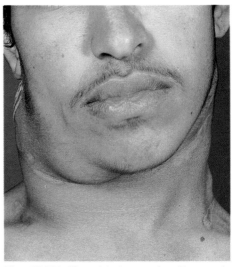

Fig. 10.94 Familial haemophagocytic syndrome: section of brain at necropsy showing (left) a collection of lymphocytes in the perivascular (Virchow-Robin) space; (right) higher magnification shows histiocytes containing both red cells (erythrophagocytosis) and lymphocytes (lymphophagocytosis) in the parenchyma. Courtesy of Dr. J.E. McLaughlin.

Fig. 10.95 Sinus histiocytosis with massive lymphadenopathy: massive painless cervical lymphadenopathy in a teenager from the Middle East. This resolved spontaneously over a 2-year period.

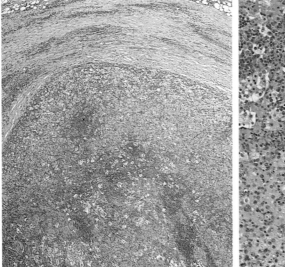

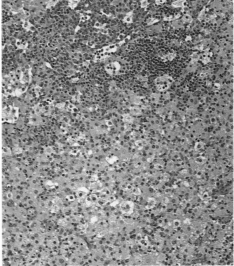

Fig. 10.96 Sinus histiocytosis with massive lymphadenopathy: lymph node biopsy showing (left) marked capsular and pericapsular fibrosis. The sinuses are distended by a proliferation of histiocytes. This condition may occasionally be confused with an histiocytic lymphoma; (right) higher power shows a confluent mass of histiocytes with abundant vacuolated cytoplasm. There is a focal collection of lymphocytes and residual medullary cords.

II
MYELOMA AND RELATED CONDITIONS

MULTIPLE MYELOMA

In multiple myeloma there is a malignant neoplastic proliferation of plasma cells in the bone marrow, usually comprising over fifteen percent of the marrow cell total in aspirates. In advanced disease the abnormal cell population may exceed half of the total cell number (Fig. 11.1). The morphology of these cells is frequently abnormal, with more primitive features and a greater variation in size than classical plasma cells (Figs. 11.2-11.4).

The majority of patients produce a monoclonal protein (M-protein or paraprotein) which may be demonstrated in the serum, urine or both. Typically, the serum protein is increased and electrophoresis shows an abnormal paraprotein in the globulin region (Fig. 11.5). Immunodiffusion techniques reveal which immunoglobulin fraction is increased, while the levels of the uninvolved classes of immunoglobulin are usually depressed. Immunoelectrophoretic techniques confirm the presence of an abnormal immunoglobulin and are able to establish the monoclonality of this protein (Fig. 11.6). The incidence of different types of M-protein produced is shown in Fig. 11.7.

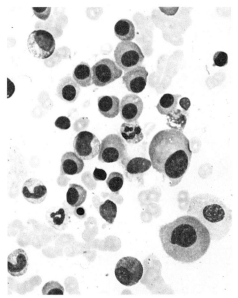

Fig. 11.1 Multiple myeloma: marrow cell trail. The majority of cells seen are atypical plasma cells.

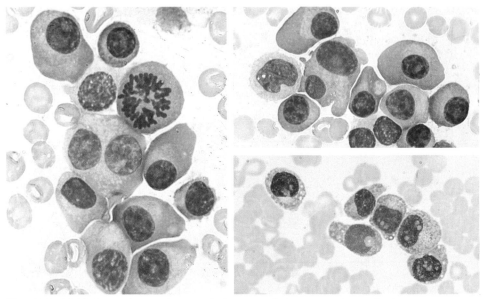

Fig. 11.2 Multiple myeloma: abnormal plasma cells in marrow in two further cases. Myeloma cells, some binuclear, with nucleoli and one with a mitotic figure (left); the nuclei of one binucleate cell vary greatly in size (upper right); abnormal cytoplasmic and nuclear vacuolation (lower right).

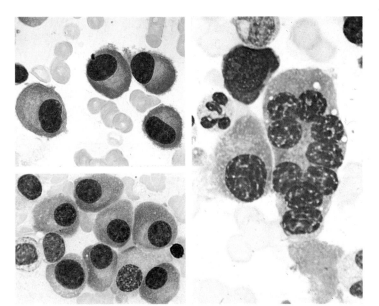

Fig. 11.3 Multiple myeloma: abnormal plasma cells in bone marrow. There is considerable variation in nuclear size and cytoplasmic volume and one of the myeloma cells is multinucleated (right).

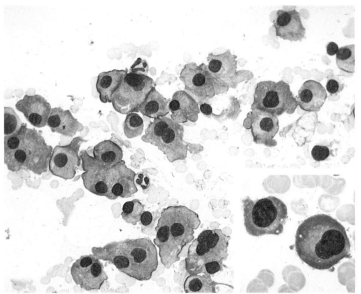

Fig. 11.4 Multiple myeloma: 'flaming' plasma cells in marrow with IgA M-protein in serum. There are numerous thesaurocytes, large plasma cells with small, sometimes pyknotic, nuclei and expanded fibrillary cytoplasm which also shows 'flaming' of the cell rim (inset). Although 'flaming' occurs most frequently with IgA production, it may also be seen with M-proteins of other classes.

In patients with complete monoclonal immunoglobulin in the serum, the synthesis of heavy and light chains in the neoplastic plasma cells is often imbalanced, with an excess production of light chains. The urine contains Bence Jones protein in two-thirds of cases; this consists of free light chains, either ϰ or λ, of the same type as the serum M-protein. In about seventeen percent of cases, Bence Jones proteinuria is the sole protein abnormality and complete abnormal immunoglobulin is not found in the serum. Occasional patients have two or more M-proteins while, in less than one percent of patients, no M-proteins are found in the serum or urine.

The advanced stage of this disease involves a normo-chromic normocytic anaemia, often with an associated neutropenia and thrombocytopenia, reflecting the development of bone marrow failure. The increased globulin in the serum is frequently associated with an increased erythrocyte sedimentation rate (ESR), and the blood may show marked red cell *rouleaux* formation and increased background staining (Fig. 11.8).

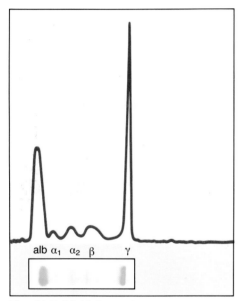

Fig. 11.5 Multiple myeloma: serum protein electrophoresis showing an M-protein in the gamma (γ) globulin region and reduced levels of background beta (β) and gamma (γ) globulins. This 'spike' and deficiency pattern is typical of patients with myeloma. *Total protein: 99g/l; IgG M-protein component: 41g/l.*

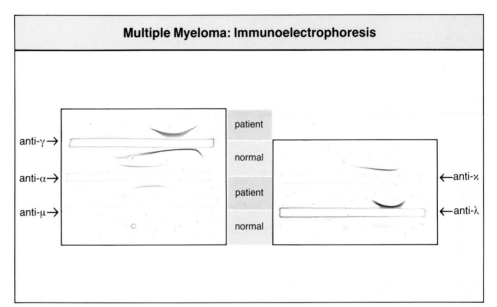

Fig. 11.6 Multiple myeloma: immunoelectrophoresis. Normal protein is recognized by characteristic arc patterns. In the reactions against anti-γ and anti-λ, the IgG-λ M-protein maintains its electrophoretic position but appears as a 'bow' or thickened arc with a smaller than usual radius. Reduced levels of IgA and IgM are reflected in small or absent arcs in the reactions with anti-α and anti-μ.

Distribution of M-Protein Types in Multiple Myeloma			
Types	Percent	Types	Percent
IgG	53	Diclonal	3
IgA	25	Light chains only	17
IgD	2		
IgE	very rare	No M-protein in serum or urine	<1

Fig. 11.7 Multiple myeloma: incidence of M-protein types. This data is taken from the results of the first British Medical Research Council Therapeutic Trial (276 cases).

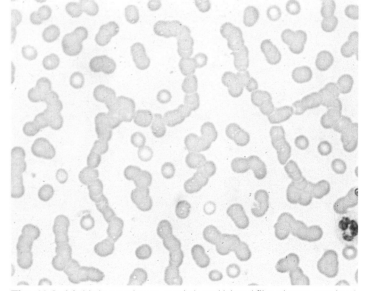

Fig. 11.8 Multiple myeloma: peripheral blood film shows marked rouleaux formation of red cells and increased background staining.

Abnormal plasma cells appear in the blood film in about fifteen percent of patients (Fig. 11.9). Sensitive gene rearrangement studies, however, reveal typical cells of the malignant clone in the peripheral blood in a higher proportion of patients.

Skeletal radiology shows osteolytic lesions in three-fifths of patients and associated pain is characteristic. The lesions include the classical 'punched-out' lesions of the skull (Figs. 11.10 & 11.11), lytic lesions and generalized bone rarefaction of the spine, ribs and pelvis, and pathological fractures (Figs. 11.12–11.15). Extensive bone resorption (Fig. 11.16) results in elevation of serum calcium in half of the patients. In occasional patients, myeloma deposits may extend beyond the skeleton into surrounding soft tissues (Figs. 11.17 & 11.18).

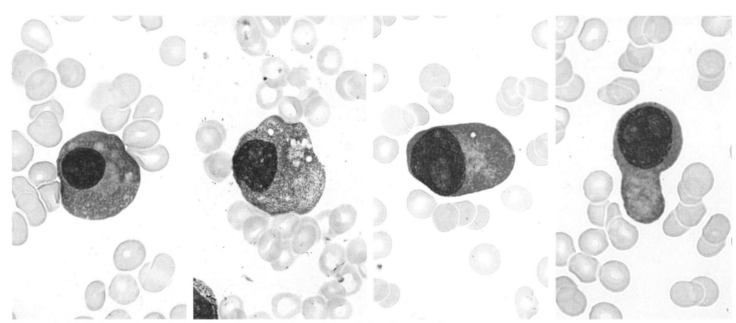

Fig. 11.9 Multiple myeloma: isolated myeloma cells in peripheral blood smears from two patients.

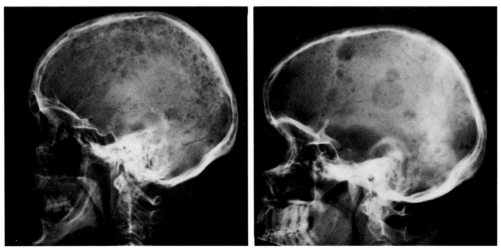

Fig. 11.10 Multiple myeloma: radiographs of skulls showing (left) typical multiple small 'punched out' osteolytic lesions; (right) the lesions vary much more in size.

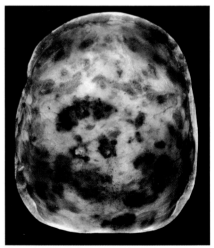

Fig. 11.11 Multiple myeloma: inside of the skull *post mortem* shows characteristic 'moth-eaten' osteolytic lesions.

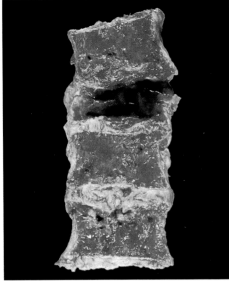

Fig. 11.12 Multiple myeloma: longitudinal section of lumbar spine *post mortem* shows a generalized replacement of normal medullary bone by vascular myeloma tissue. The body of L2 has collapsed and appears haemorrhagic.

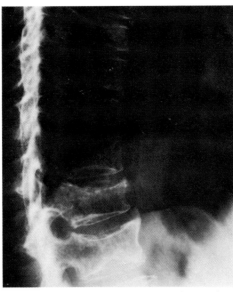
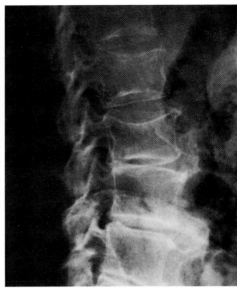

Fig.11.13 Multiple myeloma: radiographs of the lower thoracic (left) and lumbar (right) spine show severe demineralization with partial collapse of the vertebral bodies, most pronounced in T8-T12 and L3.

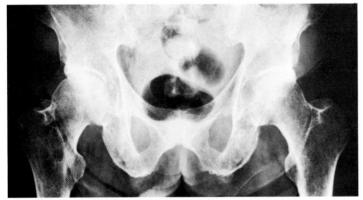

Fig.11.14 Multiple myeloma: radiograph of pelvis with osteolytic lesions in the lower pelvic girdle and in the right femur.

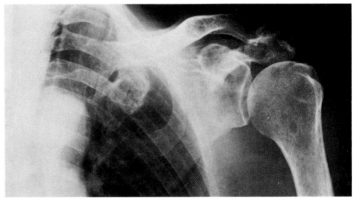

Fig.11.15 Multiple myeloma: radiograph of left shoulder region shows a pathological fracture of the acromial process of the scapula and osteolytic lesions in the humerus, clavicle and ribs.

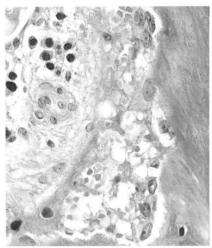

Fig.11.16 Multiple myeloma: bone biopsy. Although plasma cells are seen in the upper left, osteoclasts, the multinucleated cells at the bone-intertrabecular tissue interface, are the cells responsible for the bone absorption around the osteolytic lesion.

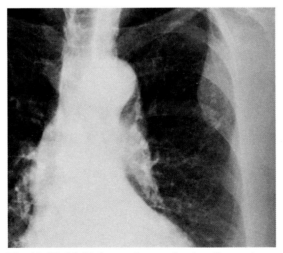

Fig.11.17 Multiple myeloma: chest radiograph showing a prominent extrapleural soft tissue mass adjacent to the third left rib.

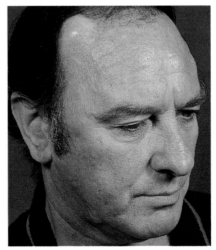

Fig.11.18 Multiple myeloma: skull deposits have invaded the soft tissues and appear as lumps on the forehead. In this case, a proportion of marrow cells were positive for the surface antigen cALLA but TdT negative. Such cells have been associated with aggressive disease.

Renal complications have an important influence on the course of multiple myeloma. Patients with persistent renal failure and blood urea in excess of 14mmol/l have a prognosis of less than a year's survival. Damage from heavy Bence Jones proteinuria (Fig. 11.19), amyloid disease (Fig. 11.20), nephrocalcinosis (Fig. 11.21) and pyelonephritis (Fig. 11.22) may be important in the pathogenesis. A more generalized amyloid disease occurs in a small number of patients, and there may be macroglossia with tongue ulceration (Figs. 11.23-11.25), 'carpal tunnel' syndrome (Fig. 11.26), skin deposits (Figs. 11.27 & 11.28) and cardiac involvement resulting in cardiomegaly and congestive heart failure (Fig. 11.29).

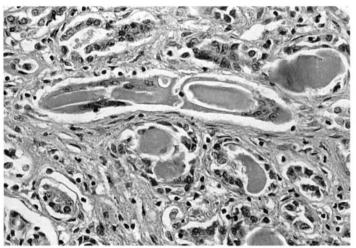

Fig.11.19 Multiple myeloma: section of kidney showing acidophilic casts of myeloma protein blocking the renal tubules. There is a surrounding giant cell reaction and interstitial fibrosis.

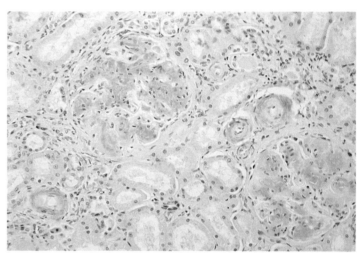

Fig.11.20 Multiple myeloma: renal amyloid disease. There is extensive amyloid deposition in the glomeruli and associated arterioles. Congo red stain.

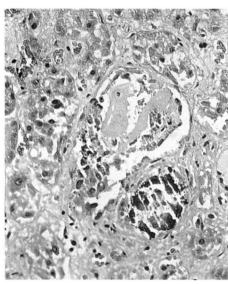

Fig.11.21 Multiple myeloma: nephrocalcinosis. Irregular fractured haematoxylinophilic deposits of calcium are seen in the fibrotic renal tissue.

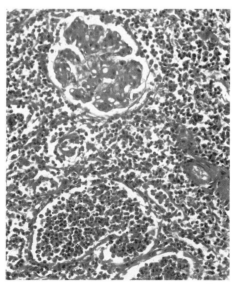

Fig.11.22 Multiple myeloma: destruction of the renal parenchyma and acute inflammatory cellular infiltration of the interstitial tissues and tubular spaces in pyelonephritis.

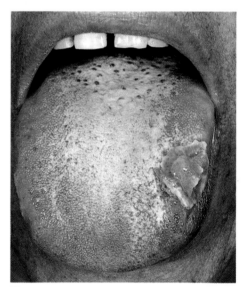

Fig.11.23 Multiple myeloma: tongue in amyloid disease shows macroglossia and a deep ulcer on the upper and lateral anterior surfaces. The floor of the ulcer has the waxy appearance typical of amyloid deposition.

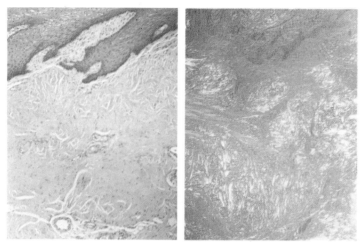

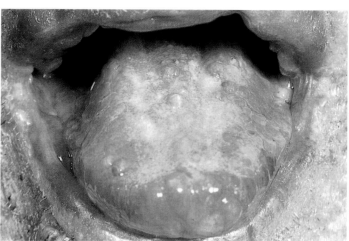

Fig.11.24 Multiple myeloma: biopsy of the ulcer seen in Fig.11.23 shows (left) extensive deposition of pale-staining acidophilic material; (right) stained with Congo red, this material shows the characteristic green birefringence of amyloid.

Fig.11.25 Multiple myeloma: gross macroglossia. These nodular deposits of amyloid contrast with the diffuse enlargement in Fig.11.23. Similar nodules are also evident in the lips.

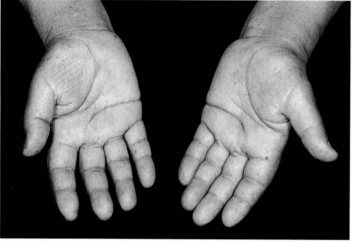

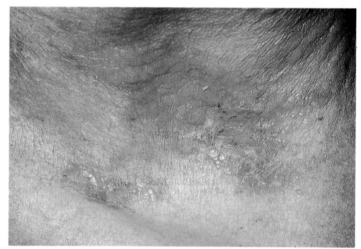

Fig. 11.26 Multiple myeloma: 'carpal tunnel' syndrome due to deposition of amyloid in the flexor retinaculum causing compression of the median nerve. There is wasting of the thenar muscles. The patient complained of paraesthesia and weakness of both hands.

Fig. 11.27 Multiple myeloma: amyloid disease of the skin. There are plaque-like hyaline infiltrations of the skin folds in the supraclavicular area.

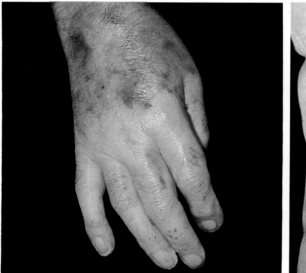

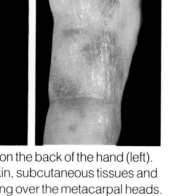

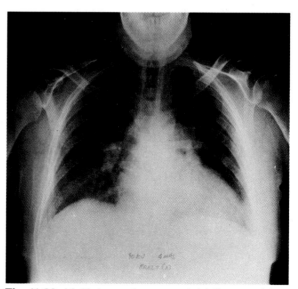

Fig. 11.28 Multiple myeloma: amyloid disease on the back of the hand (left). Extensive diffuse and nodular deposits in the skin, subcutaneous tissues and tendon sheaths have resulted in irregular swelling over the metacarpal heads. The skin surface appears hard, tense and waxy; (right) the extensive purpura, a characteristic feature, is probably due to involvement of small cutaneous blood vessels.

Fig. 11.29 Multiple myeloma: amyloid disease of the heart. This radiograph shows cardiomegaly and pulmonary congestion. Evidence of myeloma includes osteolytic lesions in the right humerus and ribs as well as pathological fractures of the left clavicle and the eighth right rib.

OTHER PLASMA CELL TUMOURS

Solitary and soft tissue plasmacytomas equally comprise the six percent of plasma cell tumours which are not multiple myeloma.

Solitary plasmacytoma of bone

In this disease (Figs. 11.30–11.35), there is no plasma cell proliferation in parts of the skeleton beyond the primary lesion; marrow aspirates distant from the primary tumour are usually normal. Associated M-proteins disappear following radiotherapy to the primary lesion.

Soft tissue plasmacytoma

These tumours are found most frequently in the submucosa of the upper respiratory and gastrointestinal tracts, in the cervical lymph nodes and in the skin. They tend to remain localized and the majority are well controlled by excision or local irradiation.

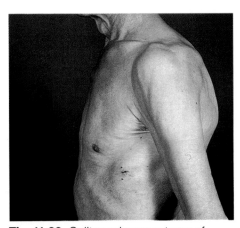

Fig. 11.30 Solitary plasmacytoma of bone: a firm ovoid mass, 9cm in diameter, over the lower lateral aspect of the left chest wall. Protein studies, blood count and bone marrow were normal. No other skeletal lesions were detected by a radiological survey. Courtesy of Dr. S. Knowles.

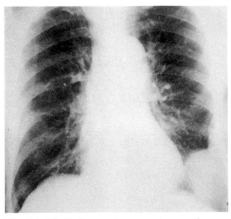

Fig. 11.31 Solitary plasmacytoma of bone: radiograph of the case in Fig. 11.30 shows a well-defined mass approximately 5cm in diameter in the lower left chest, pleural in position and arising from the ninth rib.

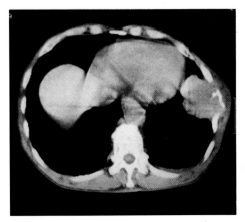

Fig. 11.32 Solitary plasmacytoma of bone: CT scan, same case as in Fig. 11.30, shows erosion of the rib with soft tissue extension into both the pleural space and external soft tissues.

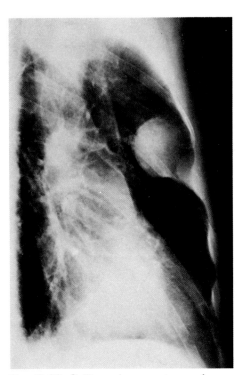

Fig. 11.33 Solitary plasmacytoma of bone: oblique radiograph of left chest. There is expansion and destruction of the left fourth rib with an overlying soft tissue mass (the tumour).

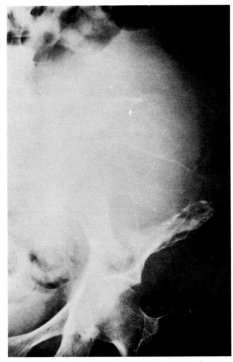

Fig. 11.34 Solitary plasmacytoma of bone: radiograph of left pelvic area shows massive destruction of the iliac bone and tumour extending into the pelvis and abdomen. Linear residual streaks of bone produce the 'soap bubble' appearance seen in this type of tumour.

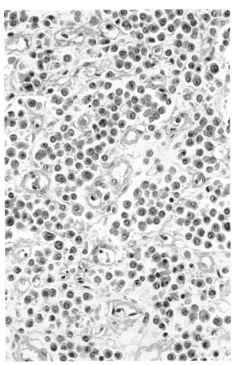

Fig. 11.35 Solitary plasmacytoma of bone: biopsy shows dense collections of plasma cells supported by a vascular stroma.

WALDENSTRÖM'S MACROGLOBULINAEMIA

This rare lymphoproliferative disorder has similarities to both multiple myeloma and lymphocytic malignant lymphoma. There is a generalized proliferation of lymphocytes, many with plasmacytoid features (Figs. 11.36 & 11.37). Frequently there is generalized lymphadenopathy and enlargement of the liver and spleen. The disease advances with extensive bone marrow involvement (Figs. 11.38 & 11.39), and patients may present with evidence of bone marrow failure.

The proliferating cells produce an IgM M-protein which increases blood viscosity more than equivalent concentrations of IgG or IgA and may result in hyperviscosity. Clinically the syndrome is characterized by loss of vision, symptoms involving the central nervous system, haemorrhagic diathesis and heart failure; the most severely affected patients may present in coma. The retina may show a variety of changes, including engorged veins, haemorrhages, exudates and a blurred disc (Fig. 11.40).

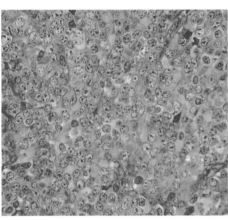

Fig. 11.36 Waldenström's macroglobulinaemia: biopsy of lymph node shows plasmacytoid lymphocytes. The nuclear chromatin has a 'clock-face' pattern with coarse chromatin blocks alternating with open areas of parachromatin clearing. Very few cells can be identified as plasma cells. Methacrylate-embedded section stained with phloxine.

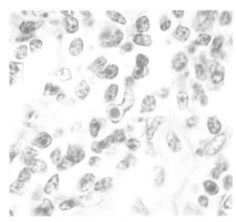

Fig. 11.37 Waldenström's macroglobulinaemia: biopsy of lymph node stained with PAS (periodic acid-Schiff) reagent. In the centre is a large PAS-positive nuclear inclusion.

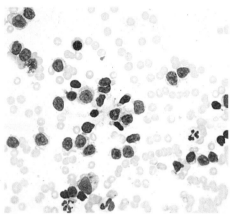

Fig. 11.38 Waldenström's macroglobulinaemia: bone marrow cell trail shows a predominance of lymphocytes and lymphoplasmacytoid cells.

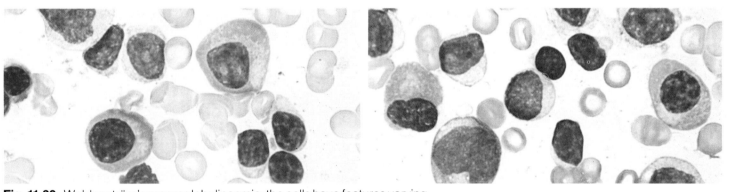

Fig. 11.39 Waldenström's macroglobulinaemia: the cells have features varying between those of classical lymphocytes and plasma cells. The chromatin patterns in the larger nuclei are more open and primitive.

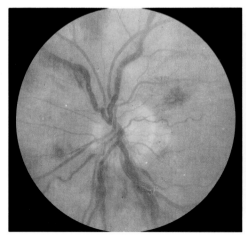
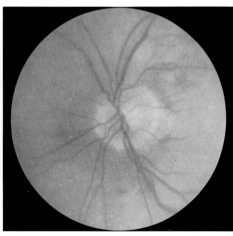

Fig. 11.40 Waldenström's macroglobulinaemia: hyperviscosity syndrome. The patient complained of blurred vision, headache and dizziness. The retina before plasmapheresis (left) shows gross distention of vessels, particularly the veins which show bulging and constriction (the 'linked sausage effect'), and areas of haemorrhage; (right) following plasmapheresis, the vascular diameters are normal and the haemorrhagic areas have cleared.

The syndrome may occur with multiple myeloma (Fig. 11.41) when there is polymerization of the abnormal immunoglobulin, and a similar syndrome is occasionally caused by increased levels of blood components other than M-proteins (Fig. 11.42). This hyperviscosity syndrome is effectively treated by plasmapheresis.

OTHER CAUSES OF SERUM M-PROTEINS

The appearance of an M-protein spike during serum electrophoresis is usually associated with more than 5g/l of that protein. Uncontrolled proliferation of an M-protein-producing clone, as in multiple myeloma or Waldenström's disease, is distinguished by a progressive increase in the serum M-protein concentration. There is a controlled or stable production of M-protein in benign monoclonal gammopathy and chronic cold agglutinin disease (cold autoimmune haemolytic anaemia). Occasionally, production of M-protein is transient, for example, following recovery from infection or during a reaction to a drug (Fig. 11.43).

Benign monoclonal gammopathy

This is the most common cause of a serum M-protein. The benign nature of this condition is distinguished by the fact that the level of M-protein in the serum (Fig. 11.44) is stable over many years. It is not associated with Bence Jones proteinuria nor with bone lesions or soft tissue plasma cell tumours. The bone marrow may have five to fifteen percent plasma cells, but patients are generally asymptomatic with no evidence of bone marrow failure. When afflicted patients are followed for periods of up to ten years, one-fifth eventually develops either myeloma or malignant lymphoma.

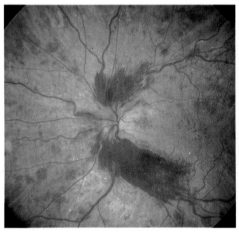 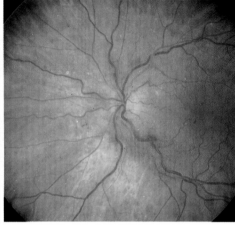

Fig. 11.41 Multiple myeloma: (left) distention of retinal veins and widespread haemorrhage in hyperviscosity syndrome; (right) two months after plasmapheresis and chemotherapy, the vessels are normal and almost all haemorrhage has cleared. The patient presented with some loss of vision and headache. Courtesy of Prof. J.C. Parr.

Causes of Hyperviscosity Syndrome

Causes	Diseases
M-proteins	Waldenström's macroglobulinaemia
	Multiple myeloma
Polycythaemia	Polycythaemia vera
	Severe secondary polycythaemia
Leucostasis	Chronic granulocytic leukaemia
	Other leukaemias with very high white cell counts
Hyperfibrino-genaemia	Following factor VIII replacement therapy with large amounts of cryoprecipitate

Fig. 11.42 Causes of the hyperviscosity syndrome: M-proteins are the dominant cause, but others of importance are polycythaemia, leucostasis and hyper-fibrinogenaemia.

Diseases Associated with Production of M-Proteins

Malignant or uncontrolled production
  multiple myeloma
  Waldenström's macroglobulinaemia
  malignant lymphoma
  primary amyloidosis
  heavy chain disease (γ, α and μ)

Benign or stable production
  benign monoclonal gammopathy
  chronic cold haemagglutinin disease
  transient M-proteins
  occasional association with carcinoma, connective tissue and skin disorders, and many other conditions

Fig. 11.43 M-proteins: uncontrolled production of M-protein occurs with plasma cell dyscrasias, lymphoproliferative disorders and primary amyloid. The most common cause is benign monoclonal gammopathy with no apparent disease association. Benign controlled M-protein production has a number of causes, including carcinoma and other tumours, 'benign' referring to the limited clone of M-protein-producing cells.

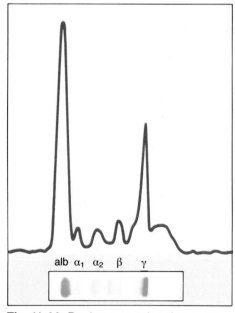

alb α_1 α_2 β γ

Fig. 11.44 Benign monoclonal gammopathy: serum protein electrophoresis shows an M-protein in the gamma region. Unlike the pattern in multiple myeloma (see Fig. 11.5), there is no reduction in the background β and γ globulins. *IgG M-protein component: 19g/l; total protein: 78g/l.*

Although usually benign paraproteinaemia is symptomless, clinical features that may be associated include peripheral neuropathy, acquired von Willebrand's syndrome, papular mucinosis, cold-haemagglutinin disease (see Chapter 4), cryoglobulinaemia and amyloid (see Chapter 15). These syndromes may also occur, however, when the disease causing the paraprotein is clearly malignant, for example, in lymphoma, myeloma or macroglobulinaemia.

Heavy-chain disease

In this rare group of disorders, the neoplastic cells secrete immunoglobulin heavy chains (γ, α or μ) without light chains attached to them. A single case of δ heavy-chain secreting disease has been described that resembled myeloma. The secreted heavy chains in all types of heavy-chain disease are usually incomplete.

Gamma-chain disease resembles a lymphoma clinically. The protein usually consists of two γ heavy chains linked together. The variable region and part of the first domain of the constant region is deleted in some cases. The disease most often occurs in males with a peak age incidence in the seventh decade with lymphadenopathy, fever and anaemia. The marrow shows a mixture of lymphocytes and plasma cells, often with eosinophilia, and the serum shows a monoclonal spike in the γ, α or β region.

Alpha-chain disease, the most common form of heavy-chain disease, has a number of special features. It occurs largely in the Mediterranean area and Africa, often in patients with an Arabic genetic background, and in areas where intestinal parasites are frequent. It commences as a relatively benign plasma cell proliferation in the gastrointestinal tract (Fig. 11.46) and, subsequently, a

Features of Paraproteinaemia		
	Benign	Malignant
Bence Jones proteinuria	Absent	May be present
Serum paraprotein concentration	Usually <20g/l and stationary	Usually >20g/l and rising
Immunoparesis	Absent	Present
Underlying lymphoproliferative disease or myeloma	Absent	Present

Fig.11.45 Distinguishing features of benign and malignant para-proteinaemia.

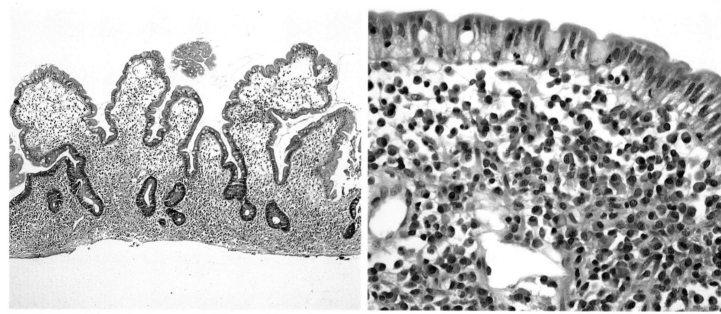

Fig.11.46 Alpha-chain disease: this 25-year old Algerian man presented in 1983 with a malabsorption syndrome, consisting of weight loss, chronic diarrhoea, steatorrhoea and hypocalcaemia, that responded to broad-spectrum antibiotics. At this stage, small intestinal biopsy (left) showed a diffuse infiltration of the lamina propria. The cells (right) were a mixture of lymphocytes, plasma cells and plasmacytoid cells. Immunocytochemical staining showed a vast majority of these cells to contain α heavy chains without $\varkappa$ or λ light chains. The serum and urine samples revealed a broad band in the α_2 region, which precipitated with an anti-IgA anti-serum but showed no reactivity to anti-$\varkappa$ or anti-λ. Courtesy of Dr. J.E. McLaughlin.

poorly differentiated lymphoma of the small bowel develops; this tumour may spread, although usually within the abdominal cavity (Fig. 11.47). The serum shows a monoclonal protein in the α_2 or β region in fifty percent of cases, and the protein may also be found in the urine. It consists of α heavy chains with an internal deletion.

A rare form of alpha-chain disease occurs sporadically outside the areas where intestinal infection is common and is characterized by a lymphoplasmacytoid infiltrate of the respiratory tract.

Mu-chain disease is the most rare; the patients are usually African and, as in alpha-chain disease, are particularly from parasite-infected zones. However, mu-chain disease presents with the clinical picture resembling chronic lymphocytic leukaemia or lymphoma with enlargement of the liver and spleen and infiltration of the marrow with plasma cells. Light chains of one type may also be found in urine but these remain separate from the μ heavy chain.

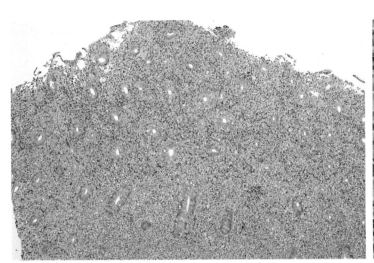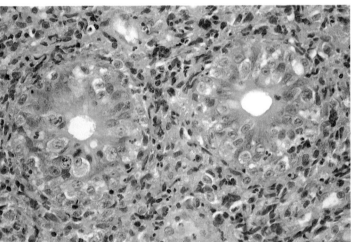

Fig.11.47 Alpha-chain disease (same case as in Fig. 11.46): two years after presentation, the patient developed small intestinal obstruction ; intestinal resection revealed the small bowel to be heavily infiltrated by a large cell 'immunoblastic lymphoma' with an additional mixed infiltrate of neutrophils, plasma cells and macrophages. Despite intensive chemotherapy, the tumour relapsed, involving the large and small bowel and intra-abdominal lymph nodes showing similar histological findings. The appearances of the rectal mucosa at low (left) and high (right) power show complete loss of normal architecture with remaining crypt cells surrounded by the diffuse infiltrate consisting of immunoblasts and mixed inflammatory cells. The α heavy chain could still be detected in serum but not in urine at this relapse. Courtesy of Dr. J.E. McLaughlin.

12

NON-LEUKAEMIC MYELOPROLIFERATIVE DISORDERS

Polycythaemia vera, myelofibrosis and essential thrombocythaemia comprise the non-leukaemic myeloproliferative disorders. The endogenous proliferative process has features which suggest a process in between benign hyperplasia and neoplasia. A clonal stem cell defect is thought to be responsible for the overlapping expansion of erythropoietic, granulopoietic and megakaryocytic components in the marrow (Fig.12.1), although no aetiological features have been identified.

POLYCYTHAEMIA VERA
In classical cases the marrow is hyperplastic. Examination of the blood reveals erythrocytosis and often a neutrophil leucocytosis and thrombocytosis; no primitive cells are seen in the peripheral blood film. The leucocyte alkaline phosphatase score is usually raised and there may be an increase in basophils. An invariable increase in total red cell volume is usually associated with mild to moderate degrees of splenomegaly and hepatomegaly, and there is minimal extramedullary erythropoiesis. The main clinical problems are related directly to the increase in total blood volume and viscosity and to the hypermetabolism associated with myeloproliferation.

Polycythaemia vera is predominantly a disease of the middle-aged and elderly. The clinical features include plethora (Figs.12.2 & 12.3), headaches, lethargy, dyspnoea, fluid retention, bleeding symptoms, weight loss, night sweats, generalized pruritus made worse by hot baths, acne rosacea (Fig.12.4) and other non-specific forms of dermatitis. There is often suffusion of the conjunctivae (Fig.12.5) and marked engorgement of the retinal vessels (Figs.12.6 & 12.7).

Mild to moderate splenomegaly is found in seventy percent of patients and the liver is palpable in fifty percent (Fig.12.8). High blood uric acid levels are accompanied by gout (Fig.12.9) in about fifteen percent of cases. Major thromboses and haemorrhages dominate the course of untreated polycythaemia. Myelofibrosis develops in about thirty percent, and death occurs in fifteen percent of patients following the development of acute leukaemia late in the course of the disease.

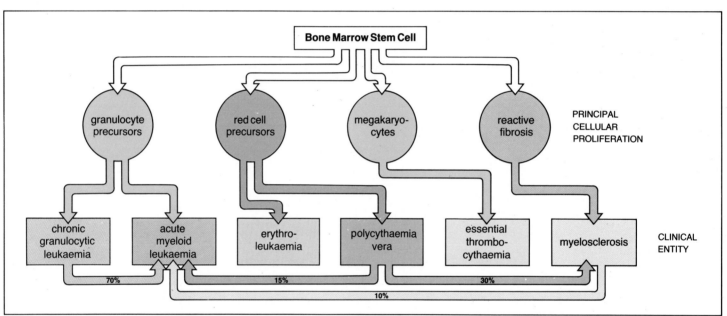

Fig.12.1 Myeloproliferative disorders and their characteristic incidence of transformation.

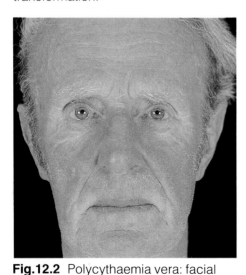

Fig.12.2 Polycythaemia vera: facial plethora in a 65-year-old man. *Hb:22g/dl; WBC:17x10⁹/l; platelets:550x10⁹/l; total RCV:65ml/kg.*

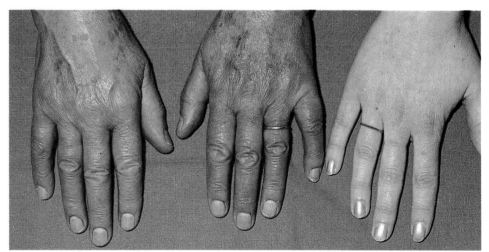

Fig.12.3 Polycythaemia vera: the hands of a 50-year-old woman (on the left) appear congested and plethoric. *Hb:20g/dl; WBC:15x10⁹/l; platelets:490x10⁹/l.* The hand on the right is of a healthy 35-year-old woman. *Hb:14.5g/dl.*

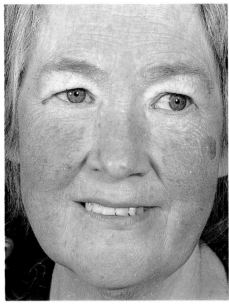

Fig.12.4 Polycythaemia vera: acne rosacea in a middle-aged woman after treatment by venesection.

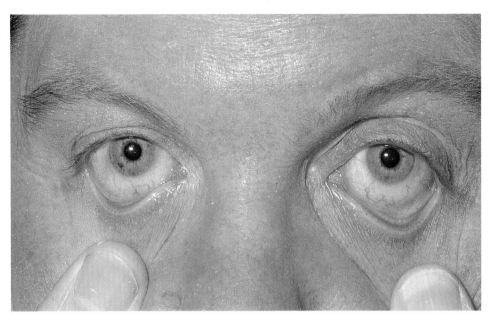

Fig.12.5 Polycythaemia vera: facial plethora and conjunctival suffusion in a 40-year-old woman. *Hb:19.5g/dl.*

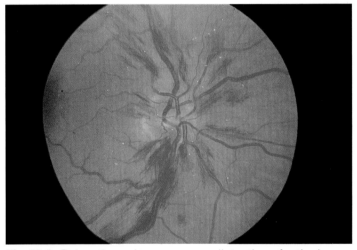

Fig.12.6 Polycythaemia vera: gross distention of retinal vessels with conspicuous haemorrhage and mild swelling of the optic disc in hyperviscosity syndrome. The patient presented with headaches, lassitude, confusion and blurred vision. *Hb:23.5g/dl; WBC:35x10⁹/l; platelets:950x10⁹/l.* Courtesy of Prof. J.C. Parr.

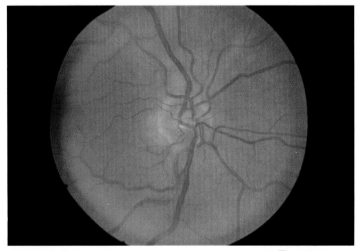

Fig.12.7 Polycythaemia vera: same retina as in Fig.12.6 following venesection. The vessels and disc have returned to normal and the areas of haemorrhage have resolved. Courtesy of Prof. J.C. Parr.

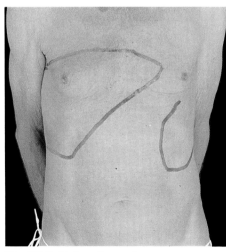

Fig.12.8 Polycythaemia vera: enlarged liver and spleen in the same patient as in Fig.12.2.

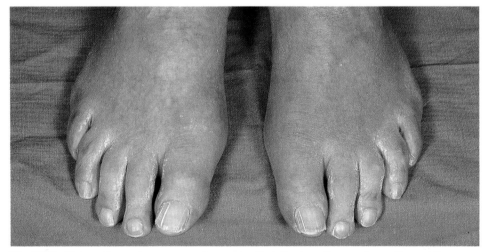

Fig.12.9 Polycythaemia vera: acute gout with inflammation and swelling of the metatarsal and interphalangeal joints of the right great toe. The skin also shows a dusky plethora. *Hb:21.5g/dl; total RCV:53ml/kg; serum uric acid:0.9mmol/l.*

Bone marrow aspirates typically show hyperplastic normoblastic erythropoiesis and granulopoiesis with increased numbers of megakaryocytes (Figs.12.10 & 12.11). Trephine biopsies confirm the hyperplastic haemopoiesis, and clusters of megakaryocytes are often prominent (Figs.12.12 & 12.13). In most patients haemopoietic tissue comprises ninety percent or more of the intertrabecular space. Silver impregnation techniques often show some increase in reticulin fibre density (Fig.12.14). Studies with radioactive iron usually demonstrate that erythropoiesis is confined to central skeletal sites without extramedullary activity (Fig.12.15). Polycythaemia vera must be differentiated from other causes of polycythaemia (Fig.12.16).

MYELOFIBROSIS
In this myeloproliferative disease, also known as myelosclerosis, agnogenic myeloid metaplasia or

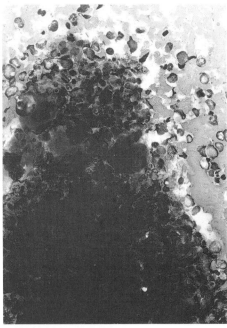

Fig.12.10 Polycythaemia vera: bone marrow aspirate showing the edge of a hypercellular fragment. There is an absence of marrow fat cells.

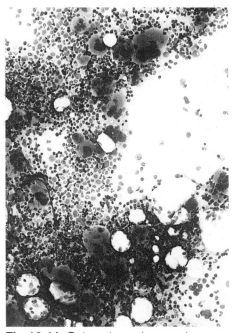

Fig.12.11 Polycythaemia vera: bone marrow aspirate with hypercellular cell trails and bone marrow fragments but incomplete replacement of marrow fat spaces. Megakaryocytes are especially prominent in the cell trails.

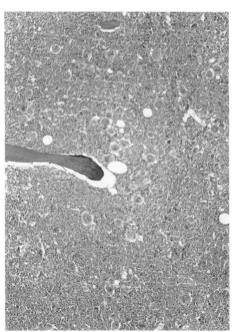

Fig.12.12 Polycythaemia vera: trephine biopsy shows almost complete filling of the intertrabecular space with hyperplastic haemopoietic tissue.

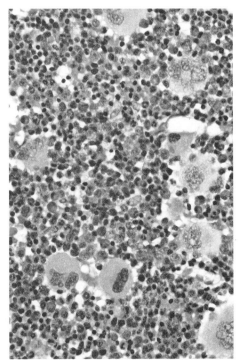

Fig.12.13 Polycythaemia vera: higher power view of Fig.12.12 shows hyperplasia of erythropoiesis, granulopoiesis and megakaryocytes.

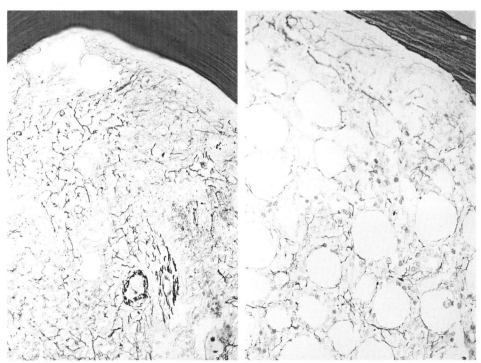

Fig.12.14 Polycythaemia vera: silver impregnation staining shows a moderate increase in the density of reticulin fibres (left) compared with normal bone marrow (right).

non-leukaemic myelosis, the haemopoietic cell proliferation is more generalized with splenic and hepatic involvement. This disorder is related closely to polycythaemia vera and a quarter of patients have a previous history of that disease. The associated increase in marrow fibre production is marked and the effectiveness of haemopoiesis decreases. Recent studies show that the fibrosis is polyclonal, suggesting that it is a reaction to the underlying monoclonal marrow stem cell disorder.

Myelofibrosis occurs in the middle-aged and elderly. Most patients present initially with symptoms caused by anaemia, splenic enlargement (Figs. 12.17 & 12.18) or hypermetabolism such as night sweats, anorexia and weight loss. Some may complain of bone pain and gout (Fig. 12.19).

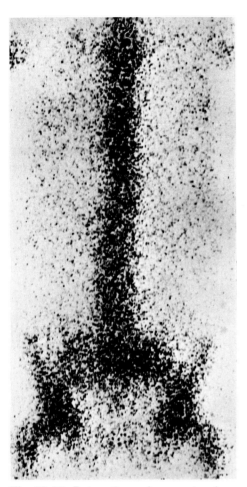

Fig.12.15 Polycythaemia vera: trunk scan showing uptake of iron-52 (^{52}Fe)-labelled transferrin in the axial skeleton indicates that erythropoiesis is confined to the bone marrow.

Causes of Polycythaemia
Primary
Polycythaemia vera
Secondary

Due to compensatory erythropoietin increase in:
    high altitudes;
    heavy smoking;
    cardiovascular disease;
    pulmonary disease & alveolar
        hypoventilation;
    increased affinity haemoglobins
        (familial polycythaemia);
    methaemoglobinaemia (rarely)
Due to inappropriate erythropoietin increase in:
    renal diseases:
        hydronephrosis,
        vascular impairment,
        cysts,
        carcinoma,
    massive uterine fibromyomata;
    hepatocellular carcinoma;
    cerebellar haemangioblastoma

Relative

'Stress' or 'spurious' polycythaemia;
Dehydration:
    water deprivation; vomiting;
    diuretic therapy
Plasma loss:
    burns;
    enteropathy

Fig.12.16 Causes of polycythaemia.

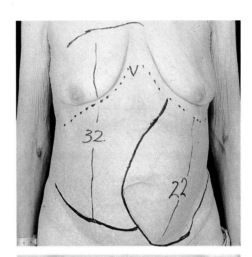
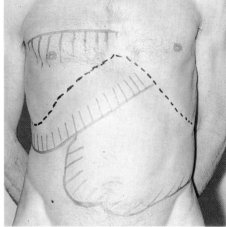

Fig.12.17 Myelofibrosis: (upper) gross splenohepatomegaly. The liver extends 32cm vertically in the midclavicular line and the spleen as far as 22cm below the left costal margin; (lower) less marked splenohepatomegaly.

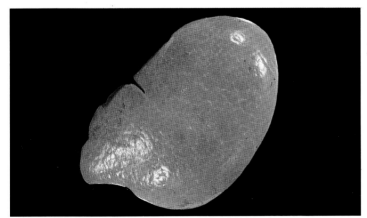

Fig.12.18 Myelofibrosis: spleen from the patient in Fig.12.17 (lower) shows a well-defined notch in the superior border. The prominent indentation in the inferior border was palpable during clinical examination.

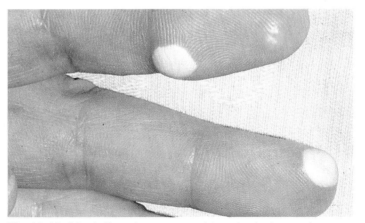

Fig.12.19 Myelofibrosis: gouty tophi on the index and middle fingers of a 55-year-old man.

As a result of a hyperkinetic portal circulation, some cases of long standing develop portal hypertension and may present with bleeding oesophageal varices or ascites (Figs. 12.20 & 12.21). Radiological surveys of the skeletal system frequently show no abnormality, although a minority does show generalized osteosclerosis (Fig. 12.22).

Most patients have a normochromic anaemia of moderate or marked severity. It may be macrocytic in those who are folate deficient or microcytic with associated iron deficiency. The peripheral blood usually shows florid leucoerythroblastic change and the number of nucleated red cells often exceeds the number of leucocytes. Marked polychromasia, anisocytosis and poikilocytosis with 'tear drop' red cells are typical changes (Fig. 12.23).

Attempts at bone marrow aspiration are usually unsuccessful; but trephine biopsy of the iliac bone reveals a variable degree of haemopoietic cell activity and marrow fibrosis (Figs. 12.24–12.26). Silver impregnation techniques show an increase in reticulin fibre density and thickness (Figs. 12.27 & 12.28); only in advanced disease is there collagen deposition and, in ten percent of cases, osteosclerosis (Fig. 12.29).

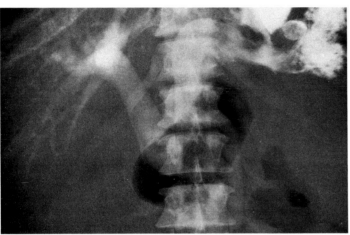
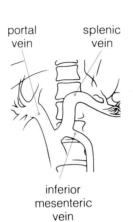
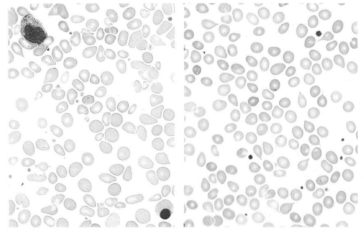

Fig.12.20 Myelofibrosis: transsplenic portal venogram showing gross dilatation of the splenic, inferior mesenteric and portal veins and increased bone density in the vertebral bodies. A great increase in splenic blood flow results in a hyperkinetic portal circulation which, together with the obstructive effects of extramedullary haemopoiesis, may be important in the pathogenesis of portal hypertension.

Fig.12.21 Myelofibrosis: gross wasting and abdominal distention from massive splenomegaly, hepatomegaly and ascites.

portal vein
splenic vein
inferior mesenteric vein

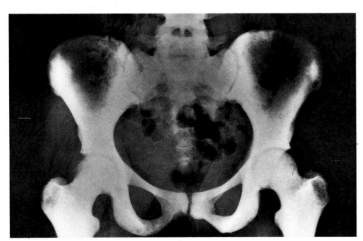
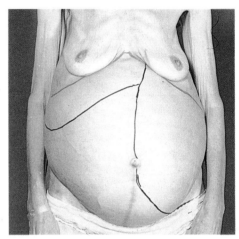

Fig.12.22 Myelofibrosis: pelvic radiograph showing a generalized increase in bone density from osteosclerosis.

Fig.12.23 Myelofibrosis: peripheral blood films showing (left) leucoerythroblastic changes with red cell polychromasia, anisocytosis and poikilocytosis including 'tear drop' forms. The nucleated cells are an erythroblast and a late myelocyte; (right) red cell anisocytosis and poikilocytosis with 'tear drop' forms in early disease.

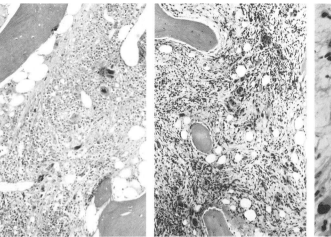
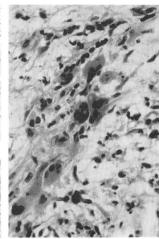

Fig.12.24 Myelofibrosis: trephine biopsies showing (left) most of the intertrabecular space occupied by cellular loose connective tissue containing scattered haemopoietic cells including prominent megakaryocytes; (middle) fat cells comprising less than fifteen percent of the intertrabecular space and extensive deposition of loose connective tissue around haemopoietic cells; (right) the prominence of megakaryocytes in the myelofibrotic tissue at higher magnification.

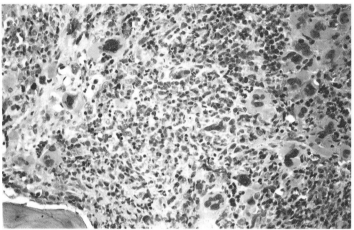

Fig.12.25 Transitional myeloproliferative disease: trephine biopsy shows complete filling of intertrabecular space by hyperplastic haemopoietic tissue with large numbers of megakaryocytes and increased stromal connective tissue between haemopoietic cells. This patient had clinical features of both polycythaemia vera and myelofibrosis. The blood film showed leucoerythroblastic features and splenic enlargement extending 20cm below the left costal margin. *Hb:18.5g/dl; WBC:120x10⁹/l;platelets:450x10⁹/l; total RCV:49ml/kg.*

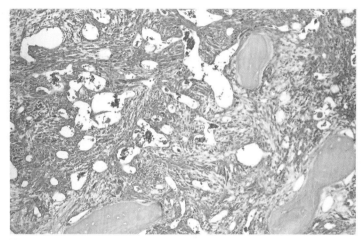

Fig.12.26 Transitional myeloproliferative disease: trephine biopsy shows prominent dilated venous sinuses surrounded by hyperplastic and fibrotic haemopoietic tissue. The blood film showed leucoerythroblastic change. *Hb:19.5g/dl; WBC:38x10⁹/l; platelets:850x10⁹/l; total RCV:44ml/kg.*

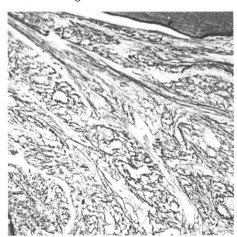

Fig.12.27 Myelofibrosis: silver impregnation staining of the biopsy in Fig.12.24, middle shows a gross increase in reticulin fibre density and thickness.

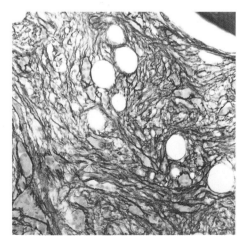

Fig.12.28 Transitional myeloproliferative disease: silver impregnation staining of the biopsy in Fig.12.26 shows a marked increase in reticulin fibre density.

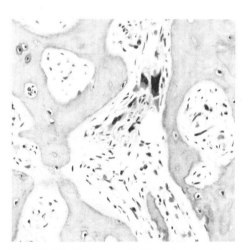

Fig.12.29 Osteomyelofibrosis: trephine biopsy showing replacement of normal intertrabecular tissue by a fibrous connective tissue containing only isolated haemopoietic cells (the larger central cells are megakaryocytes). There is an increased amount of trabecular bone with an irregular lamellar pattern.

12.7

Radioisotope investigations are used to determine the severity of the disease and may also help to elucidate the mechanism of the anaemia. Whole body scanning techniques use cyclotron-produced iron-52 to assess the distribution of the injected radioiron in the body (Figs.12.30 & 12.31). Extramedullary haemopoiesis may also be confirmed by liver biopsy or after splenectomy (Fig.12.32). Myelofibrosis must be differentiated from other causes of reactive marrow fibrosis (Fig.12.33).

ESSENTIAL THROMBOCYTHAEMIA

A diagnosis of essential thrombocythaemia is considered when there is a sustained rise in platelet count in excess of $1000 \times 10^9/l$. There are usually abnormalities of platelet function and the clinical course may be dominated by recurrent haemorrhage and thrombosis. In many patients this disorder is not easily distinguished from myelosclerosis and particularly polycythaemia vera, of which many consider thrombocythaemia to be merely a variant. The dominant clinical problem is bleeding from

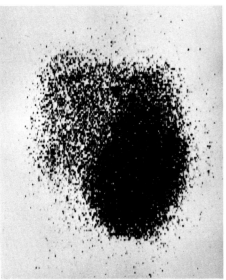

Fig.12.30 Myelofibrosis: trunk scan showing dominant uptake of iron-52 (^{52}Fe)-labelled transferrin into the enlarged spleen and liver with no evidence of skeletal concentration, a pattern consistent with predominant extramedullary haemopoiesis.

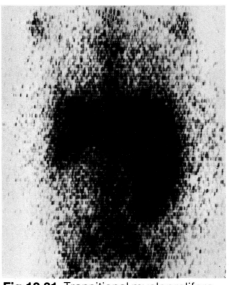

Fig.12.31 Transitional myeloproliferative disease: trunk scan showing obvious uptake of ^{52}Fe-labelled transferrin in the liver and spleen as well as in the central skeleton.

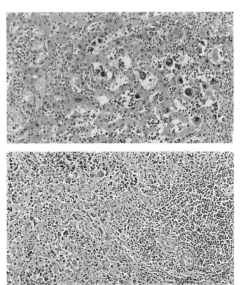

Fig.12.32 Myelofibrosis: extramedullary haemopoiesis. Liver biopsy (upper) shows groups of erythroblasts, granulopoietic cells and multinucleated megakaryocytes in the sinuses; (lower) section of spleen following splenectomy shows similar groups of haemopoietic cells in the reticuloendothelial cords and sinuses.

Causes of Marrow Fibrosis

Myelosclerosis

Infections:
  tuberculosis (see Chapter 15),
  osteomyelitis (focal fibrosis)

Malignant lymphoma,
  including Hodgkin's disease (see Chapter 10)

Occasionally in chronic granulocytic
  leukaemia (see Chapter 9)
  & other leukaemias (see Chapter 8)

Metastatic carcinoma,
  especially breast & prostate (see Chapter 15)

Excess irradiation

Benzene poisoning

Excess fluorine

Paget's disease
  (focal fibrosis; see Chapter 15)

Osteopetrosis (see Chapter 15)

Fig.12.33 Causes of reactive marrow fibrosis.

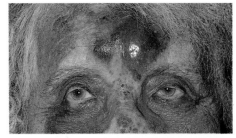
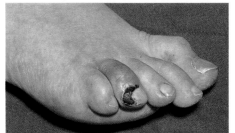

Fig.12.34 Essential thrombocythaemia: (upper) haemorrhage into subcutaneous tissues following minor trauma. There were gross defects of platelet aggregation with ADP, adrenalin and thrombin. *Platelets:2300×10⁹/l*; (lower) gangrene of the left fourth toe. *Platelets:1900×10⁹/l.*

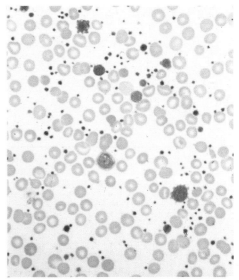

Fig.12.35 Essential thrombocythaemia: peripheral blood film showing a gross increase in platelet numbers.

the gastrointestinal tract and, less frequently, epistaxis, menorrhagia, haematuria or haemoptysis. Spontaneous bruising often appears (Fig.12.34, upper) and cerebrovascular accidents are common complications. Blockage of peripheral blood vessels may result in ischaemia and gangrene (Fig.12.34, lower).

The peripheral blood film shows a distinctive increase in platelet count and the platelets are often of abnormal morphology with many giant forms. Howell–Jolly bodies and other stigmata of splenic atrophy are found in

a third of cases and careful search may reveal the presence of megakaryocyte fragments (Figs.12.35–12.37).

Aspiration of bone marrow may be difficult. There is usually a general hyperplasia of haemopoietic cells with a striking increase in the number of megakaryocytes (Fig.12.38) which are often found in cohesive clusters (see Fig.12.41, upper). They tend to show many nuclear lobes and their average cell volume is greater than normal (Figs.12.39–12.40).

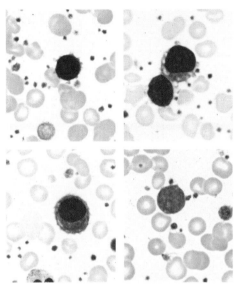

Fig.12.36 Essential thrombocythaemia: peripheral blood films showing circulating megakaryocyte fragments.

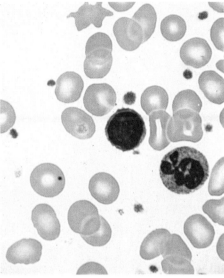

Fig.12.37 Essential thrombocythaemia: peripheral blood film at high magnification shows features of splenic atrophy including a Howell–Jolly body, red cell targetting, crenation and acanthocytosis.

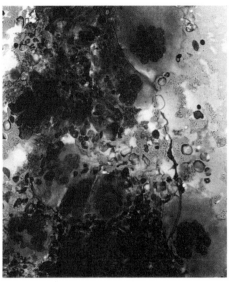

Fig.12.38 Essential thrombocythaemia: bone marrow aspirate fragment shows a marked increase in the number of megakaryocytes.

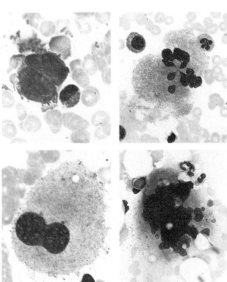

Fig.12.39 Essential thrombocythaemia: bone marrow aspirate showing (upper left) binucleate megakaryoblast; (lower left) binucleate megakaryocyte with cytoplasmic differentiation; (upper right) relatively low and (lower right) high nuclear ploidy in hypersegmented megakaryocytes.

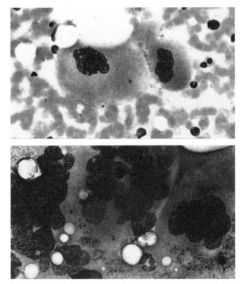

Fig.12.40 Essential thrombocythaemia: bone marrow aspirates showing clumping of megakaryocytes with (upper) definite cell borders and (lower) lack of cytoplasmic separation.

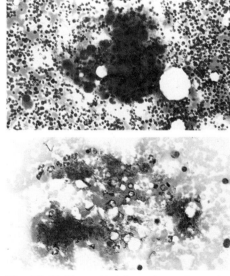

Fig.12.41 Essential thrombocythaemia: bone marrow aspirate cell trails showing (upper) a prominent cluster of megakaryocytes and (lower) large masses of aggregated platelets.

In many patients the dominant feature is masses of adherent platelets which may be confused with marrow fragments (see Fig.12.41,lower). Trephine biopsy preparations reflect the dramatic increase in the megakaryocyte population; large numbers of abnormal megakaryocytes are seen at all stages of development (Fig.12.42) Silver impregnation techniques demonstrate an increase in reticulin patterns intermediate to those of polycythaemia vera and myelofibrosis.

Splenic atrophy (Fig.12.43) often increases the severity of platelet elevation in the peripheral blood as obliteration of the splenic red pulp areas, where platelet pooling normally occurs, results in the entire marrow platelet production being accommodated in the general circulation. Essential thrombocythaemia must be differentiated from other causes of a high platelet count (Fig.12.44).

LEUKAEMIC TRANSFORMATION OF POLYCYTHAEMIA VERA AND MYELOFIBROSIS

It is generally accepted that transformation is part of the natural history of the myeloproliferative syndrome. Transition to myelofibrosis from polycythaemia vera occurs in approximately thirty percent and to acute leukaemia in about half that number. This is usually acute myeloblastic leukaemia but acute lymphoblastic leukaemia has been described. There is a similar incidence of leukaemia in those treated with either ^{32}P or chemotherapy. Ten percent of patients with myelofibrosis develop a terminal leukaemia (Figs.12.45–12.48). Survival beyond leukaemic transformation in either condition is brief.

ACUTE MYELOFIBROSIS

Patients with this syndrome present acutely with symptoms due to anaemia, neutropenia or thrombocytopenia and show leucoerythroblastic changes in the peripheral blood. Attempts at marrow aspiration are unsuccessful but trephine biopsies reveal evidence of myelofibrosis (Figs.12.49 & 12.50). This is usually due to the megakaryoblastic type of acute myeloid leukaemia, but may also be caused by lymphoma.

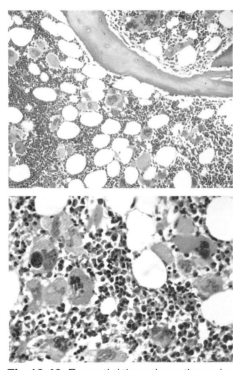

Fig.12.42 Essential thrombocythaemia: trephine biopsy shows (upper) that the overall cellularity of haemopoietic tissue is not greatly increased but (lower) there are large numbers of megakaryocytes, seen particularly well at higher magnification.

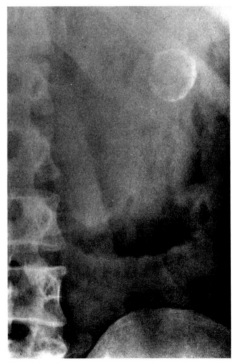

Fig.12.43 Essential thrombocythaemia: abdominal radiograph showing a small spherical calcified mass (at upper left). The blood film showed features of splenic atrophy. At post-mortem the fibrotic remnant of spleen weighed only 30g and had extensive areas of dystrophic calcification.

Causes of High Platelet Count
Reactive:
Haemorrhage
Trauma
Postoperative
Chronic iron deficiency
Malignancy
Chronic infections
Connective tissue diseases: rheumatoid arthritis, etc.
Postsplenectomy with continuing anaemia and active marrow
Endogenous:
Essential thrombocythaemia
In some cases of polycythaemia vera, myelosclerosis & chronic granulocytic leukaemia

Fig.12.44 Causes of thrombocytosis.

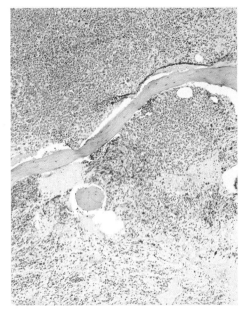

Fig.12.45 Myelofibrosis transformed into acute leukaemia: trephine biopsy shows areas (lower) that are consistent with myelofibrosis but the intertrabecular space (upper) contains sheets of closely packed mononuclear cells without obvious stromal connective tissue.

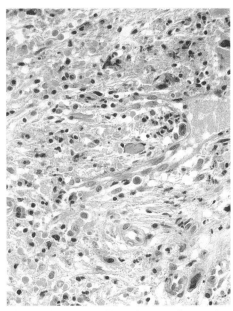

Fig.12.46 Myelofibrosis transformed into acute leukaemia: higher power view of the lower area Fig.12.45 shows isolated haemopoietic cells surrounded by a loose fibrous connective tissue.

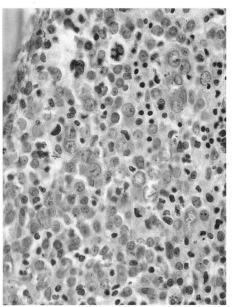

Fig.12.47 Myelofibrosis transformed into acute leukaemia: higher power view of upper area in Fig.12.45 shows predominantly primitive myeloid blast cells and promyelocytes. Following a nine-year history of myelofibrosis, the patient had presented with a fever and bronchopneumonia. *Hb:7.1g/dl; WBC:6x10⁹/l; blasts:4.5x10⁹/l;neutrophils:0.6x10⁹/l;platelets:40x10⁹/l.*

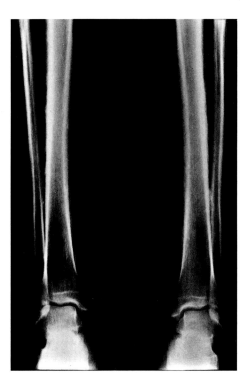

Fig.12.48 Myelofibrosis transformed into acute leukaemia: radiograph of the lower legs of a middle-aged man shows extensive periosteal elevation due to infiltration by myeloid blast cells from underlying medullary bone. Although the medullary cavities of these bones in adults usually contain only fat, there may be extension of haemopoietic tissue to distal skeletal tissues in longstanding myeloproliferative disease.

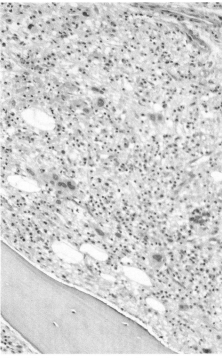

Fig.12.49 Acute myelofibrosis: trephine biopsy shows abnormal haemopoietic tissue with predominant mononuclear cells, isolated megakaryocytes and an abundant fibrous stroma.

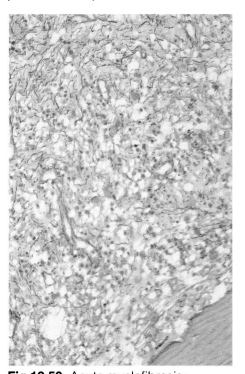

Fig.12.50 Acute myelofibrosis: trephine biopsy with silver impregnation staining shows a marked increase in reticulin fibre density.

In typical cases the features of the blast cells indicate that the condition is a megakaryoblastic variant of acute leukaemia (Fig. 12.51). The majority of patients do not have gross splenomegaly. This acute syndrome has a poor prognosis.

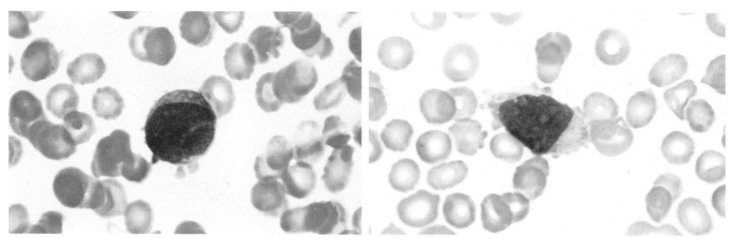

Fig.12.51 Acute myelofibrosis: peripheral blood films showing blast cells which are somewhat larger than classical myeloblasts and have irregular cytoplasmic borders. Electronmicroscopic studies and detection of factor VIIIR:AG in their cytoplasm using monoclonal antibodies confirmed that they were megakaryoblasts. *Hb:6.3g/dl; WBC:3x10^9/l; blasts:1.2x10^9/l; neutrophils:0.9x10^9/l; platelets:65x10^9/l.*

13

VASCULAR AND PLATELET BLEEDING DISORDERS

HAEMOSTASIS AND BLEEDING DISORDERS

The mechanism of normal haemostasis involves the interaction of blood vessels, platelets and coagulation factors (Fig.13.1). The initial arrest of haemorrhage is the result of vasoconstriction and the elastic recoil of severed blood vessels together with the formation of platelet plugs. This is followed by activation of the blood coagulation factors which converts the fluid blood into an insoluble fibrin clot, reinforcing the sealing effect. The coagulation cascade is detailed in Chapter 14.

The main function of the intact vessel wall is to prevent haemostasis and platelet aggregation (Fig.13.2). A number of substances are produced by the endothelium which inhibit platelet aggregation (for example, prostacyclin) or blood coagulation (for example, antithrombin III and protein C activator), or activate fibrinolysis (for example, tissue plasminogen activator). Von Willebrand's factor, necessary for platelet–cell wall interaction, is also produced. A break in the vessel wall exposes clotting factors and platelets to the subendothelial connective tissue.

The platelet has a trilamellar surface membrane which invaginates into the cytoplasm to form an open canalicular system, giving a large surface (platelet factor 3) to which clotting factors may adsorb (Fig.13.3). A mucopolysaccharide coat outside the membrane is important in platelet adhesion to the vessel wall and in aggregation and adsorption of clotting factors, especially fibrinogen and factor VIII. Glycoproteins on the platelet surface include Ib (defective in Bernard-Soulier syndrome), and IIb and IIIa (defective in thrombasthaenia). Both sites are important in attachment of platelets to the von Willebrand's factor and, hence, to vascular endothelium (Fig.13.4). The binding site for IIb-IIIa is also the receptor for fibrinogen and leads to platelet-platelet aggregation.

A submembranous microtubular system maintains the platelet shape; microfilaments distributed throughout the cytoplasm (including a complex mixture of muscle proteins) are involved in changes in platelet contraction and secretion, and clot retraction. The platelets also contain a number of organelles, including α-granules which contain a variety of proteins (Fig.13.3), dense bodies (δ-granules) which contain calcium, adenine nucleotides and serotonin, lysosomes which contain acid hydrolases, peroxisomes which contain catalase, mitochondria and a dense tubular system that contains substantial quantities of calcium and may be a site of synthesis of prostaglandins and thromboxane A_2.

The platelet attaches to subendothelial structures of damaged vessels, probably via attachment to von Willebrand's factor (factor VIII-antigen; Fig.13.4). Von Willebrand's factor itself has binding sites for collagen microfibrils in the exposed subendothelium.

Bleeding disorders may be the result of abnormalities of blood vessels, or qualitative or quantitative defects of blood platelets (dealt with in this chapter), or of deficiencies of blood coagulation factors (dealt with in Chapter 14). They may present as excessive post-traumatic bleeding, epistaxis, haematemesis, melaena, rectal bleeding or haematuria.

Disorders of platelets and small blood vessels present as purpuras with pronounced cutaneous and mucosal bleeding. Prolonged bleeding from superficial cuts

and abrasions is a feature of thrombocytopenia and disorders of platelet function. Menorrhagia is often the dominant clinical problem of women with severe thrombocytopenia or von Willebrand's disease. Repeated haemarthroses, deep dissecting haematomas and serious delayed excessive post-traumatic bleeding are more characteristic of severe deficiencies of blood coagulation factors. Initial haemostasis, in these cases, may be accomplished by vascular reaction and platelet plugs.

VASCULAR BLEEDING DISORDERS

Disorders associated with vascular bleeding are listed in Fig.13.5.

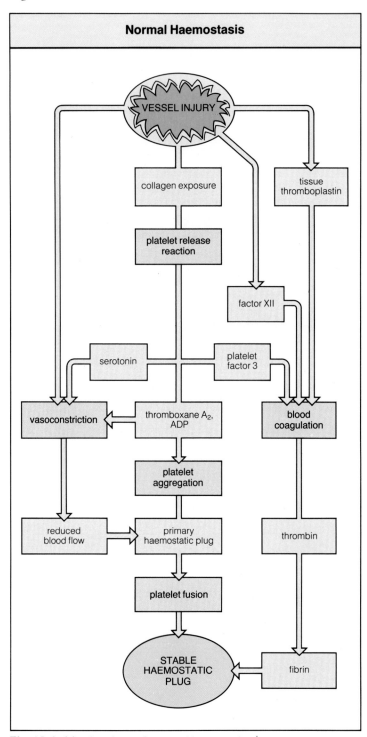

Fig.13.1 Mechanism of normal haemostasis.

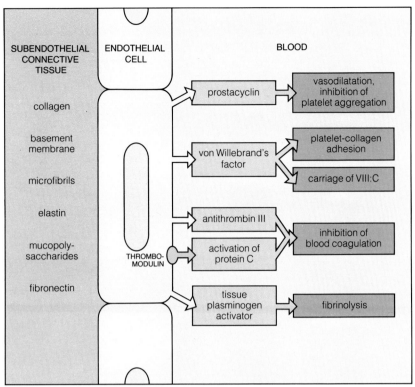

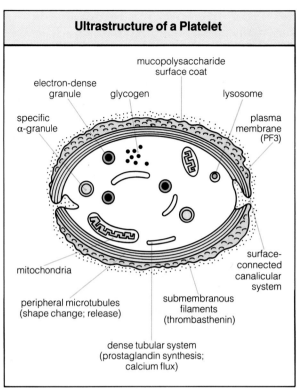

Fig.13.2 The endothelial cell forms a barrier between platelet and plasma clotting factors, and subendothelial connective tissues. Endothelial cells produce a variety of substances which inhibit haemostasis or platelet aggregation, or activate fibrinolysis.

Fig.13.3 Ultrastructure of a platelet: electron-dense granules contain adenine nucleotides, calcium and serotonin; specific α-granules contain growth factor, fibrinogen, factors V and VIII:VWF, fibronectin, β-thromboglobulin, heparin antagonist (PF4) and thrombospondin; lysosomes contain acid hydrolases; the plasma membrane (PF3) is the site of receptors for clotting factors and aggregating agents. Courtesy of Dr. R. A. Hutton.

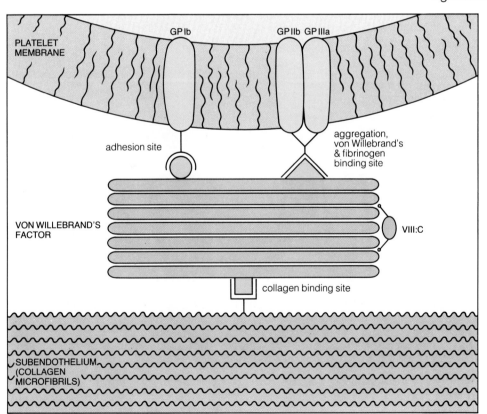

Fig.13.4 The adhesion of platelets to vascular endothelium is mediated by von Willebrand's factor [VIII-antigen (Ag)] which also carries factor VIII coagulation factor (VIII-C). There are two binding sites on the platelet membrane for von Willebrand's factor, glycoprotein (GP) Ib and GP IIb-IIIa complex. Courtesy of Dr. R. A. Hutton.

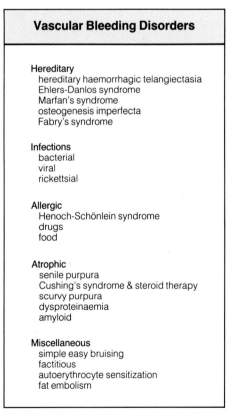

Fig.13.5 Disorders associated with abnormal vascular bleeding.

Hereditary haemorrhagic telangiectasia

The small vascular malformations which are the essential lesion in this condition may be confused with petechiae. These bright red or purple spots are permanent and most noticeable on the face, nose, lips and tongue, and on plantar and palmar surfaces (Figs.13.6–13.8). Usually the lesions do not appear until adulthood, becoming more numerous with advancing age. Bleeding from the telangiectasia of the gastrointestinal mucosa produces a state of chronic severe iron deficiency.

Ehlers–Danlos syndrome

In this syndrome the purpura is due to deficiency in platelet aggregation by skin collagen. It is most marked in type IV Ehlers-Danlos syndrome (Fig.13.9) in which there is a deficiency of type III collagen.

Senile purpura

Relatively indolent purpuric ecchymoses are found frequently in the elderly, particularly on areas of skin exposed to sunlight, for example, on the backs of the hands and wrists (Fig.13.10), the extensor surfaces of the forearms and the back of the neck. This condition may be caused by atrophy of dermal collagen and loss of subcutaneous fat, weakening the supporting tissue of the small blood vessels of the skin which then become more susceptible to shear strain.

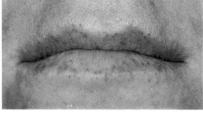

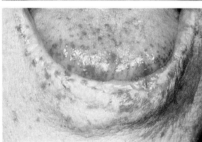

Fig.13.6 Hereditary haemorrhagic telangiectasia: the characteristic small vascular lesions are obvious on the lips (upper & lower) and tongue (lower).

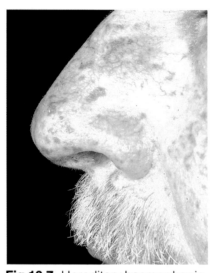

Fig.13.7 Hereditary haemorrhagic telangiectasia: characteristic vascular malformations in the skin of the nose.

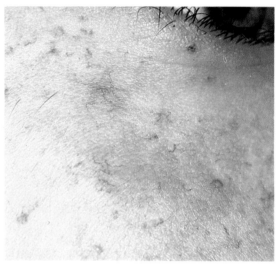

Fig.13.8 Hereditary haemorrhagic telangiectasia: close-up view of the linear and punctate vascular lesions.

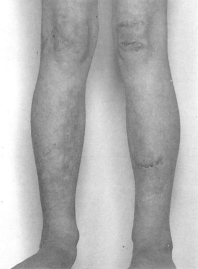

Fig.13.9 Ehlers-Danlos syndrome: purpura into scars of the skin especially around the knees of a 16-year-old boy who also display-ed hyperextensible joints, thin, easily torn, skin and poor healing. The scars are raised into folds by the underlying bulging subcutaneous tissues. Courtesy of Dr. I Sarkany.

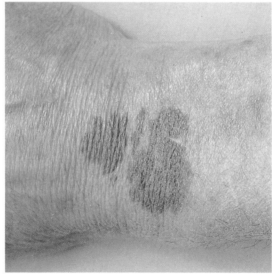

Fig.13.10 Senile purpura: typical ecchymoses on the extensor surface of the wrist of an elderly man.

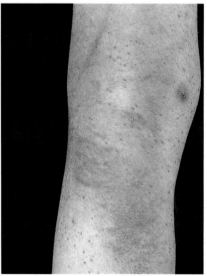

Fig.13.11 Scurvy: widespread petechial perifollicular haemorrhages becoming confluent. Deeper haematomata were also present.

Scurvy

Petechiae of perifollicular distribution (Fig.13.11) are a feature of scurvy, probably due to a defect in the microvascular supporting tissue. Disordered platelet function may also be present.

Purpura associated with abnormal proteins

Petechiae and ecchymoses may be seen in patients with multiple myeloma (Fig.13.12), Waldenström's macroglobulinaemia, benign monoclonal gammopathy, cryoglobulinaemia or cryofibrinogenaemia. Many of the proteins involved in these conditions interfere with platelet function and fibrin formation. Small vessel haemorrhages may also result from hyperviscosity of blood or from damage to the vessel upon precipitation of these proteins in the cooler parts of the skin. Similarly, patients with amyloidosis may show purpura due to deposition of amyloid in the microcirculation (Fig.13.13).

Allergic purpuras

The skin lesions in the allergic purpuras are more variable. Petechiae and ecchymoses associated with the Henoch-Schönlein syndrome may be accompanied by itching, tingling sensations, erythema and urticarial swelling. The lesions occur most commonly on the buttocks and legs (Fig.13.14). In this syndrome there may be associated submucosal haemorrhage in the intestines (Fig.13.15), haematuria and joint pain.

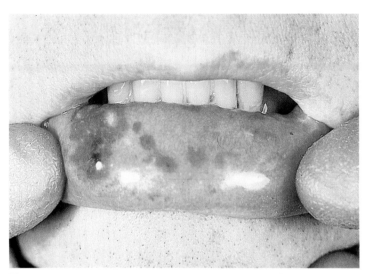

Fig.13.12 Multiple myeloma: purpuric haemorrhages in the mucosal surface of the lower lip.

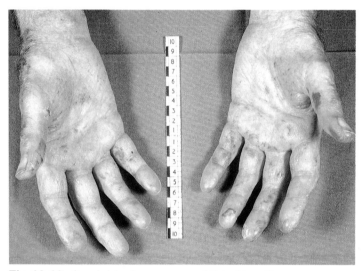

Fig.13.13 Amyloidosis: purpura of the skin with characteristic smooth yellowish deposits secondary to multiple myeloma.

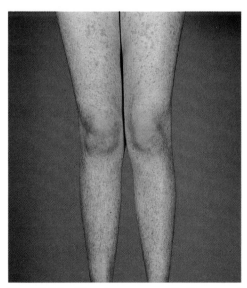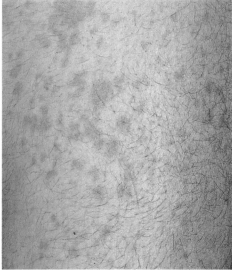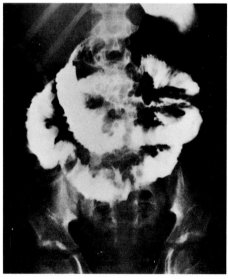

Fig.13.14 Allergic purpura: (left) extensive purpura of the skin of the legs in Henoch-Schönlein syndrome; (right) the early lesions are more an urticarial erythema than true petechial haemorrhage.

Fig.13.15 Allergic purpura: radiograph of Henoch-Schönlein syndrome and mucosal bleeding in the small intestine, evidenced by the characteristic 'thumbprinting' appearance of the barium pattern.

Some allergic drug reactions present as erythematous and purpuric skin eruptions (Fig.13.16). The lesions may be generalized or may have a symmetrical proximal distribution. Extensive purpuric bleeding may also accompany severe vasculitis as in fulminant systemic lupus erythematosus (Fig.13.17) and other connective tissue disorders.

Purpura associated with infection
This may be the result of toxic damage to the endothelium or of immune complex-type hypersensitivity. In some conditions, for example, meningococcal septicaemia (Fig.13.18), there is often associated disseminated intravascular coagulation. There may be extensive bleeding into the vesicular lesions of herpes zoster in patients with leukaemia (Fig.13.19), and petechial haemorrhage of the palate in infectious mononucleosis (Fig.13.20).

The rare condition known as purpura fulminans is characterized by the widespread development of painful large, confluent and necrotic ecchymoses (Fig.13.21). Almost any area of skin may be involved, but the face, extremities, buttocks and lower back are often the worst affected. When seen it is usually in children who are recovering from scarlet fever, varicella or other infections. Some patients have shown evidence of associated disseminated intravascular coagulation with thrombocytopenia and coagulation factor deficiencies.

PLATELET BLEEDING DISORDERS
The most common cause of abnormal bleeding is a platelet disorder as a result of either reduced numbers of platelets (thrombocytopenia; Fig.13.22) or defective platelet function (see Fig.13.34). It is characterized by spontaneous skin purpura (Figs.13.23 & 13.24), mucosal haemorrhage and prolonged bleeding after trauma (Fig.13.25).

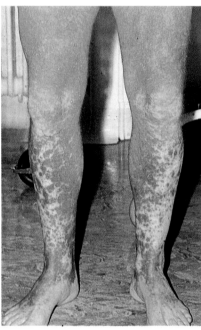

Fig.13.16 Allergic purpura: symmetrical widespread erythematous and purpuric eruption as a hypersensitivity reaction to allopurinol.

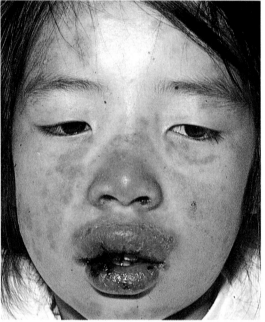
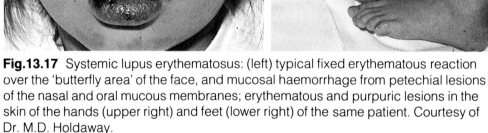

Fig.13.17 Systemic lupus erythematosus: (left) typical fixed erythematous reaction over the 'butterfly area' of the face, and mucosal haemorrhage from petechial lesions of the nasal and oral mucous membranes; erythematous and purpuric lesions in the skin of the hands (upper right) and feet (lower right) of the same patient. Courtesy of Dr. M.D. Holdaway.

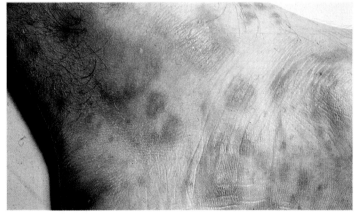

Fig.13.18 Meningococcal septicaemia: typical purpuric skin lesions around the ankle in acute fulminating disease with disseminated intravascular coagulation.

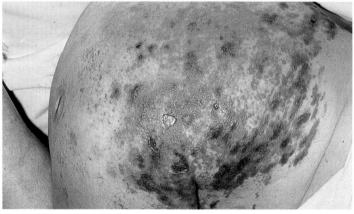

Fig.13.19 Herpes zoster: haemorrhagic herpetic skin eruption over the buttock in a patient with acute leukaemia.

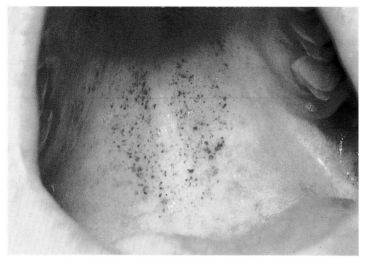

Fig.13.20 Infectious mononucleosis: extensive petechiae in the mucosa of the palate.

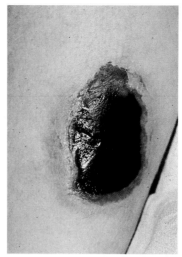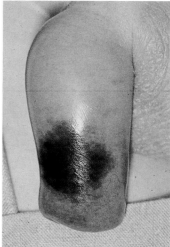

Fig.13.21 Purpura fulminans: large necrotic ecchymoses of the skin of the leg (left) and penis (right) of an infant, following varicella infection. Courtesy of Dr. M.D. Holdaway.

Causes of Thrombocytopenia

Failure of platelet production
Generalized bone marrow failure:
leukaemia; myelodysplasia; aplastic anaemia; myelofibrosis; megaloblastic anaemia; uraemia; multiple myeloma; marrow infiltration, e.g. carcinoma, lymphoma
Selective megakaryocyte depression:
drugs; alcohol; chemicals; viral infections
Hereditary thrombocytopenias:
May-Hegglin, Wiskott-Aldrich, Bernard-Soulier syndromes & others

Abnormal distribution of platelets
Splenomegaly

Increased destruction of platelets
Immune:
alloantibodies: neonatal, post-transfusion;
autoantibodies: primary; secondary, e.g. systemic lupus erythematosus, chronic lymphocytic leukaemia, post-infection, AIDS, post-bone marrow transplantation
Drug-induced:
immune or due to platelet aggregation
Disseminated intravascular coagulation:
microangiopathic processes: haemolytic-uraemic syndrome; thrombotic thrombo-cytopenic purpura; extracorporeal circulation;
giant haemangioma (Kasabach-Merritt syndrome)

Dilutional loss
Massive transfusion of stored blood

Fig.13.22 Common causes of thrombocytopenia.

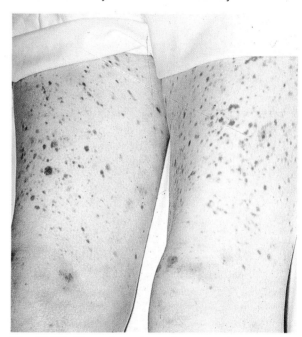

Fig.13.23 Thrombocytopenia: extensive purpura of the skin in marrow failure from disseminated carcinoma.

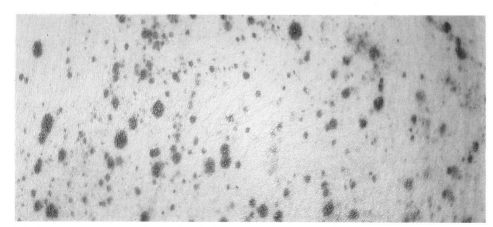

Fig.13.24 Thrombocytopenia: abdominal skin purpura in myelodysplastic syndrome. The platelets are often functionally abnormal as well as reduced in number.

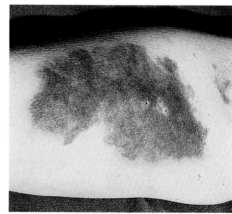

Fig.13.25 Thrombocytopenia: large ecchymosis following performance of the Ivy bleeding time test. The puncture marks of the stylet cutter are clearly seen.

Thrombocytopenia

Failure to produce platelets is the most common cause of thrombocytopenia. Drug toxicity or viral infections may result in selective megakaryocyte depression while in aplastic anaemia, leukaemia, myelosclerosis, cytotoxic chemotherapy or marrow infiltrations, decreased numbers of megakaryocytes may be part of a generalized bone marrow failure. There can be congenital deficiency of megakaryocytes, in many cases with associated skeletal, renal or cardiac malformations, bilateral aplasia of the radii being the most common associated abnormality (Fig.13.26).

Neonatal thrombocytopenia occurs in newborn infants due to intrauterine rubella or other infections, platelet antibodies, disseminated intravascular coagulation, hereditary thrombocytopenias, giant haemangioma or congenital absence of megakaryocytes. Among the variety of hereditary thrombocytopenias, in the Wiskott-Aldrich syndrome there is associated immunodeficiency and eczema (Fig.13.27); in some, such as the Bernard-Soulier syndrome, there are also abnormalities of platelet morphology and function while other syndromes are better known for their associated abnormalities (May-Hegglin; Chédiak-Higashi; see Chapter 7).

Immune thrombocytopenic purpura

In this relatively common disorder, platelet sensitization with autoantibodies (usually IgG) leads to their premature removal from the circulation by cells of the reticuloendothelial system. Patients present with petechial haemorrhage, easy bruising and, in women, menorrhagia. The blood film shows reduced numbers of

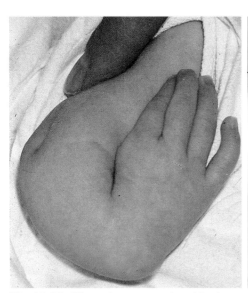

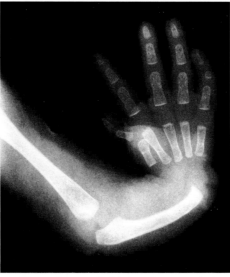

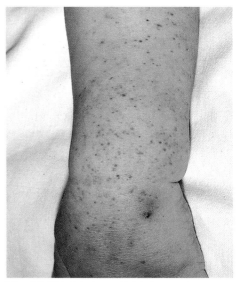

Fig.13.26 Thrombocytopenia with absent radii syndrome: (left) the characteristic flexion deformity; (right) radiography shows complete absence of the radius.

Fig.13.27 Wiskott-Aldrich syndrome: eczema and skin purpura in an infant. Courtesy of Dr. U. O'Callaghan.

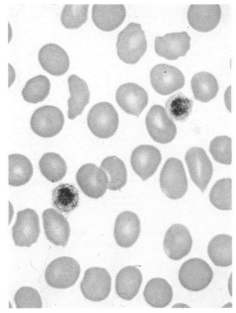

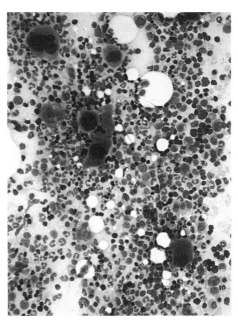

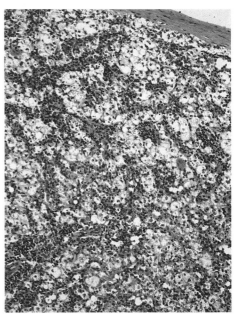

Fig.13.28 Immune thrombocytopenia (ITP): blood film showing two large platelets.

Fig.13.29 Immune thrombocytopenia (ITP): bone marrow aspirate showing increased numbers of megakaryocytes.

Fig.13.30 Immune thrombocytopenia (ITP): histological section of spleen showing prominent collections of lipid-filled macrophages due to excessive breakdown of platelets in the splenic pulp.

platelets which are often large (Fig.13.28); the bone marrow has increased numbers of megakaryocytes (Fig.13.29), and sections of splenic tissue may show prominent collections of lipid-laden macrophages (Fig.13.30). Splenectomy is frequently performed in patients who do not respond to corticosteroids.

Drug-induced immune thrombocytopenia

An allergic mechanism has been demonstrated to be the cause of many drug-induced thrombocytopenias. Rapid removal of platelets from the circulation may result in severe thrombocytopenia and many patients present with mucosal haemorrhage (Fig.13.31) in addition to skin purpura.

Disseminated intravascular coagulation and thrombotic thrombocytopenic purpura

In these conditions, thrombocytopenia is the result of increased consumption of platelets. Disseminated intravascular coagulation is discussed in detail in Chapter 14. In thrombotic thrombocytopenic purpura there is widespread platelet aggregation and accretion in small blood vessels. The clinical course is often fulminant and fatal with confluent purpura and ischaemic damage to many organs, for example, the brain, kidneys and skin (Figs.13.32 & 13.33). The majority of patients have an associated microangiopathic haemolytic anaemia.

Disorders of platelet function

Many of the conditions associated with abnormal platelet function are listed in Fig.13.34.

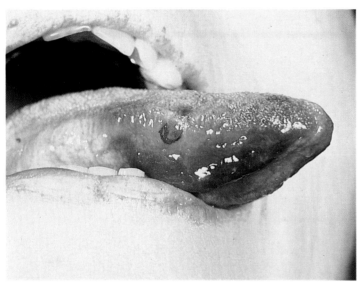

Fig.13.31 Drug-induced thrombocytopenia: sublingual mucosal haemorrhage.

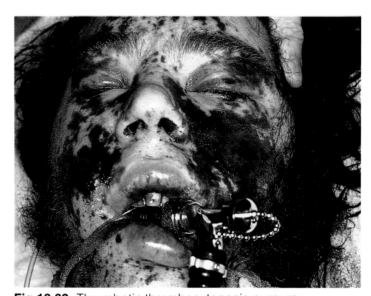

Fig.13.32 Thrombotic thrombocytopenic purpura: widespread confluent and necrotic ecchymoses of the facial skin.

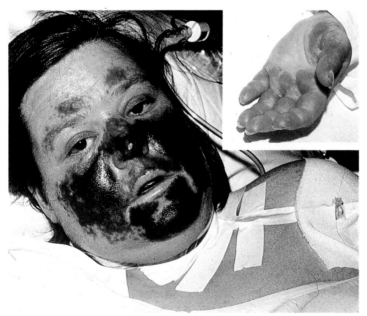

Fig.13.33 Thrombotic thrombocytopenic purpura: massive area of haemorrhagic necrosis of the facial skin and extensive confluent ecchymoses on the hand (inset).

Disorders of Platelet Function
Inherited
Plasma membrane defects: thrombasthenia; Bernard-Soulier syndrome; PF3 deficiency
Storage organelle deficiency: dense body deficiency: idiopathic storage pool disease; Hermansky-Pudlak, Wiskott-Aldrich & Chédiak-Higashi syndromes α-granule deficiency: grey platelet syndrome
Cyclooxygenase & thromboxane synthetase deficiencies
von Willebrand's disease
Acquired
Myeloproliferative disorders
Myelodysplastic syndromes
Acute myeloblastic leukaemia
Dysproteinaemias
Uraemia
Acquired storage pool deficiency: disseminated intravascular coagulation; haemolytic-uraemic syndrome; TTP; disseminated autoimmune disease
Acquired von Willebrand's disease
Drugs: aspirin; dipyridamole; sulphinpyrazone; prostacyclin; carbenicillin; imipramine; non-steroidal anti-inflammatory; etc.

Fig.13.34 Causes of abnormal platelet function.

Hereditary disorders

The rare inherited disorders of platelet function may produce defects at different phases of the reactions leading to the formation of the haemostatic plug. In thrombasthenia there is failure of primary platelet aggregation (Fig. 13.35). The platelet count, size and morphology are normal. There is deficiency of two closely associated membrane glycoproteins, GP IIb and IIIa, on which receptors for fibrinogen and von Willebrand's factor are normally exposed during aggregation (see Fig. 13.4).

In Bernard–Soulier syndrome the platelets are larger than normal (Fig. 13.36) and are deficient in a surface

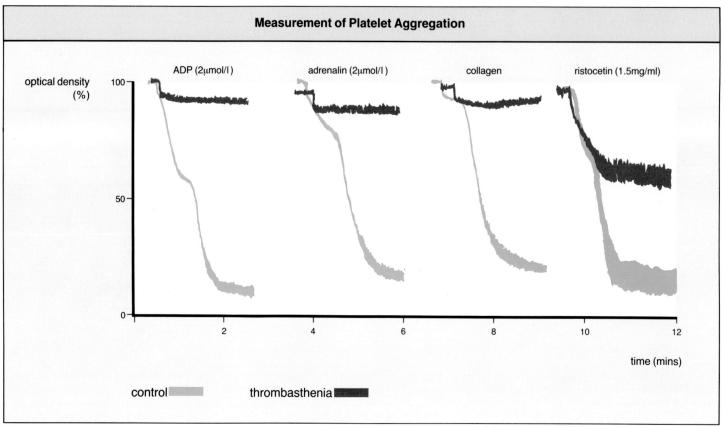

Fig.13.35 Hereditary thrombasthenia: platelet aggregation studies show defective primary and secondary aggregation with adenosine diphosphate (ADP), and defective aggregation with adrenalin and collagen, but not with ristocetin. Courtesy of Dr. R.A. Hutton.

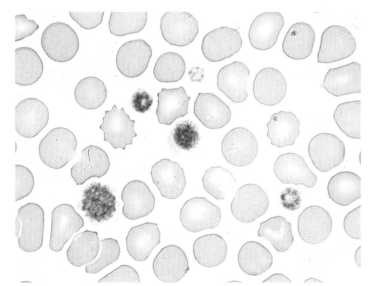

Fig.13.36 Bernard-Soulier syndrome: blood film showing abnormally large platelets.

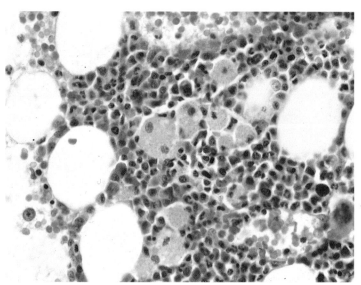

Fig.13.37 Hermansky-Pudlak syndrome: bone marrow trephine biopsy showing prominent macrophages with ceroid-like pigment-laden cytoplasm. Courtesy of Dr. E.G.D. Tuddenham.

glycoprotein I necessary for interaction between platelets and von Willebrand's factor (see Fig. 13.4); there is defective adhesion and diminished availability of platelet phospholipid. In the Hermansky-Pudlak syndrome, defective platelet aggregation is associated with oculocutaneous albinism and the accumulation of ceroid-like pigment in marrow macrophages (Fig. 13.37).

In storage pool disorders (SPD), there is defective platelet aggregation (Fig. 13.38) due to intrinsic deficiency in the number of dense granules (δ-SPD). One type of storage pool disorder, the grey platelet syndrome (Fig. 13.39), is characterized by variable thrombocytopenia and large platelets which have a specific deficiency of α-granules (α-SPD).

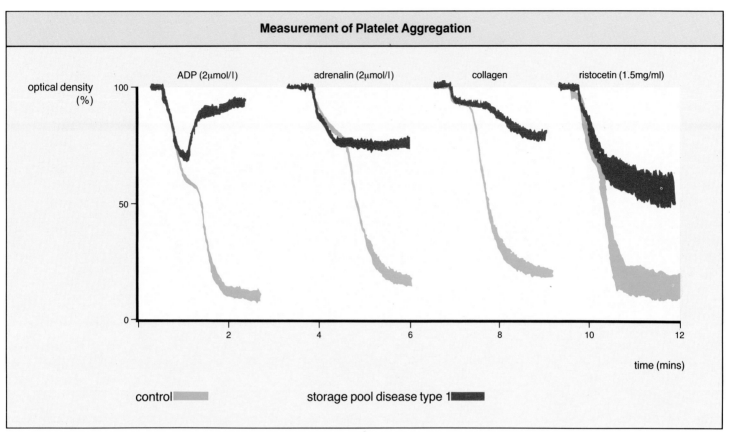

Fig. 13.38 Platelet storage pool disease: platelet aggregation studies show defective aggregation patterns with ADP (no secondary phase), adrenalin and collagen. Courtesy of Dr. R.A. Hutton.

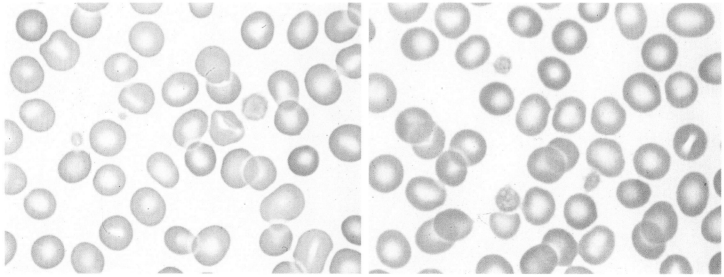

Fig. 13.39 Grey platelet syndrome: typical large platelets which lack normal α-granules. Courtesy of Dr. P.C. Shrivastava.

In von Willebrand's disease, in addition to a platelet function defect there is low factor VIII clotting activity. The primary defect appears to be reduced synthesis of the major structural component of the factor VIII molecules, VIII–Ag, resulting in defective platelet adhesion and defective *in vitro* aggregation activity with ristocetin (Fig.13.40).

Acquired disorders

Intrinsic abnormalities of platelet function are found in many patients with essential thrombocythaemia (see Fig.12.34) and other myeloproliferative diseases, uraemia, liver disease and hyperglobulinaemia. Aspirin and other non–steroidal anti–inflammatory drugs produce a platelet functional defect which often manifests as abnormal bleeding time; however, spontaneous haemorrhage during therapy, except for gastric mucosal bleeding due to erosions, is not common.

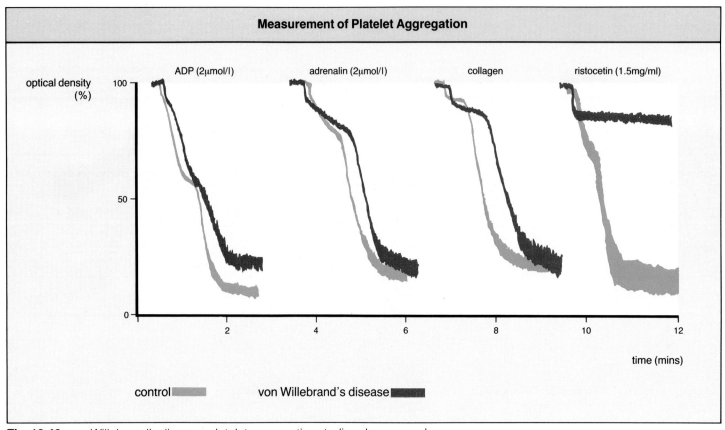

Fig.13.40 von Willebrand's disease: platelet aggregation studies show normal aggregation patterns with ADP, adrenalin and collagen but no aggregation with ristocetin. Courtesy of Dr. R.A. Hutton.

14
COAGULATION DISORDERS

Following the initiation of blood coagulation, the coagulation factor enzymes are activated sequentially. There are a number of essential cofactors and the final steps involve the conversion of soluble plasma fibrinogen into fibrin by thrombin (Fig. 14.1).

HEREDITARY COAGULATION DISORDERS
Most inherited coagulation disorders involve deficiency of a single factor, deficiencies of factor VIII (haemophilia A; von Willebrand's disease) and IX (haemophilia B) being the most common. All other hereditary disorders are rare.

Haemophilia
In haemophilia A there is an absence or a low level of plasma factor VIII clotting activity (VIII:C) due either to defective synthesis of the clotting component of the factor VIII molecule or to synthesis of a structurally abnormal molecule (Fig. 14.2). At this time, six different genetic lesions have been detected in various haemophilia kindreds. These include three different single point mutations, in all of which the stop codon TGA (thymine-guanine-adenine) has been introduced by substitution of the base cytosine (C) with thymine (T) and three different types of deletion. In two of

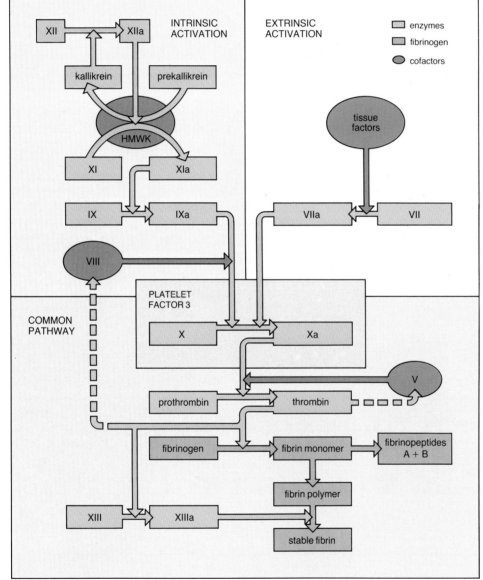

Fig. 14.1 The coagulation pathway.

HMWK = high molecular weight
               kininogen.

The interrupted arrows indicate feedback-inhibitory pathways.

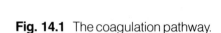

Fig. 14.2 Gene for factor VIII clotting factor: there are 26 exons which code for the active protein separated by 25 non-coding sequences (introns) and a total of 189 kilobases, producing a protein of 2332 amino acids of molecular weight 360,000. The initial RNA transcript is from both the exons and introns; the latter are then removed by excision and ligation (splicing) so that mature mRNA represents only the exons. This transfers to ribosomes via transfer RNA in the cytoplasm. Courtesy of Dr. E.G.D. Tuddenham.

14.2

the cases with single point mutations and two with deletions, the patients had developed a factor VIII inhibitor in plasma. Normal amounts of the major structural component of the molecule (VIIIR:AG) are present and the part concerned with platelet vessel wall interaction is unaffected.

In haemophilia B (Christmas disease) there is either absence of factor IX or a structurally abnormal factor IX molecule. The inheritance of both haemophilias is sex-linked (Fig. 14.3).

Major haemorrhage of the joints is the dominant problem in severe haemophilia A or B and most frequently affects the knees, elbows, ankles and wrists, but other synovial joints may also be involved. There is usually severe pain and the affected joint is tender, warm and may be grossly distended (Figs. 14.4 & 14.5). Chronic joint haemorrhage results in degenerative joint changes and mechanical derangement of articular surfaces (Figs. 14.6 & 14.7).

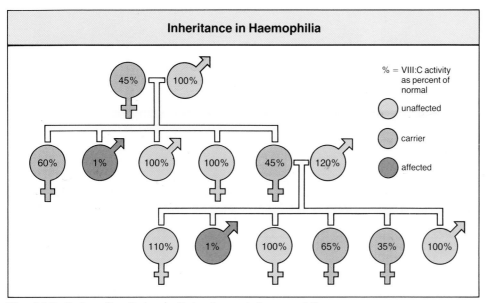

Fig. 14.3 Pattern (family tree) of inheritance in haemophilia.

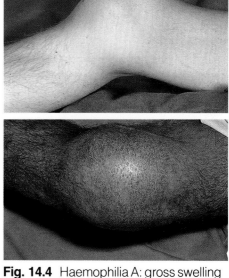

Fig. 14.4 Haemophilia A: gross swelling due to acute haemarthroses of the right (upper) and left (lower) knee joints.

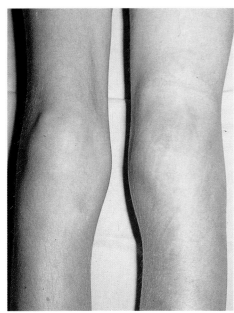

Fig. 14.5 Haemophilia A: acute haemarthroses of the left knee joint with swelling of the suprapatellar area. There is wasting of the quadriceps muscles particularly on the right.

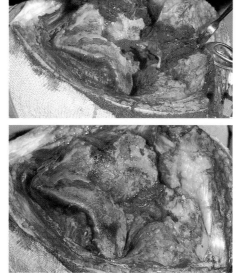

Fig. 14.6 Haemophilia A: (upper) opened knee joint showing the femoral condyles and hypertrophied haemosiderin-stained synovium. Widespread erosion of the articular cartilage has exposed large areas of haemosiderin-stained bone; (lower) removal of the synovium of the suprapatellar pouch and of the patella exposes the grossly damaged femoral articular surface.

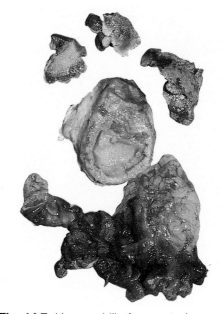

Fig. 14.7 Haemophilia A: resected material from the knee in Fig. 14.6 included (from top to bottom) osteophytes from the arthritic femoral condyles, the patella which shows haemosiderin-stained articular cartilage and secondary arthritic changes, and a portion of grossly haemosiderin-stained synovium of the suprapatellar pouch.

Demineralization, loss of articular cartilage, bone lipping and osteophyte formation produce deformity and crippling (Figs. 14.8 & 14.9). The end result in poorly treated patients is permanent fixation of the affected joint or flexion deformities (Figs. 14.10 & 14.11).

Traumatic and spontaneous soft tissue haemorrhage is another feature of haemophilia (Figs. 14.12-14.15). Dissecting haematomas may involve large areas of muscle or deep fascial layers (Fig. 14.16). Haemorrhage into retroperitoneal fascial spaces or into the psoas muscle may produce consider-

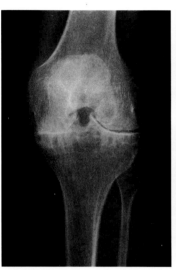
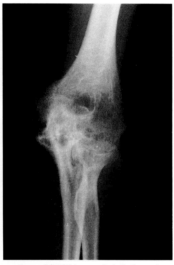

Fig. 14.8 Haemophilia A: radiographs of (left) knee joint showing marked narrowing of the joint space, particularly medially, a widened intercondylar notch, prominent osteoarthritic changes and subchondral cyst formation. There is erosion of the upper lateral border of the tibial plateau; (right) elbow joint showing marked joint space narrowing, enlargement of the radial head, secondary osteoarthritic features and subchondral cyst formation.

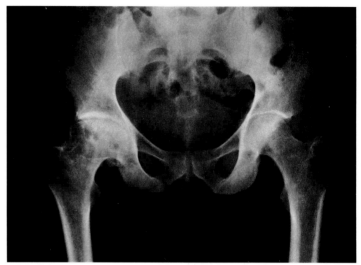

Fig. 14.9 Haemophilia A: radiograph of pelvis showing marked destruction and deformation of the right acetabulum and femoral head. There are numerous subchondral cysts, and shortening and widening of the right femoral neck.

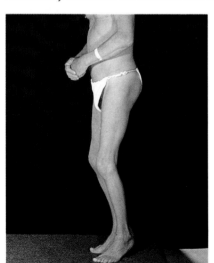

Fig. 14.10 Haemophilia A: flexion deformities of the elbow, hip, knee and ankle joints following a 35-year history of multiple haemarthroses.

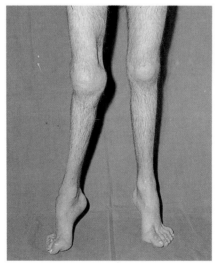

Fig. 14.11 Haemophilia A: gross crippling. The right knee is swollen with posterior subluxation of the tibia on the femur. The ankles and feet show residual deformities of talipes equinus and some degree of cavus and associated toe clawing. Generalized muscle wasting is most marked on the right. The scar on the medial side of the right lower thigh is the site of a previously excised 'pseudotumour'.

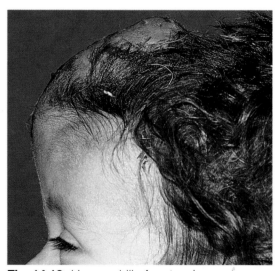

Fig. 14.12 Haemophilia A: extensive post-traumatic haematoma of the forehead in an infant.

able problems in differential diagnosis (Figs. 14.17–14.20) as associated pain, tenderness and fever may suggest other causes of the acute abdomen.

Haemophilic 'pseudotumours' are a serious complication of extensive fascial or subperiosteal haemorrhage. These blood-filled multiloculated cysts may cause extensive destruction of both soft tissue (Fig. 14.21) and bone (Figs. 14.22 & 14.23) as their size increases.

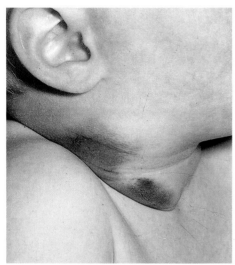

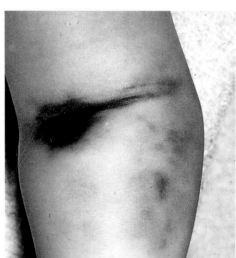

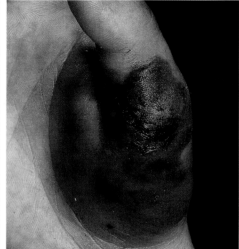

Fig. 14.13 Haemophilia B: extensive haemorrhage into the soft tissues of the neck following venepuncture of the external jugular vein.

Fig. 14.14 Haemophilia B: (left) extensive subcutaneous haemorrhage about the elbow joint of an infant following venepuncture; (right) extensive bleeding into the thenar muscles and overlying subcutaneous tissue.

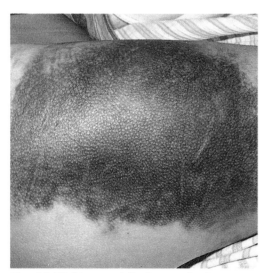

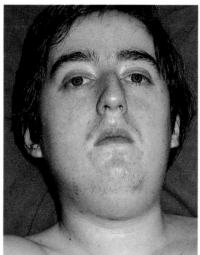

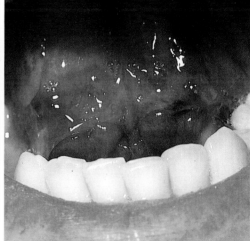

Fig. 14.15 Haemophilia A: massive haemorrhage in the area of the right buttock following an intramuscular injection.

Fig. 14.16 Haemophilia A: (left) marked submandibular swelling due to a large haemorrhage in the sublingual tissues; (right) the most superficial part of the sublingual haemorrhage shows clearly beneath the mucosa of the floor of the mouth.

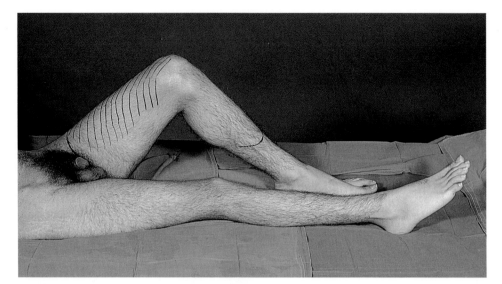

Fig. 14.17 Haemophilia A: acute retroperitoneal haemorrhage into the left psoas muscle. The lines indicate an area of anaesthesia over the distribution of the femoral nerve. There was also weakness of the quadriceps muscle and a flexion contracture at the left hip.

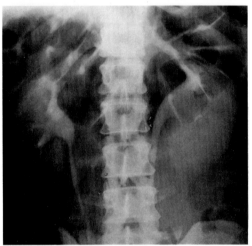

Fig. 14.18 Haemophilia A: IVP (intravenous pyelogram) showing acute retroperitoneal haemorrhage. A soft tissue mass in the left flank has caused medial rotation of the left kidney and anteromedial displacement of the ureter.

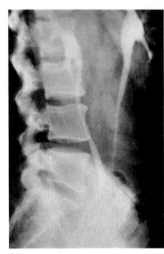

Fig. 14.19 Haemophilia A: lateral view IVP (same patient as in Fig. 14.18) confirms the anterior displacement of both the kidney and ureter.

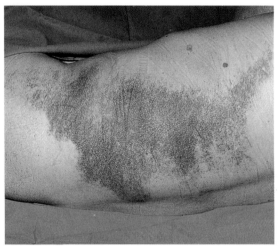

Fig. 14.20 Haemophilia A: acute retroperitoneal haemorrhage (same patient as in Fig. 14.18). The extensive subcutaneous bruising of the left flank appeared 24 hours after presentation.

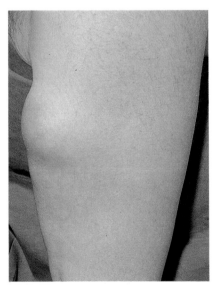

Fig. 14.21 Haemophilia A: 'pseudotumour' of the biceps. This is, in fact, a hard residual encapsulated swelling following incomplete resolution and repair of previous muscle haemorrhage.

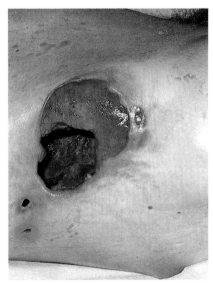

Fig. 14.22 Haemophilia A: large ulcer overlying the entrance to a multiloculated and cavernous pseudotumour of the right iliac bone and overlying soft tissues.

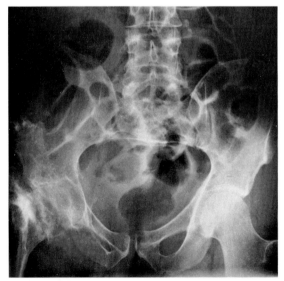

Fig. 14.23 Haemophilia A: pelvic radiograph (same patient as in Fig. 14.22). The pseudotumour has destroyed a large area of the wing of the right iliac bone, including the anterior crest. There is obliteration of the hip joint space on the right and an ununited fracture of the femoral neck with resultant pseudoarthrosis, gross deformity and shortening.

Ischaemic contractures may follow extensive haemorrhage into the muscles of the limbs (Fig. 14.24), for example, Volkmann's contracture of the forearm (Fig. 14.25). Prolonged bleeding occurs after dental extractions and operative haemorrhage is life-threatening in both severely and mildly affected patients. Spontaneous intracranial haemorrhage (Fig. 14.26), although an infrequent cause of bleeding in individuals, remains the most common cause of death in severe haemophilia.

von Willebrand's disease

There is defective synthesis of the high molecular weight fraction of factor VIII, factor VIII-antigen (von Willebrand's factor). This protein is an oligomer of units, each of molecular weight 210,000. It carries factor VIII-coagulation factor and is itself essential for adhesion of platelets to damaged vessel walls (see Fig. 13.4).

The inheritance pattern of von Willebrand's disease in most patients is autosomal dominant. The disorder is characterized by operative and post-traumatic haemorrhage (Fig. 14.27), mucous membrane bleeding and excessive blood loss from superficial cuts and abrasions. Spontaneous haemarthroses and arthritic changes are rare, occurring only in homozygous patients (Fig. 14.28).

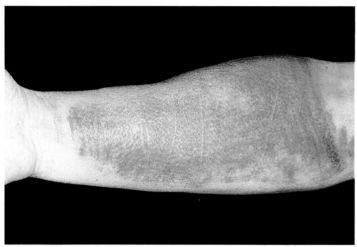

Fig. 14.24 Haemophilia B: subcutaneous bruising and extensive haemorrhage into the flexor muscles and associated soft tissues of the right forearm.

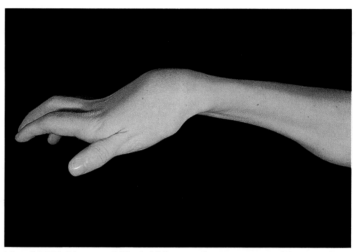

Fig. 14.25 Haemophilia A: Volkmann's contracture. The wasting and flexion deformities are a result of extensive repair and stricture formation in muscles damaged by repeated haematomas.

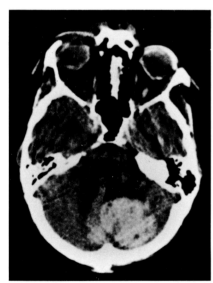

Fig. 14.26 Haemophilia A: CT (computerized tomographic) scan showing a large haematoma of the right cerebellum.

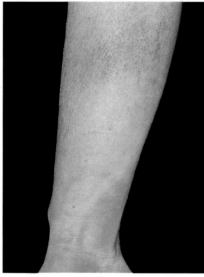

Fig. 14.27 von Willebrand's disease: subcutaneous bruising overlying haemorrhage into the muscles and soft tissues of the left forearm.

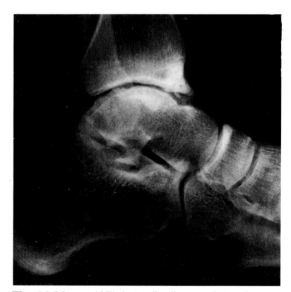

Fig. 14.28 von Willebrand's disease: lateral radiograph of ankle joint showing loss of joint space, marginal sclerosis and a small subchondral cyst in the tibial epiphysis.

Other hereditary coagulation disorders

Patients with inherited defects of coagulation factors other than VIII or IX often show easy bruising and spontaneous and excessive post-traumatic bleeding. Spontaneous haemarthroses and soft tissue haematomas are, however, most unusual.

INHERITED THROMBOTIC DISORDERS
Protein C deficiency

Protein C is a vitamin K-dependent plasma protein synthesized by the liver. Its active form inhibits the active forms of coagulation factor V and VIII, and also increases lysis of clots by inactivating a protein which normally destroys tissue plasminogen activator. Activation of protein C occurs via thrombin bound to a protein thrombomodulin on the surface of the endothelial cell (Fig. 14.29).

Partial protein C deficiency predisposes affected individuals to recurrent venous thromboses, which tend to present at an early age, usually below the age of thirty. Homozygous protein C deficiency results in neonatal purpura fulminans, characterized by superficial thromboses. The skin lesions are initially swollen and red or purple; they become blue–black and may necrose (Fig. 14.30). The blood shows features of disseminated intravascular coagulation with low levels of factors V and VIII, antithrombin III, fibrinogen and platelets.

Protein S deficiency

Activation of protein C requires a cofactor, protein S. This is also vitamin K-dependent and exists in plasma as free and bound forms. Protein S deficiency, inherited probably as a dominant gene, presents as recurrent venous thromboses.

Antithrombin III deficiency

Antithrombin III is a potent inhibitor of the activated (a) serum proteases factor XIIa, XIa, Xa and IXa, VIIa and thrombin. It forms high molecular weight inactive complexes with these proteins. Deficiency of antithrombin III leads to recurrent venous thromboses which tend to be severe and present early in the homozygous form. The action of antithrombin III is potentiated by heparin.

ACQUIRED COAGULATION DISORDERS

In clinical practice the acquired coagulation disorders (Fig. 14.31) are seen more often than the inherited disorders. Unlike the inherited diseases, there are usually multiple clotting factor deficiences. Bleeding episodes due to vitamin K deficiency, overdosage with oral anticoagulants or in association with liver disease and with disseminated intravascular coagulation are seen most frequently.

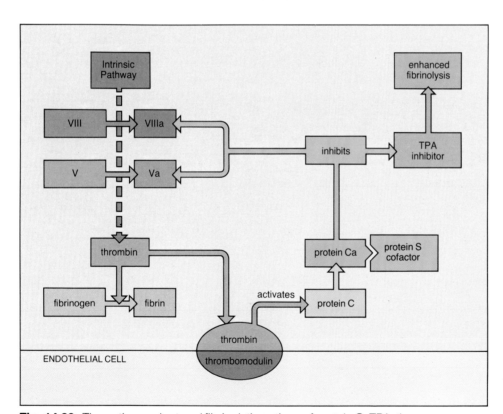

Fig. 14.29 The anticoagulant and fibrinolytic actions of protein C: TPA, tissue plasminogen activator; a, activated.

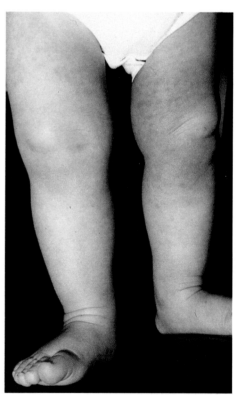

Fig. 14.30 Homozygous protein C deficiency: this 15-month-old infant presented in the first year of life with superficial discolored areas over the buttocks and lower limbs which disappeared with infusions of fresh plasma. In this case the lesions are milder than usual as, typically, there is purpura fulminans with skin necrosis (see Fig. 14.36). Courtesy of Dr. A. Awidi.

Liver disease

Liver cell immaturity and lack of vitamin K synthesis in the gut are the principal causes of haemorrhagic disease of the newborn. In adults, vitamin K deficiency may be the result of obstructive jaundice, pancreatic or small bowel disease. Multiple haemostatic abnormalities contribute to increased surgical bleeding and may exacerbate haemorrhage from oesophageal varices. Biliary obstruction results in impaired absorption of vitamin K and decreased synthesis of factors II, VII, IX and X by the liver parenchymal cells. The hypersplenism associated with portal hypertension frequently results in thrombocytopenia. Patients in liver failure have deficiency of factor V, variable abnormalities of platelet function and often produce functionally abnormal fibrinogen. As well as variceal bleeding and increased loss of blood during surgery, patients with severe liver disease may also suffer from spontaneous superficial haemorrhage (Figs. 14.32 & 14.33).

Overdosage with anticoagulants

Overdosage with oral anticoagulants which are vitamin K antagonists results in severe deficiencies of coagulation factors II, VII, IX and X. Patients may present with extensive skin bruising (Fig. 14.34) or severe internal bleeding (Fig. 14.35).

Acquired Coagulation Disorders

Liver disease

Deficiency of vitamin K-dependent factors:
 haemorrhagic disease of the newborn;
 biliary obstruction;
 malabsorption of vitamin K, e.g. sprue, coeliac disease;
 vitamin K-antagonist therapy, e.g. coumarins, indanediones

Disseminated intravascular coagulation

Inhibition of coagulation:
 specific inhibitors. e.g. antibodies against factor VIII components;
 non-specific inhibitors, e.g. antibodies found in systemic lupus erythematosus, rheumatoid arthritis

Miscellaneous:
 diseases with M-protein production;
 L-asparaginase;
 therapy with heparin, defibrinating agents or thrombolytics;
 massive transfusion syndrome

Fig. 14.31 The acquired coagulation disorders.

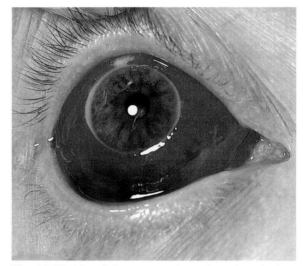

Fig. 14.32 Liver failure: extensive subconjunctival haemorrhage.

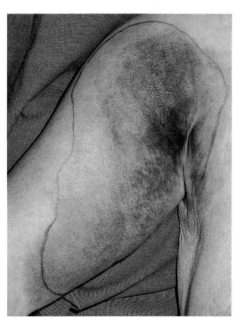

Fig. 14.33 Liver failure: subcutaneous haemorrhage of the upper arm following minor trauma. Laboratory tests revealed deficiences of factors II, VII, IX and X as well as dysfibrinogenaemia.

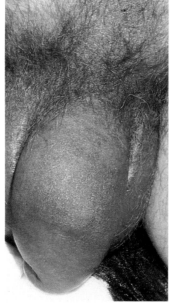

Fig. 14.34 Warfarin overdose: massive subcutaneous haemorrhage over the penis, scrotal and pubic areas following sexual intercourse.

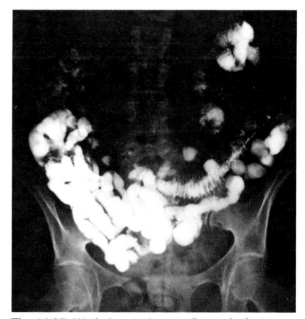

Fig. 14.35 Warfarin overdose: radiograph shows intramural bleeding in the small intestine with the characteristic 'stacked coin' pattern of barium distribution. Courtesy of Dr. D. Nag.

Similar skin lesions to those seen in homozygous protein C deficiency may occur in patients commencing anticoagulant therapy with coumarin drugs. Temporarily there may be selective severe protein C deficiency before the levels of the vitamin K-dependent clotting factors fall (Fig. 14.36).

Disseminated intravascular coagulation

Disseminated intravascular coagulation (DIC) is a consequence of many disorders causing widespread endothelial damage, platelet aggregation or release of procoagulant material into the circulation (Fig. 14.37). It is associated with widespread intravascular deposition of fibrin and consump-

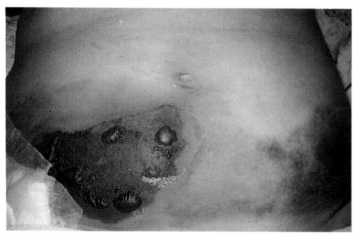

Fig. 14.36 Warfarin skin necrosis: these lesions over the abdomen and chest developed in the first few days of warfarin therapy in a 40-year-old female. Her protein C level was not measured but, in more recent examples of coumarin-induced skin necrosis, patients subsequently have been found to have reduced plasma levels of protein C. Courtesy of Dr. S. J. Machin.

Conditions Associated with Disseminated Intravascular Coagulation	

Infections:
    Gram-negative & meningococcal
      septicaemia;
    septic abortion & *Clostridium*
      welchii septicaemia;
    severe falciparum malaria;
    viral infection (purpura fulminans)
 	
 Malignancy:
    widespread mucin-secreting
      adenocarcinoma;
    acute promyelocytic leukaemia
 	
 Obstetric complications:
    amniotic fluid embolism;
    premature separation of placenta;
    eclampsia; retained placenta
	Hypersensitivity reactions:
	    anaphylaxis;
	    incompatible blood transfusion
	
	 Widespread tissue damage:
	    following surgery or trauma
	
	 Miscellaneous:
	    liver failure;
	    snake & invertebrate venoms;
	    severe burns;
	    hypothermia;
	    heat stroke;
	    hypoxia;
	    vascular malformations
	      (Kasabach-Merritt syndrome)

Fig. 14.37 Causes of disseminated intravascular coagulation.

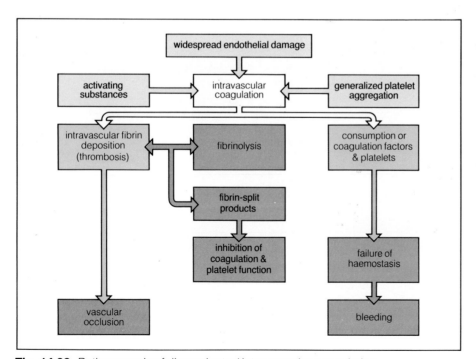

Fig. 14.38 Pathogenesis of disseminated intravascular coagulation.

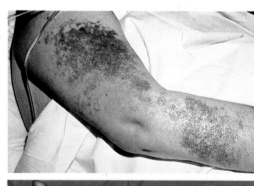
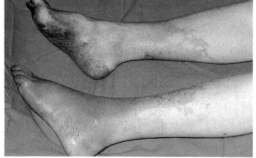

Fig. 14.39 Disseminated intravascular coagulation: (upper) indurated and confluent purpura of the arm; (lower) peripheral gangrene with swelling and discoloration of the skin of the feet in fulminant disease.

tion of coagulation factors and platelets (Fig. 14.38). This may lead to both abnormal bleeding and widespread thrombosis which is often fulminant (Figs. 14.39–14.42; see also Chapter 13), although it can run a less severe and chronic course.

In the Kasabach-Merritt syndrome, a congenital haemangioma is associated with DIC (Fig. 14.43). The stimulus to intravascular coagulation is local but the enhanced proteolytic activity of both coagulation and fibrinolytic systems probably becomes disseminated throughout the blood.

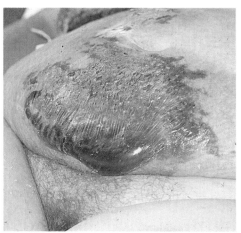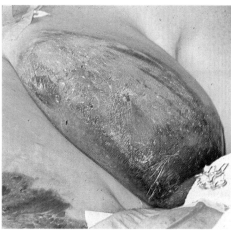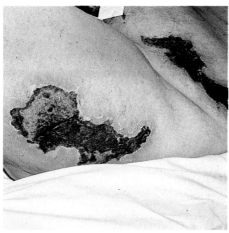

Fig. 14.40 Disseminated intravascular coagulation: extensive necrosis of the skin and subcutaneous tissues of the (left) lower abdominal wall and (right) the breast in a grossly obese patient. Courtesy of Dr. B. B. Berkeley.

Fig. 14.41 Disseminated intravascular coagulation: later stages of skin necrosis (same patient as in Fig. 14.40). Loss of superficial necrotic tissue over the thigh and lateral abdominal wall has left large deep irregular ulcers with haemorrhagic areas of exposed tissue. Courtesy of Dr. B.B. Berkeley.

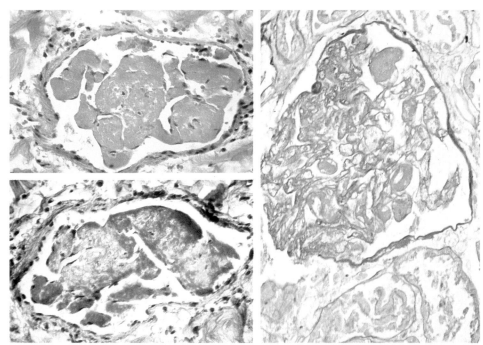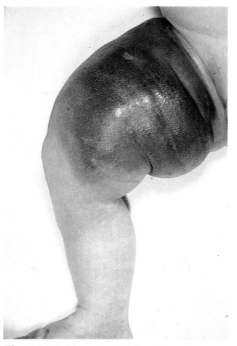

Fig. 14.42 Disseminated intravascular coagulation: sections through a skin venule deep to an area of necrosis shows occlusion by a thrombus composed mainly of fibrin. Haematoxylin and eosin (upper left) and Martius scarlet-blue (lower left) stains; (right) necrosis of the glomerulus and the surrounding tubules with variable amounts of fibrinous material in the glomerular blood vessels. Periodic acid-Schiff stain.

Fig. 14.43 Kasabach-Merritt syndrome: this giant congenital haemangioma of the thigh was associated with disseminated intravascular coagulation.

Acquired coagulation factor inhibitor

Occasionally, patients present with a bleeding syndrome (Fig. 14.44) caused by circulating antibodies to coagulation factor VIII or to other clotting factors. These antibodies usually occur *post partum*, in systemic lupus erythematosus (SLE) and in old age.

Patients with SLE and other autoimmune disorders and, rarely, infections may also develop a less specific inhibitor, IgG or IgM, which is directed against phospholipid and is associated with a prolongation of the partial thromboplastin time which is not corrected by normal plasma. The patient with this 'lupus anticoagulant' may have no clinical symptoms, or may thrombose or bleed excessively.

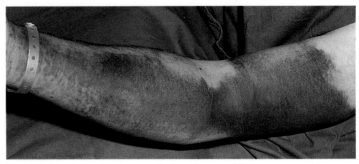

Fig. 14.44   Acquired coagulation factor inhibitor: extensive subcutaneous and deep soft tissue haemorrhage in the arm due to an acquired circulating autoantibody to factor VIII.

15

BONE MARROW IN NON-HAEMOPOIETIC DISEASES

The bone marrow may be involved in a number of disorders which are not primary diseases of the haemopoietic system. Bone marrow aspirates or trephine biopsies may be used to assess bone marrow involvement after the primary diagnosis has been made from material taken from other sites or may be responsible for the primary diagnosis itself.

METASTATIC BONE TUMOURS

The most common malignant tumours of bone are metastatic deposits from primary sites elsewhere in the body. Carcinomas of the breast, lung, kidney, thyroid and prostate are very likely to involve the marrow (Figs.15.1-15.3); involvement of the stomach (Fig.15.4), pancreas, colon (Fig.15.5) and rectum occur less frequently, but virtually any malignant tumour may metastasize to bone. The initial diagnosis may be made during bone marrow examination particularly when the primary site of malignancy is not obvious.

In advanced disease, leucoerythroblastic changes may be found in the blood film; there may also be evidence of bone marrow failure. The skeletal lesions are predominantly osteolytic, presenting as radiolucent areas on radiographic examination (Fig.15.6). Extensive osteoclastic resorption of bone is often found in trephine biopsies (Fig.15.7). Almost all tumours provoke some degree of bone healing and sometimes new bone deposition; osteoblastic activity is most pronounced in metastatic spread from carcinoma of the prostate (Fig.15.8) and the breast (Fig.15.9).

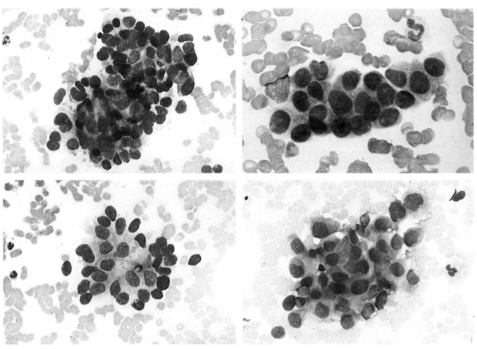

Fig. 15.1 Metastatic carcinoma: (left) clusters of malignant epithelial cells in bone marrow. Further investigation revealed a primary tumour in the prostate; (upper right) an isolated group of small, fairly uniform, malignant epithelial cells. The primary lung tumour was an 'oat cell' carcinoma; (lower right) a clump of epithelial cells with features of a large undifferentiated cell carcinoma. The primary carcinoma was of the breast.

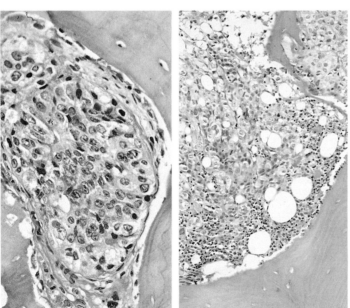

Fig. 15.2 Metastatic carcinoma: replacement of normal haemopoietic tissue in the intertrabecular areas (left) by nests of malignant epithelial cells (same case as in Fig.15.1, left) and (right) by sheets of pleomorphic neoplastic epithelial cells. The primary carcinoma was of the kidney.

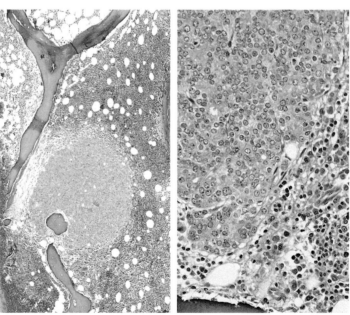

Fig. 15.3 Metastatic carcinoma: (left) a prominent paratrabecular deposit of neoplastic epithelial cells. The patient had chronic lymphocytic leukaemia and a primary carcinoma of the prostate; (right) higher power shows a clear separation of malignant epithelial tissue from haemopoietic tissue containing increased numbers of lymphocytes.

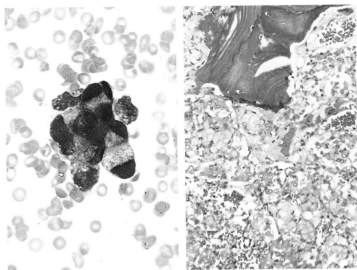

Fig. 15.4 Metastatic carcinoma: (left) a clump of distended and vacuolated neoplastic epithelial cells in a patient with micro-angiopathic haemolytic anaemia and laboratory evidence of disseminated intravascular coagulation; (right) sheets and acini of mucin-secreting adenocarcinoma in the same patient with a primary tumour of the stomach.

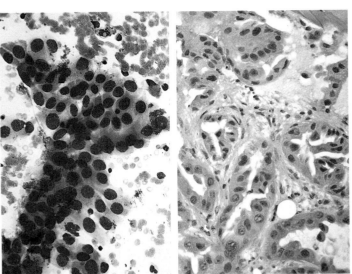

Fig. 15.5 Metastatic carcinoma: (left) a sheet of neoplastic columnar cells in bone marrow; (right) replacement of normal haemopoietic tissue by acini of neoplastic columnar cells. The primary carcinoma was of the ascending colon.

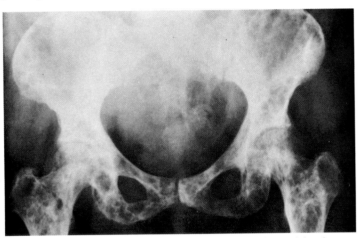

Fig. 15.6 Metastatic carcinoma: radiograph of the pelvis of a 58-year-old man with carcinoma of the lung. Metastatic deposits from the tumour have produced widespread lytic lesions, most marked in the lower pelvis and upper parts of the femurs.

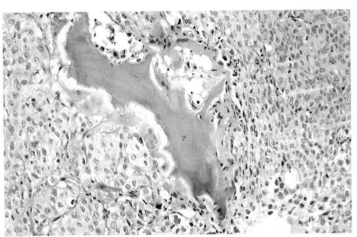

Fig. 15.7 Metastatic carcinoma: metastatic deposits from a carinoma of the kidney. Sheets of neoplastic epithelial cells surround residual trabecular bone with osteoclasts adjacent to the scalloped edges.

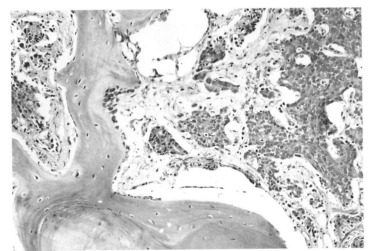

Fig. 15.8 Metastatic carcinoma: there is thickening of medullary trabecular bone and osteoblasts are prominent along the right-hand margin of the vertical trabecula. The intertrabecular space contains nests of malignant epithelial cells supported by an abundant fibrous stroma. The patient had carcinoma of the prostate.

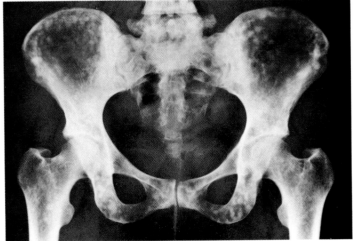

Fig. 15.9 Metastatic carcinoma: radiograph of the pelvis of a 45-year-old woman with carcinoma of the breast. The widespread foci of increased bone density are the result of osteoblastic activity surrounding metastases.

15.3

Occasionally, fragments of skin epidermis are carried into the marrow cavity during trephine biopsy (Fig. 15.10), but the well differentiated nature of such fragments allows easy distinction from metastatic carcinoma.

Involvement of bone marrow by tumours other than carcinomas also occurs. Figs. 15.11 to 15.13 demonstrate involvement by malignant melanoma, neuroblastoma and medulloblastoma. Bone marrow involvement due to malignant lymphomas and histiocytic proliferative disorders is discussed in Chapter 10. Although the majority of primary bone tumours do not metastasize to parts of the skeleton distant from their origin, bone marrow examination may reveal evidence of dissemination in Ewing's tumour of bone (Fig. 15.14).

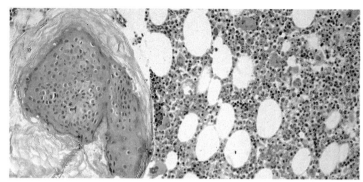

Fig. 15.10 Artefact on trephine biopsy: a small fragment of well differentiated keratinized squamous epithelium has been carried into the bone marrow cavity. Normal haemopoietic tissue is on the right.

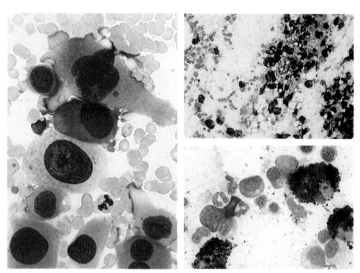

Fig. 15.11 Metastatic malignant melanoma: (left) large malignant melanoma cells of variable size with primitive chromatin patterns and nucleoli; (upper right) low and (lower right) higher power show no malignant cells but numerous melanin-filled macrophages are evident. The patient had a malignant melanoma on the skin of the back.

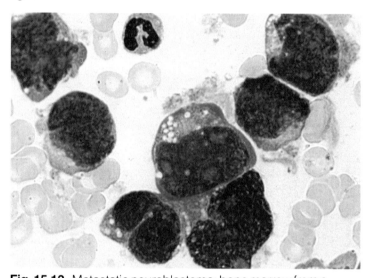

Fig. 15.12 Metastatic neuroblastoma: bone marrow from a 3-year-old boy with neuroblastoma in the right thorax shows malignant 'neuroblasts'. These are somewhat larger and more pleomorphic than haemopoietic blast cells and have fine chromatin patterns and prominent nucleoli. Neuroblastoma cells are often seen as small clumps in a 'rosette' arrangement (not shown).

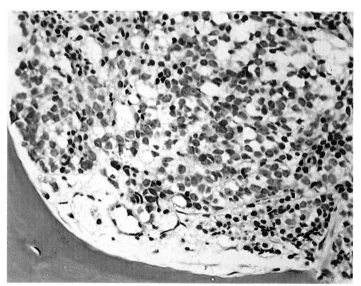

Fig. 15.13 Metastatic medulloblastoma: extensive replacement of haemopoietic tissue by a sheet of small primitive cells with round nuclei, open chromatin patterns and scanty cytoplasm. The young patient presented with a midline cerebellar tumour diagnosed as a medulloblastoma.

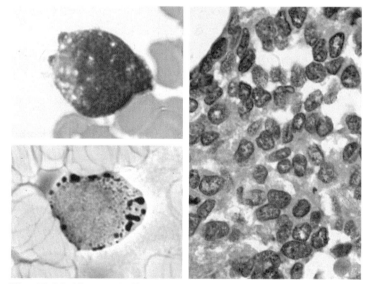

Fig. 15.14 Metastatic Ewing's sarcoma of the femur: (left) isolated tumour cells with fine open chromatin patterns and thin rims of vacuolated basophilic cytoplasm. The lower cell shows coarse granules of PAS-positive material; (right) a sheet-like deposit of rather uniform primitive cells with poorly defined nucleoli and inconspicuous cytoplasmic outlines. Two mitotic figures are seen.

MAST CELL DISEASE

Systemic mastocytosis is a rare disease of adults in which a persistent and progressive cutaneous eruption is a characteristic presentation (Fig. 15.15). Radiography usually reveals multiple, irregularly rounded, lytic lesions or new bone formation in the skeleton. In severe cases there may be lymphadenopathy, hepatosplenomegaly and extensive infiltration of the bone marrow by mast cells (Fig. 15.16). Evidence of disease may also be found at splenectomy (Fig. 15.17). Disease confined to the skin and bone is frequently associated with prolonged survival; but patients who develop extensive reticuloendothelial involvement often die soon after diagnosis.

GRANULOMATOUS DISEASE
Sarcoidosis

This granulomatous disorder of unknown aetiology most frequently affects the middle-aged. It is characterized by widespread epithelioid cell granulomas, depression of delayed hypersensitivity and lymphoproliferation. Multisystemic involvement is characteristic with intrathoracic disease affecting ninety percent of patients, ocular and skin involvement in about twenty-five percent each, and erythema nodosum in up to a third of cases. In different series, the reticuloendothelial system was involved in up to forty percent of patients. Evidence of disease may be found during bone marrow examination (Fig. 15.18) or at splenectomy (Fig. 15.19).

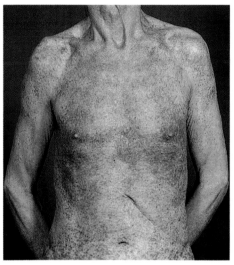

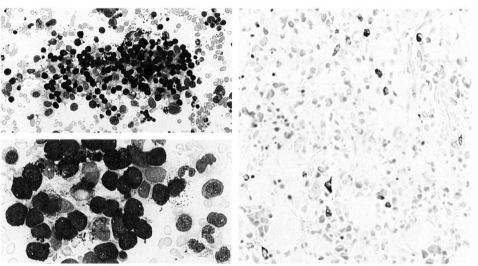

Fig. 15.15 Systemic mastocytosis: generalized pigmented and nodular cutaneous eruption seen after splenectomy (see Fig.15.17) and PUVA (psoralen and ultraviolet light activation) therapy.

Fig. 15.16 Systemic mastocytosis: (left) an extensive accumulation of mast cells at low and higher power; (right) the characteristic metachromatic staining reaction of the mast cells in the cytoplasm. Toluidine blue stain.

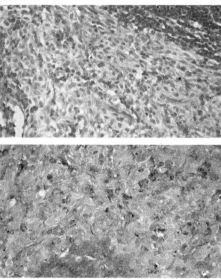

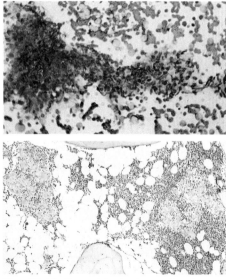

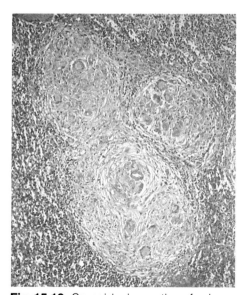

Fig. 15.17 Systemic mastocytosis: sections of spleen showing mononuclear histiocyte-like cells on staining with (upper) haematoxylin and eosin and (lower) toluidine blue to demonstrate the cytoplasmic metachromasia. Courtesy of Dr. J.E. McLaughlin.

Fig. 15.18 Sarcoidosis: (upper) a sheet of epithelioid histiocytic cells, scattered lymphocytes and myeloid cells; (lower) two small granulomas comprising epithelioid cells and lymphocytes.

Fig. 15.19 Sarcoidosis: section of spleen showing granulomatous collections of epithelioid cells including prominent multinuclear forms and peripheral lymphoid cells.

Tuberculosis

Blood-borne tubercle bacilli may lodge in the bone marrow; aspirates from patients with suspected miliary or other atypical haematogenous forms of tuberculosis may show characteristic epithelioid granulomas (Fig. 15.20). If left untreated the disease will become extensive, particularly in the anterior aspects of the vertebral bodies and in the metaphyseal areas of the long bones. The tuberculous foci may progress, producing cystic areas of osteomyelitis which erode the end plates and involve the nearby joint spaces. Tuberculous spondylitis (Pott's disease) involves the anterior aspects of the vertebral bodies with subsequent wedging and eventual collapse (Fig. 15.21).

Other granulomas

Evidence of other granulomatous disease is occasionally found during bone marrow examination. Subsequent investigations may reveal the cause of the granulomas, for example brucellosis, while, in many others, no cause is found (Fig. 15.22). Rarely, foreign body granulomas are found during routine examination of trephine biopsies (Fig. 15.23).

KALA-AZAR (VISCERAL LEISHMANIASIS)

Kala-azar is distributed widely throughout tropical and warm regions of the world. The causal organism, *Leishmania donovani*, is transmitted by the bite of sandflies of the genus *Phlebotomus*. The non-flagellated amastigote forms of the

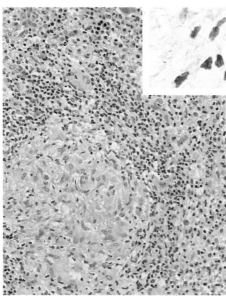

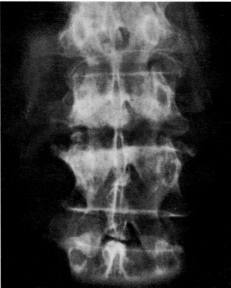

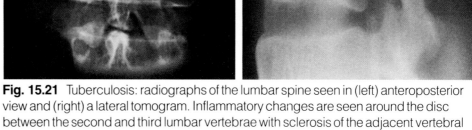

Fig. 15.20 Tuberculosis: a small granuloma surrounded by hyperplastic haemopoietic tissue; (inset) small numbers of acid-fast bacilli (Ziehl-Neelsen stain).

Fig. 15.21 Tuberculosis: radiographs of the lumbar spine seen in (left) anteroposterior view and (right) a lateral tomogram. Inflammatory changes are seen around the disc between the second and third lumbar vertebrae with sclerosis of the adjacent vertebral end plates. Courtesy of Dr. R. Dick.

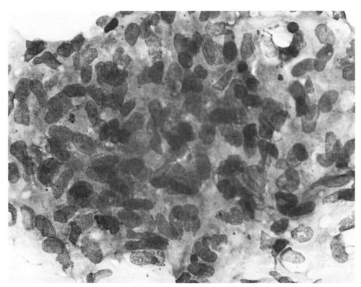

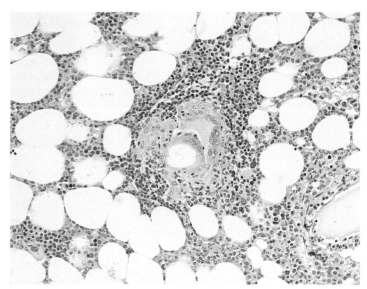

Fig. 15.22 Non-specific marrow granuloma: this small collection of epithelioid cells was found in a bone marrow cell trail which showed no other abnormality. No specific diagnosis was made.

Fig. 15.23 Foreign body granuloma: an isolated granuloma with a central large vacuole containing a refractile body of uncertain origin is surrounded by giant cells.

organism are distributed widely through reticuloendothelial macrophages in the bone marrow, spleen and liver. Diagnosis is made usually by examining bone marrow (Fig. 15.24), splenic aspirates or biopsy specimens. Clinical features include prolonged fever, lassitude, weight loss, splenomegaly, hepatomegaly, anaemia, leucopenia and polyclonal increases in immunoglobulin.

OTHER INFECTIONS

Bone marrow examination has little part to play in the diagnosis and management of osteomyelitis although, occasionally, initial evidence of a disseminated fungal infection may be uncovered (Fig. 15.25).

GAUCHER'S DISEASE

This relatively common familial disorder is characterized by the accumulation of glucocerebrosides (especially glucosylceramide) in reticuloendothelial cells because the enzyme ß-glucocerebrosidase is deficient. The chronic adult nonneuropathic form of the disease is accompanied by hepatosplenomegaly (Fig. 15.26) and bone lesions, and sometimes lymphadenopathy, skin pigmentation and pingueculae (Fig. 15.27). The most acute neuropathic forms present in infancy and survival beyond the first three years of life is rare. A juvenile form may present in childhood with features of the chronic adult form as well as progressive neurological dysfunction.

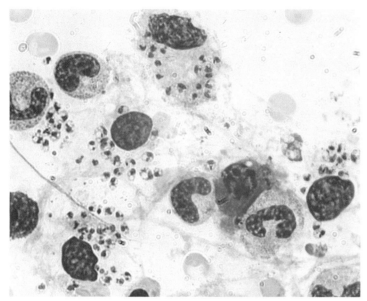

Fig. 15.24 Kala-azar (visceral leishmaniasis): bone marrow shows macrophages containing Leishman-Donovan bodies. Also seen are neutrophil metamyelocytes and a plasma cell.

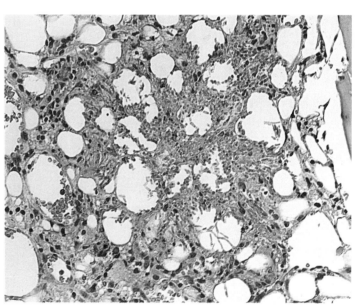

Fig. 15.25 Disseminated aspergillosis: biopsy taken after bone marrow transplantation shows hyphae of *Aspergillus* in an area of necrosis. There was also evidence of lung and liver infection.

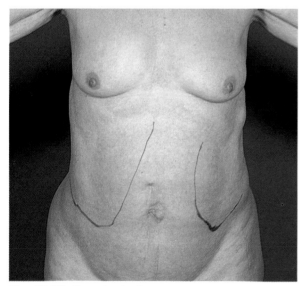

Fig. 15.26 Gaucher's disease: moderate enlargement of both the spleen and liver.

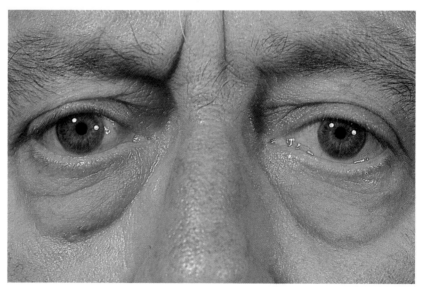

Fig. 15.27 Gaucher's disease: pingueculae, the brownish-yellow wedge-shaped thickenings of the bulbar conjunctiva.

A presumptive diagnosis of this disease may be made when Gaucher's cells are detected in marrow aspirates (Fig.15.28, left) and trephine biopsies (Fig.15.28, upper right). Diagnosis can be confirmed by demonstration of the absence or severe deficiency of the enzyme glucosylceramide ß-glucosidase in fibroblast cultures. Occasionally the diagnosis is suspected when Gaucher's cells are found after splenectomy (Fig.15.28, lower right). Most patients with this condition have elevated plasma acid phosphatase activity (which is not inhibited by L-tartrate). Over half of the adult patients have usually asymptomatic radiographic changes, such as cortical expansion of the lower end of the femur which produces a characteristic radiolucent area (Fig.15.29).

NIEMANN-PICK DISEASE

Niemann-Pick disease is a sphingomyelin lipidosis which is rarer than Gaucher's disease and is characterized by extensive tissue storage of sphingomyelin, hepatic and splenic enlargement and large lipid-filled macrophages in the bone marrow. In its best defined forms there is an inherited deficiency of the enzyme sphingomyelinase, and sphingomyelin concentration in the tissues is up to one hundred times higher than normal. As in Gaucher's disease, there are acute neuropathic and chronic non-neuropathic forms.

This diagnosis is suspected in young children with hepato-splenomegaly when bone marrow aspirates show the presence of foam cells (Fig.15.30). Confirmation is by showing low levels of sphingomyelinase in fibroblasts cultured from skin or bone marrow. In less severe adult forms of the disease, large numbers of sea-blue histiocytes may be found in bone marrow aspirates in addition to the classical foam cells (Fig.15.31).

CYSTINOSIS

In this recessively inherited disease there is deposition of cystine crystals in the reticulendothelial and corneal tissues. In its most severe form (cystinosis with Fanconi's syndrome or the de Toni-Fanconi-Lignac syndrome) there is progressive renal degeneration which is fatal during early childhood. Children with this syndrome usually present with anorexia, thirst, polyuria, failure to thrive, rickets or photophobia. Laboratory tests reveal glycosuria, proteinuria, low serum bicarbonate, hypokalaemia or hypophosphataemia. The diagnosis is established by the demonstration of cystine crystals in macrophages in bone marrow aspirates (Fig.15.32).

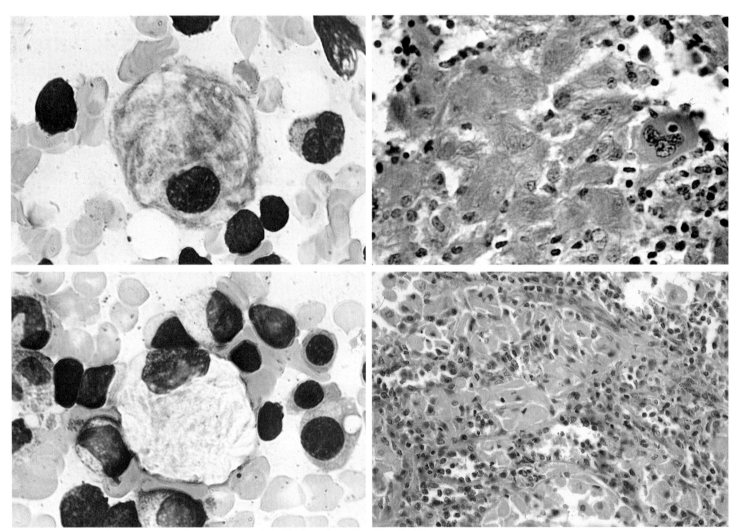

Fig. 15.28 Gaucher's disease: (left) characteristic histiocytic cells with a fibrillar or 'onion-skin' pattern of unstained inclusion material. In biopsy (upper right) these cells appear as bland histiocytes with a finely granular cytoplasmic PAS reaction. The markedly PAS-positive cell is a megakaryocyte. In the spleen (lower right) they appear as pale clusters in the reticuloendothelial cords between the venous sinuses.

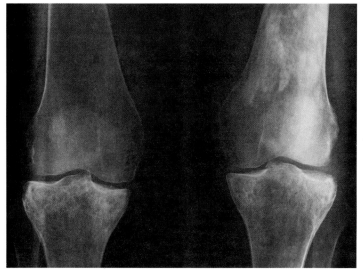

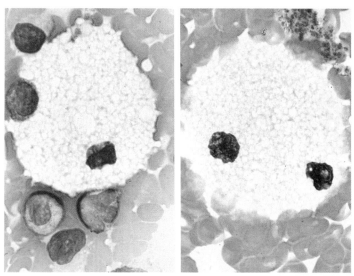

Fig. 15.29 Gaucher's disease: radiograph of the knee joints in a 45-year-old woman shows failure of correct modelling with expansion of the lower ends of the femurs. Bone thinning and loss of trabecular pattern is seen particularly in the right femur. The sclerosis in the left femur and right tibia are due to bone infarcts.

Fig. 15.30 Niemann-Pick disease: bone marrow showing histiocytic cells with foamy deposits in the cytoplasm due to lipid accumulation.

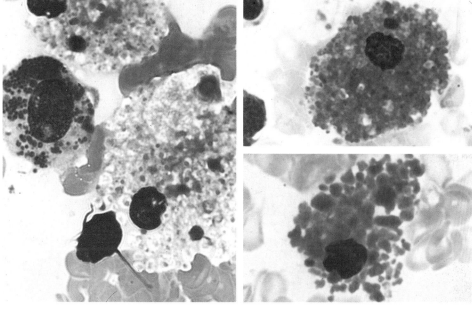

Fig. 15.31 Niemann-Pick disease (adult): bone marrow showing, in addition to the typical foam cells, prominent histiocytes with sea-blue cytoplasm (the sea-blue histiocyte syndrome)

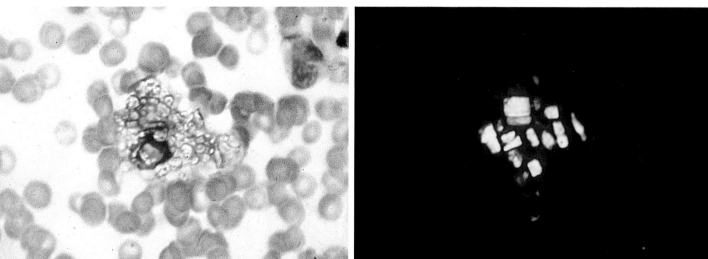

Fig. 15.32 Cystinosis: bone marrow containing (left) histiocytic cells which under polarized light (right) show the characteristic birefringence of cystine crystals.

OSTEOPETROSIS (ALBERS-SCHÖNBERG OR MARBLE BONE DISEASE)

This rare familial disorder is characterized by an increase in density of all bones due to a functional defect in osteoclasts with failure of bone resorption and remodelling. Severe forms of the disease present in infancy with anaemia and hepatosplenomegaly. These children have little or no bone marrow; haemopoiesis is chiefly extramedullary and blood transfusions are required to sustain life. The typical radio-graphic appearances are seen in Fig. 15.33; characteristic microscopic abnormalities are found in trephine bone biopsies (Figs. 15.34 & 15.35) and leucoerythroblastic changes are seen in the blood (Fig. 15.36). Failure to resorb bone results in optic atrophy, deafness and hydrocephalus. Milder cases may present later in childhood or in adult life with retarded growth, anaemia and splenomegaly (Figs. 15.37 & 15.38).

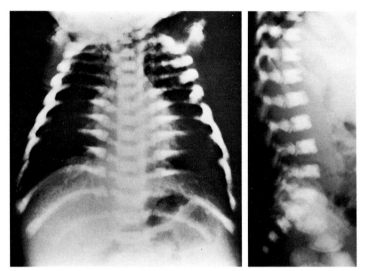

Fig. 15.33 Osteopetrosis: radiographs of the chest (left) and lower spine (right) of an infant with a gross generalized increase in bone density. The changes are most marked at the upper and lower margins of the vertebral bodies.

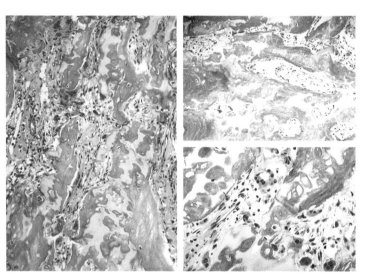

Fig. 15.34 Osteopetrosis: (left) compacted intramedullary osseous tissue and relatively little haemopoietic tissue. Cores of cartilaginous matrix are bordered by areas of primitive bone; (upper right) persistence of cartilage and lack of bone modelling; (lower right) primitive osseous tissue at the edges of and within the cartilage. Picro-Mallory stain (right).

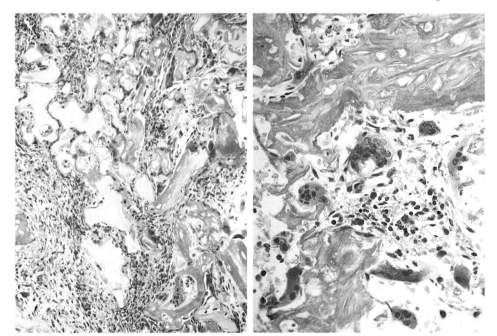

Fig. 15.35 Osteopetrosis: biopsy (same case as in Fig. 15.34) shows (left) large numbers of osteoclasts, better seen at higher power (right). There is little evidence of bone resorption, and no trabeculae or haemopoietic marrow spaces are seen. Picro-Mallory stain.

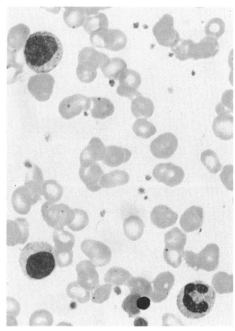

Fig. 15.36 Osteopetrosis: leucoerythro-blastic changes. The red cells show anisocytosis and poikilocytosis; the nucleated cells include a myelocyte and an erythroblast.

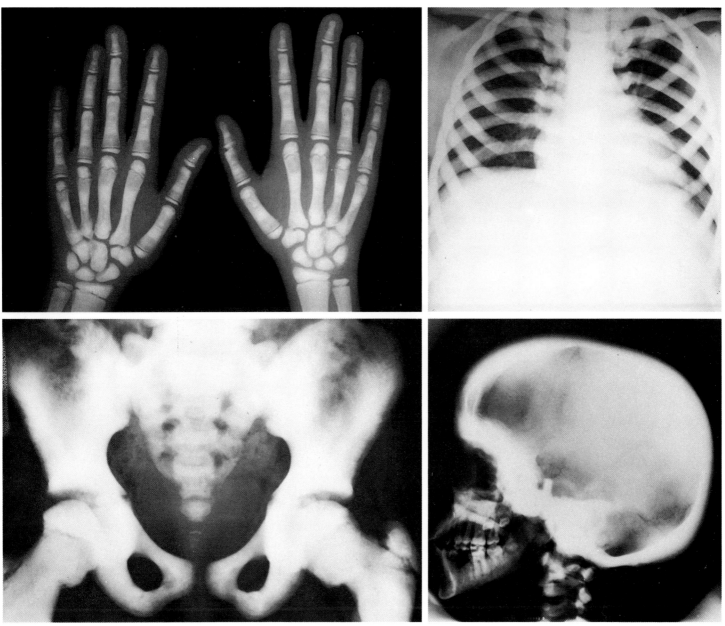

Fig. 15.37 Osteopetrosis: radiographs of the hands, chest, pelvis and skull of a 14-year-old girl who presented with retarded growth, leucoerythroblastic anaemia and massive splenomegaly. The bones are dense with coarse trabeculation and lack the usual corticomedullary demarcation. The mandible appears normal.

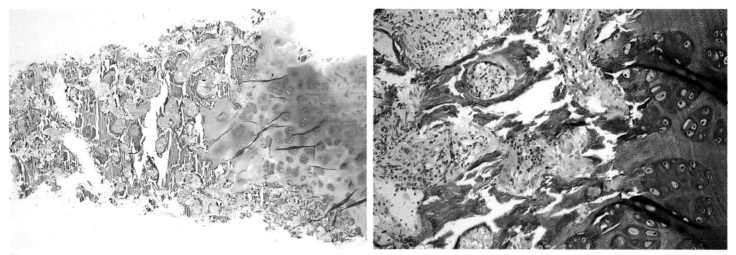

Fig. 15.38 Osteopetrosis: biopsy of the posterior iliac crest (same case as in Fig.15.37) seen at (left) low and (right) high power shows persistence of cartilage in the cortex and medulla, and architecturally disordered marrow with islands of haemopoietic tissue surounded by sheets of primitive osteochondroid material. Courtesy of Dr. J.E. McLaughlin.

AMYLOIDOSIS

Amyloidosis is a deposit of linear, non-branching, protein fibrils laid down in a pleated structure. Polysaccharides may form complexes with the protein. It occurs in a number of conditions (Fig.15.39). In cases associated with immunocyte proliferation, immunoglobulin light chains appear to be the principal protein component (see Chapter 11); in the reactive type the major protein is not derived from immunoglobulins. Polymerization of the protein subunits involved in both types yields a characteristic fibrillary structure, visible by electron microscopy, with a distinct yellow-green dichroic birefringence under polarization microscopy after Congo red staining. In some patients, particularly those with reactive systemic amyloidosis, a trephine bone marrow biopsy may reveal the first evidence of amyloidosis (Fig.15.40).

RENAL OSTEODYSTROPHY AND OSTEOMALACIA

In uraemia there is resistance to the action of vitamin D and a compensatory parathyroid hyperplasia. Characteristic changes are found in the bony architecture on trephine biopsy examination (Figs.15.41 & 15.42). In mild disease the lesions are predominantly osteomalacic. Microscopically the trabeculae are increased in thickness and in number, and the osteoid seams have defective mineralization. A similar picture is seen in dietary vitamin D deficiency. In severe disease there is also evidence of osteitis fibrosa.

PAGET'S DISEASE OF BONE (OSTEITIS DEFORMANS)

In this disease of unknown aetiology, there is rapid bone formation and resorption in the involved regions of the skeleton. The lesions are essentially local and asymmetrical in the early stages and frequently involve the weight-bearing bones, especially the sacrum and pelvis. Unsuspected disease may be found during trephine bone marrow biopsy examination (Figs.15.43 & 15.44). The plasma calcium and phosphorus levels are usually normal while the alkaline phosphatase level is invariably high.

The bony trabeculae may have a striking mosaic appearance created by the pattern of cement lines. In areas of extensive repair the bone may be osteomalacic with wide osteoid seams. Where there is extremely rapid absorption, areas of fibrosis and intensive osteoclastic activity may resemble the microscopical appearances of osteitis fibrosa.

Classification of Amyloidosis		
Type	Chemical Nature	Organs Involved
Immunocyte-related: myeloma; Waldenström's macroglobulinaemia; heavy-chain disease; etc. also, primary amyloidosis	Ig light chains and/ or parts of their variable regions (AL)	tongue; skin; heart; nerves; connective tissue; kidneys; liver; spleen
Reactive systemic: rheumatoid arthritis; tuberculosis; bronchiectasis; Hodgkin's disease; Mediterranean fever; etc. also, familial	protein (acute reactive; AA)	liver; spleen; kidneys; bone marrow
Localized: tumours; old age; also, in skin	hormones; protein A with other constituents	around endocrine tumours; skin

Fig. 15.39 Amyloidosis: classification of types, structure and organ involvement.

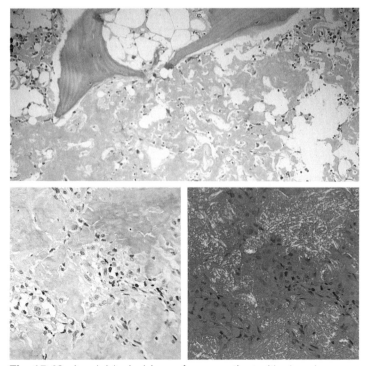

Fig. 15.40 Amyloidosis: biopsy from a patient with chronic bronchiectasis shows (upper) extensive replacement of haemopoietic tissue by pale acidophilic material; (lower) higher power shows the characteristic yellow-green birefringence of amyloid. Congo red stain.

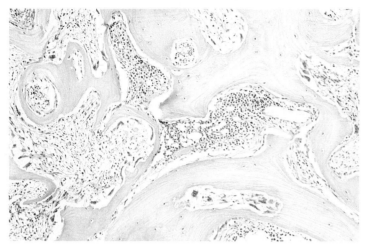

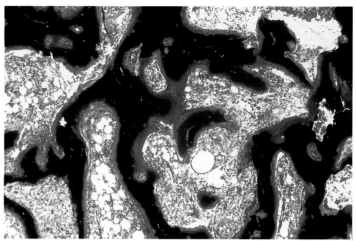

Fig. 15.41 Renal osteodystrophy/osteitis fibrosa cystica: extensive resorption of bone trabeculae with fibrous replacement. Osteoclasts lie adjacent to areas of active resorption.

Fig. 15.42 Osteomalacia: thickened trabeculae with prominent layers of uncalcified osteoid on their outer borders. von Kossa stain. Courtesy of P.G. Bullough & V.J. Vigorita (1984), *Atlas of Orthopaedic Pathology*. New York: Gower Medical Publishing.

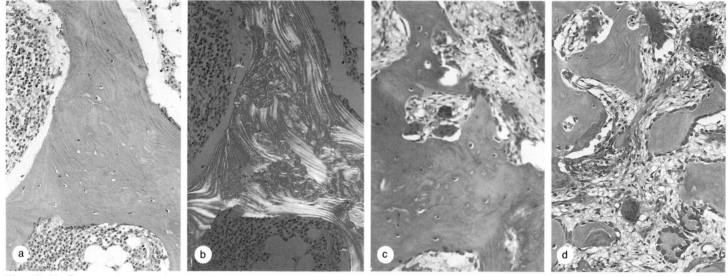

Fig. 15.43 Paget's disease of bone: thickened and irregular trabecular bone (a) seen under polarized light (b); intense bone resorption by osteoclasts (c) and bone apposition by osteoblasts during the active phase of this disease (d). The normal intertrabecular haemopoietic tissue has been extensively replaced by vascular loose connective tissue.

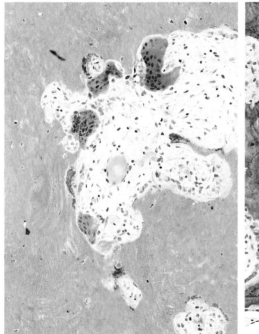

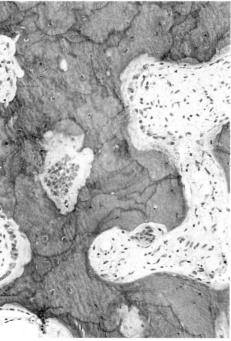

Fig. 15.44 Paget's disease of bone: (left) autopsy section shows increased osteoclastic and osteoblastic activity with scalloping of the bone surface (green) adjacent to the osteoclasts; (right) biopsy of more advanced disease. The disturbed bone (undecalcified) architecture is obvious. Irregular cement lines separate the uneven bone sections, and osteoblasts and osteoclasts are prominent. Goldner's stain (left). Courtesy of P.G. Bullough & V.J. Vigorita (1984), *Atlas of Orthopaedic Pathology*. New York: Gower Medical Publishing.

ANOREXIA NERVOSA

These patients suffer from severe deficiency of carbo-hydrates, fats and calories but little protein deficiency. The peripheral blood may reveal mild anaemia and thrombo-cytopenia with acanthocytes; the marrow is hypocellular with fat cells replaced by acid mucopolysaccharides appearing as pink-staining extracellular material (Fig. 15.45).

PRIMARY OXALURIA

In this fatal autosomal recessive metabolic disorder, there is widespread deposition of calcium oxalate crystals in the kidneys and elsewhere in the body, including the liver, spleen and bone marrow (Figs. 15.46 & 15.47). A number of different enzyme deficiencies have been implicated as causal factors.

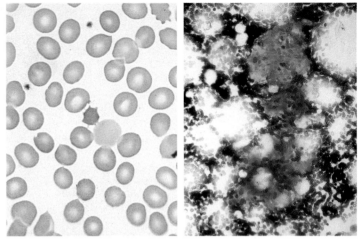

Fig. 15.45 Anorexia nervosa: (left) peripheral blood film showing occasional acanthocytes and a central, densely staining, micro-cyte with spicules; (right) bone marrow showing extracellular homogeneous pink- and purple-staining material replacing fat spaces and composed of acid mucopolysaccharide.

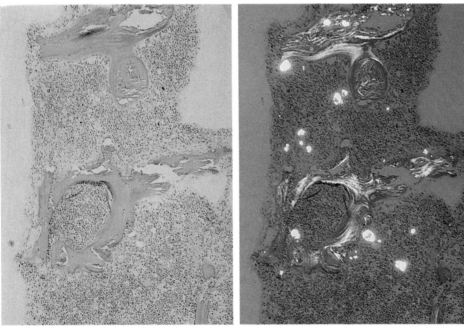
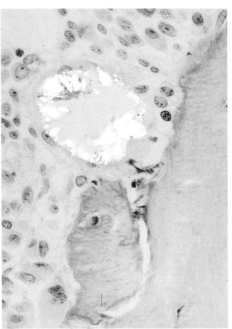

Fig. 15.46 Primary oxaluria: (left) normal and (right) polarizing microscopy shows birefringent calcium oxalate monohydrate crystals (and normal birefringent cortical bone). The patient, a 3-month-old boy, presented with renal failure. Courtesy of Dr. S. Milkins.

Fig. 15.47 Primary oxaluria: higher power (polarized) of Fig. 15.46 shows the oxalate crystals.

16

PARASITIC INFECTIONS DIAGNOSED IN BLOOD

MALARIA

This protozoal disease has a distribution which is essentially world-wide in tropical and warm temperate regions. Mosquito-borne infection is caused by four species of the genus *Plasmodium*: *P. vivax* (benign tertian); *P. falciparum* (malignant tertian); *P. malariae* (quartan); and *P. ovale* (ovale tertian). Infections due to *P. vivax* and *P. falciparum* are the most common and the latter is much more likely to progress to infections of life-threatening severity.

The malarial life cycle begins in the female mosquito after ingestion of human blood containing the sexual forms (gametocytes) of the causal organisms. The resultant conjugate develops into infective forms (sporozoites) within the mosquito which are then transmitted to humans by the insect bite.

The sporozoites pass to the liver parenchymal cells where they multiply and divide, producing merozoites in this pre-erythrocytic phase. When the liver cell ruptures, the parasites enter the red cells. Except for *P. falciparum*, the liver phase persists.

In the red cells, the parasites pass from early trophozoite or ring forms to an actively amoeboid form with malarial pigment (haemozoin), which then undergoes chromatin division to form a merozoite. The mature parasite is called a schizont. The red cell ruptures, releasing merozoites into plasma which may then enter other red cells and repeat the cycle, or form male and female sexual forms (gametocytes).

The four types of malaria organisms may be distinguished by their characteristic appearances within red cells (Fig.16.1). With infection by *P. vivax* (Fig.16.2), the red cells are large (as they are young), Schuffner dots (degraded red cell microtubules) are present and ring forms are large, as are the schizonts, with up to twenty-four merozoites.

In *P. falciparum* infections (Fig.16.3), there is usually a heavy parasitaemia with small ring forms, often with double chromatin dots and multiple ring forms, some on the margins, within individual red cells. The red cells may contain blue-staining Maurer's clefts. The gametocytes have a characteristic crescentic (elliptical or banana) shape and schizonts are rarely seen.

Identification of Malaria in Peripheral Blood				
Feature	Plasmodium falciparum	Plasmodium malariae	Plasmodium vivax	Plasmodium ovale
Red cells:				
Enlargement	none	none	yes	yes; oval shape; fimbriated edge
Inclusions (not always present)	Maurer's clefts	none	Schuffner dots (coarse red granules)	James dots (similar to Schuffner)
Ring form:				
Size	<⅓ of RBC	>⅓ of RBC	>⅓ of RBC	>⅓ of RBC
Multiple parasites in RBC	common; often at margins	rare	rare	rare
Shape	delicate; often double chromatin dot	tends to be compact; inverted chromatin dot	rough; single chromatin dot	rough; single chromatin dot
Amoeboid forms	absent	common; often as band across RBC	common	common
Schizont:				
Frequency	very rarely seen	common; dense, central, yellow/black haemozoin pigment	common; with haemozoin pigment	common
Configuration	random	daisy-head	random	daisy-head
Merozoite number	8-24	8-12	12-24	8-12
Gamete:	crescent forms (sausage-shaped); centrally placed chromatin	small & round; eccentrically placed chromatin; occupies ½-⅔ of RBC	large & round; eccentrically placed chromatin; fills RBC	small & round; eccentrically placed chromatin; occupies ½-⅔ of RBC

N.B. Infections with two types of malarial parasite are common.

Fig.16.1 Identification of the different forms of malaria in the peripheral blood.

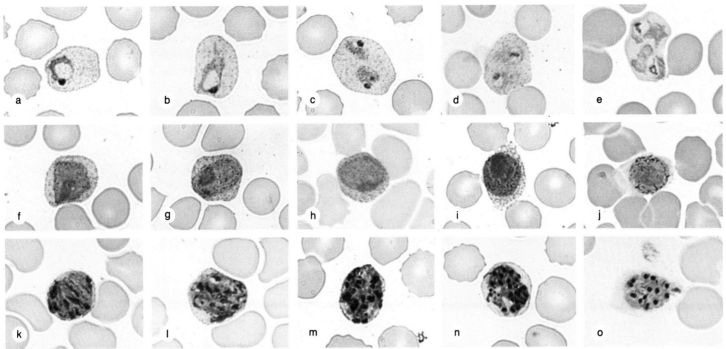

Fig.16.2 Malaria: peripheral blood films showing various stages of *P. vivax*; (a) early trophozoite or ring form; (b-c) young amoeboid trophozoites with Schuffner dots; (d-e) developing trophozoites which have undergone asexual binary fission; (f-h) female gametocytes with localized eccentric chromatin; (i-j) male gametocytes with more diffuse chromatin; (k-o) early and late schizonts with haemozoin pigment densities and many merozoites randomly distributed.

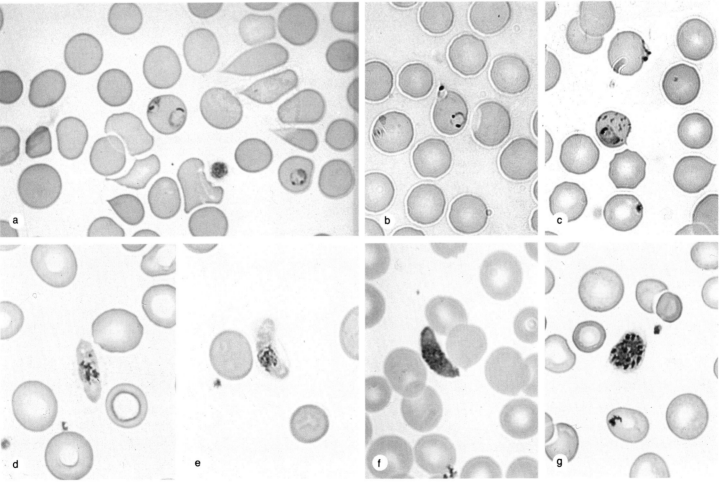

Fig.16.3 Malaria: peripheral blood films showing various stages of *P. falciparum*; (a-b) small ring forms; (c) Maurer's clefts, which are denatured red cell microtubules; (d-f) crescentic gametocytes with centrally placed chromatin; (g) rarely seen schizont with randomly distributed merozoites. Courtesy of Dr. S. Knowles (b & c).

As in *P. falciparum* infections, with *P. malariae* (Fig.16.4) the red cells are not enlarged; the red cells do not contain pigment and the ring form tends to have an inverted chromatin dot. The amoeboid trophozoites often show band forms and the merozoites may show a 'daisy-head' distribution.

P. ovale (Fig.16.5) infections are distinguished by the parasitized red cells being enlarged and oval-shaped but with fimbriated edges. The red cells show James dots (similar to Schuffner dots) and the schizonts have a daisy-head distribution.

BANCROFTIAN FILARIASIS

This widespread disease occurs throughout tropical and subtropical regions of the world and is caused by *Wuchereria bancrofti* or the related *Brugia malayi*. The organism is transmitted by infected mosquitoes. Larvae pass into the lymphatic vessels and lymph nodes where they mature into adult worms (Fig.16.6). The fertilized females release microfilariae via the lymphatic vessels into the bloodstream. Many patients are asymptomatic, but others develop a febrile illness with headaches, muscle pains and lymphadenitis. Chronic inflammatory changes in the infected lymphoid system may lead to lymphatic obstruction and elephantiasis of the scrotum or lower extremities. Diagnosis is usually made by demonstrating microfilariae in the blood (Fig.16.7). Greatest numbers are found usually during the middle of the night.

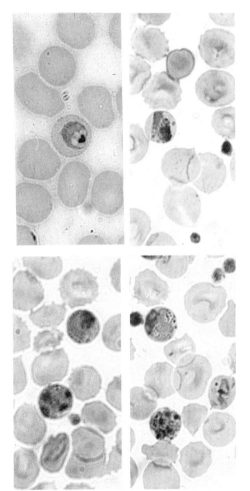

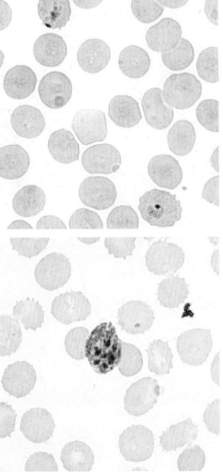

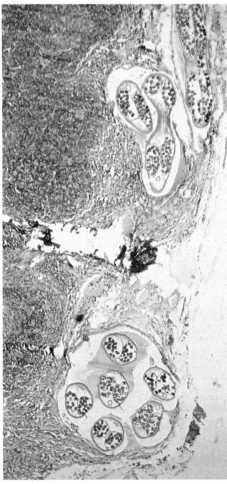

Fig.16.4 Malaria: peripheral blood films showing various stages of *P. malariae*; (upper left) ring form with inverted chromatin dot; (upper right) band-form amoeboid trophozoite; (lower left) developing trophozoite and female gamete; (lower right) from top left clockwise, male gamete, ring form and developing schizont with daisy-head merozoite distribution.

Fig.16.5 Malaria: peripheral blood films showing various stages of *P. ovale*; (upper) ring forms in enlarged red cells with fimbriated margins and faint James dots; (lower) schizont with daisy-head merozoite distribution. Courtesy of Dr. S. Knowles and Mr. J. Griffiths.

Fig.16.6 Bancroftian filariasis: section of lymph node showing adult forms of *Wuchereria bancrofti* in the peripheral sinus area.

LOIASIS

Infection from *Loa loa* occurs in Central and West Africa. The adult worm causes subcutaneous swellings, but occasionally its passage through the subconjunctival tissues produces local pain and acute conjunctivitis. Microfilariae are found in the blood (Fig.16.8) and infestation is through tabanid flies.

TRYPANOSOMIASIS

The East African and West African variants of trypanosomiasis are caused by *Trypanosoma rhodesiense* and *Trypanosoma brucei gambiense* respectively. Both are transmitted by tsetse flies of the genus *Glossina*. The dominant clinical problems are related to involvement of the central nervous system. In the acute phase of the disease, organisms are found in the blood (Fig.16.9).

American trypanosomiasis or Chagas' disease occurs widely in Mexico and in many countries in Central and South America. The causative organism, *Trypanosoma cruzi*, is transmitted by the triatomid beetle. During the acute febrile stage of the illness, flagellated parasites may be found in the blood (Fig.16.9, right). In the chronic stage of the illness, which is associated with myocarditis, megacolon or megaoesophagus, nests of amastigote forms are found within the tissues.

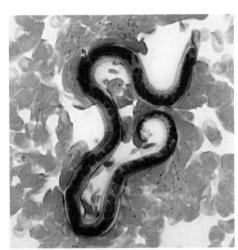

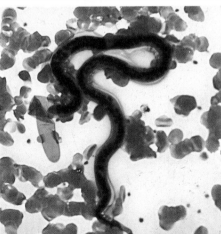

Fig.16.7 Bancroftian filariasis: peripheral blood films showing sheathed microfilariae of *Wuchereria bancrofti*.

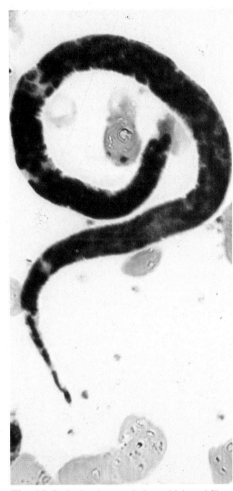

Fig.16.8 Loiasis: peripheral blood film showing sheathed microfilariae of *Loa loa*.

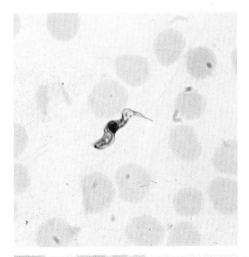

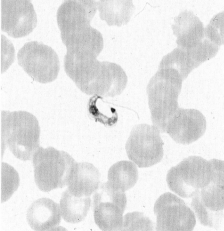

Fig.16.9 Trypanosomiasis: peripheral blood films showing the flagellated protozoa of African and American trypanosomiasis, (upper) *Trypanosoma rhodesiense* and (lower) *Trypanosoma cruzi*. Courtesy of Mr.J. Williams, Department of Medical Protozoology, London School of Hygiene and Tropical Medicine (upper).

RELAPSING FEVER

Various spirochaetes of the genus *Borrelia* are the cause of relapsing fever. Louse-borne relapsing fever is a human disease caused only by *Borrelia recurrentis*, but tick-borne relapsing fever is a zoonosis caused by a number of different species. It is during the febrile period of the disease that the organisms are present in the blood (Fig.16.10). With the production of antibodies, the *Borrelia* disappear and the patient becomes afebrile. Relapses occur after seven to ten days with the production of new antigenic variants of the organisms. In louse-borne relapsing fever there is usually a single relapse while, in the tick-borne forms of the disease, multiple relapses may occur.

BABESIOSIS

Babesiosis is a tick-borne disease caused by protozoan parasites of the genus *Babesia*. The disease affects a number of animal species and is only occasionally transmitted to man. In most patients the illness is mild and characterized by fever, malaise, myalgia, mild hepatosplenomegaly and haemolytic anaemia. Occasional patients who have had previous splenectomy are known to have developed a more fulminating infection with massive intravascular haemolysis which has sometimes proved fatal.

The majority of human infections have been caused by *Babesia microti*, a species which usually infects rodents. Several cases in splenectomized patients have been due to *Babesia bovis*, a species associated with red water fever in cattle. Diagnosis is made by finding the trophozoites, which resemble small ring forms of *Plasmodium falciparum*, in the red cells (Fig.16.11).

BARTONELLOSIS

Bartonella bacilliformis causes a severe febrile haemolytic anaemia. The disease occurs in inhabitants of the Andes mountains in Peru, Colombia and Equador. The characteristic rod-shaped coccobacilli are found in red cells (Fig.16.12). The infection is also known as Oroya fever and Carrión's disease and is transmitted by *Phlebotomus* sandflies.

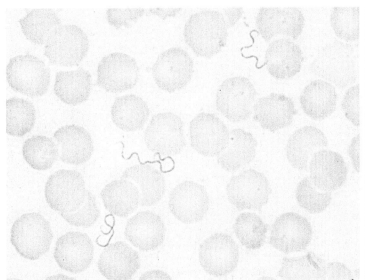

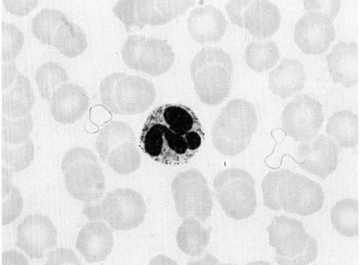

Fig.16.10 Relapsing fever: peripheral blood films showing coiled spirochaetes of *Borrelia recurrentis*.

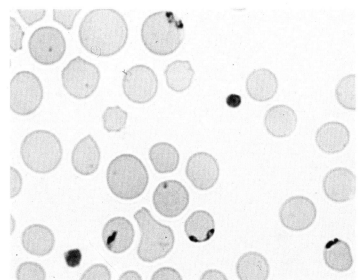

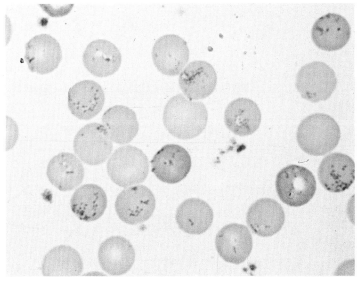

Fig.16.11 Babesiosis: peripheral blood film showing red cell infestation with the typical small coccoid and dumb-bell-shaped *Babesia* organisms. Courtesy of Mr. P.J. Humphries.

Fig.16.12 Bartonellosis: peripheral blood film showing rod-shaped coccobacilli of *Bartonella bacilliformis* in the red cells in Oroya fever. Courtesy of Mr. H. Furze.

Bibliography

Begemann, H. & Rastetter, J. (1979) *Atlas of Clinical Hematology, 3rd Edition*. Berlin: Springer Verlag.

Catovsky, D. (Ed.) (1981) *The Leukaemic Cell*. Edinburgh: Churchill Livingstone.

Chanarin, I. (1979) *The Megaloblastic Anaemias, 2nd Edition*. Oxford: Blackwell Scientific Publications.

Dacie, J.V. & Lewis, S.M. (1984) *Practical Haematology, 6th Edition*. Edinburgh: Churchill Livingstone.

Hann, I.M., Rankin, A., Lake, B.D. & Pritchard, J. (1983) *Colour Atlas of Paediatric Haematology and Oncology*. Oxford: Oxford Medical Publications.

Hardisty, R.M. & Weatherall, D.J. (1982) *Blood and Its Diseases, 2nd Edition*. Oxford: Blackwell Scientific Publications.

Hayhoe, F.G.J. & Flemans, R.J. (1982) *A Colour Atlas of Haematological Cytology, 2nd Edition*. London: Wolfe Medical Publishers.

Hoffbrand, A.V. & Pettit, J.E. (1984) *Essential Haematology, 2nd Edition*. Oxford: Blackwell Scientific Publications.

Hoffbrand, A.V. & Lewis, S.M. (Eds.) (1981) *Postgraduate Haematology*. London: Heinemann Medical Books.

Kaplan, H.S. (1980) *Hodgkin's Disease, 2nd Edition*. Cambridge, MA: Harvard University Press.

Linch, D. & Yates, A.P. (1986) *Colour Aids Haematology*. Edinburgh: Churchill Livingstone.

McDonald, G.A., Dodds, T.C. & Cruickshank, B. (1978) *Atlas of Haematology, 4th Edition*. Edinburgh: Churchill Livingstone.

Roitt, I.M., Brostoff, J. & Male, D.K. (1985) *Immunology*. Edinburgh-London: Churchill Livingstone-Gower Medical Publishing.

Serjeant, G.R. (1985) *Sickle Cell Disease*. Oxford: Oxford University Press.

Undritz, E. (1973) *Sandoz Atlas of Haematology, 2nd Edition*. Basle: Sandoz.

Weatherall, D.J. & Clegg, J.B. (1981) *The Thalassaemia Syndromes, 3rd Edition*. Oxford: Blackwell Scientific Publications.

Wickramasinghe, S.N. (Ed.) (1986) *Blood and Bone Marrow*. Edinburgh: Churchill Livingstone.

Williams, W.J., Beutler, E., Erslev, A.J. & Rundles, R.W. (1983) *Hematology, 3rd Edition*. New York: McGraw-Hill.

Wintrobe, M.M., Lee, G.R., Boggs, D.R., Bithell, T.C., Foerster, J., Athens, J.W. & Lukens, J.M. (1981) *Clinical Hematology, 8th Edition*. Philadelphia: Lea & Febiger.

Zucker-Franklin, D., Greaves, M.F., Grossi, C.E., Marmont, A.M. (1980) *Atlas of Blood Cells*. Philadelphia: Lea & Febiger.

Appendix I

Cytogenetic Abnormalities in Acute and Chronic Leukaemias, and Myelodysplasia (for abbreviations, see text).

Acute Myeloid Leukaemia (AML)
Relatively specific:
M_2 t(8; 21) (q22: q22)
M_3 t(15; 17) (q22; q11)
M_4 inv(16) (p13; q22) or del (16) (q22)*
M_5 t(9; 11) (p21; q23)
Others:
t(9; 22) (q34; q11)
t(6:9) (p22; q34)†
t(3;3) (q21; q29) inv(3) (q21; q26)††
+8
+21
5q–/–5;
7q–/–7
12p11–p13 (del or t)†

* associated with abnormal eosinophils
† with increased basophils
†† associated with thrombocytosis

Acute Lymphoblastic Leukaemia (ALL)
L_1 and/or L_2 (cALL or null-ALL)
t(9;22) (q34; q11)
t(4; 11) (q21; q23)
t(1;19) (q22; p13)
del (6) (9)
t(11; 14) (q13; q32)
t or del (12) (p12)
9p–
+21
B-ALL
t(8; 14) (q24; q32)
t(8; 22) (q24; q11)
t(2; 8) (p11-13; q24)
T-ALL
14q+(q32) or 14q–(q11)
t(11; 14) (p13; q11)
9p–

Myelodysplasia (MDS)
t(1;3) (p36; q21)
21q–
5q–
7q– or –7

9q–
12p–
20q–
+8

Chronic Granulocytic Leukaemia (CGL)
t(9; 22) (q34; q11)
CGL (at presentation or blast transformation):
+Ph
+8
i(17q)
–Y

B-Cell Chronic Lymphocytic Leukaemia (B-CLL)
+12
14q+
t(11; 14) (q13; q32)

T-CLL, T-Lymphomas
inv (14) (q11; q32)
t(11; 14) (p13; q11)

Follicular Lymphomas
t(14; 18) (q32; q21)

APPENDIX II

Electronmicroscopic Appearances of Acute and Chronic Leukaemia Cells

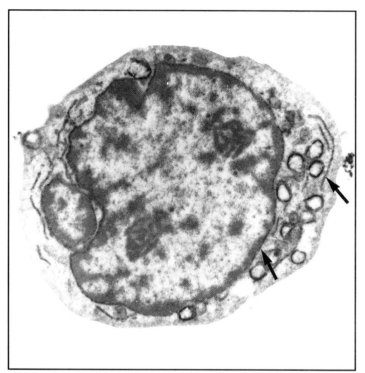

Fig. A1 Megakaryoblast: morphologically, this cell resembles a lymphoblast but is identified by the reactivity with the platelet-peroxidase reaction (linear black areas) in the endoplasmic reticulum and nuclear membrane (arrows). Mitochondria are non-specifically positive. x 9250. Courtesy of Dr. E. Matutes and Dr. D. Catovsky.

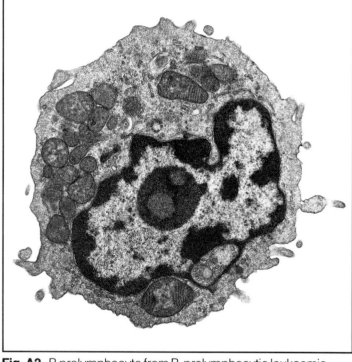

Fig. A2 B prolymphocyte from B-prolymphocytic leukaemia (B-PLL): the cell is characterized by its relatively large size, moderately abundant cytoplasm, chromatin condensed in the periphery of the nucleus and a prominent nucleolus. x11,000. Courtesy of Mrs. D. Robinson and Dr. D. Catovsky.

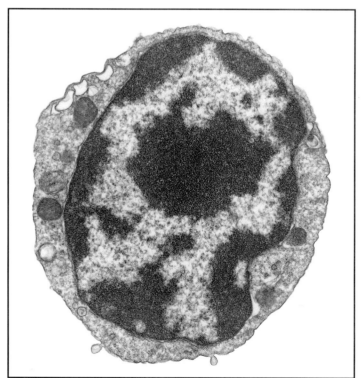

Fig. A3 B-CLL lymphocyte: compared with Fig.A2, this cell is smaller, has less cytoplasm [high nuclear/cytoplasmic (N/C) ratio] and more marked nuclear chromatin without a visible nucleolus. x18,350. Courtesy of Mrs. D. Robinson and Dr. D. Catovsky.

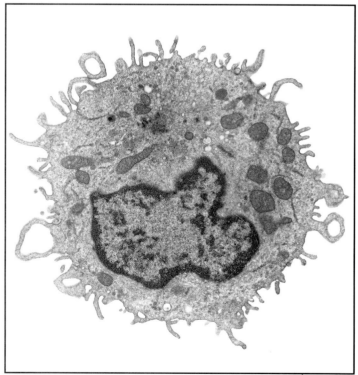

Fig. A4 Hairy cell: from the peripheral blood of a patient with hairy cell leukaemia. Typical features are the abundant cytoplasm, low N/C ratio, and the cytoplasmic projections or villi which give the cell a 'hairy' appearance. x9200. Courtesy of Mrs. D. Robinson and Dr. D. Catovsky.

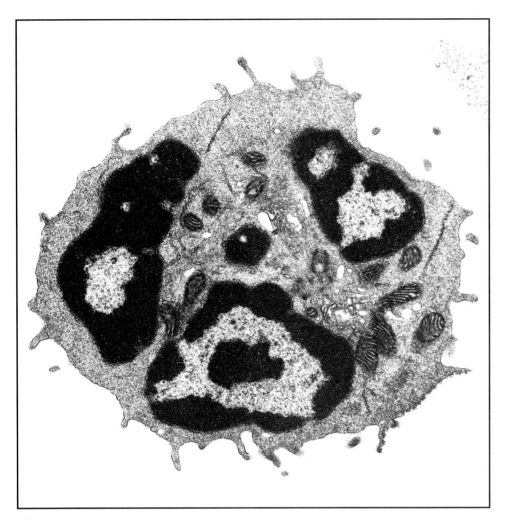

Fig. A5 Polylobed T-lymphocyte: from the peripheral blood of a patient with adult T-cell leukaemia/lymphoma. This nuclear configuration is characteristic of this disease. x17,250. Courtesy of Dr. E. Matutes and Dr. D. Catovsky.

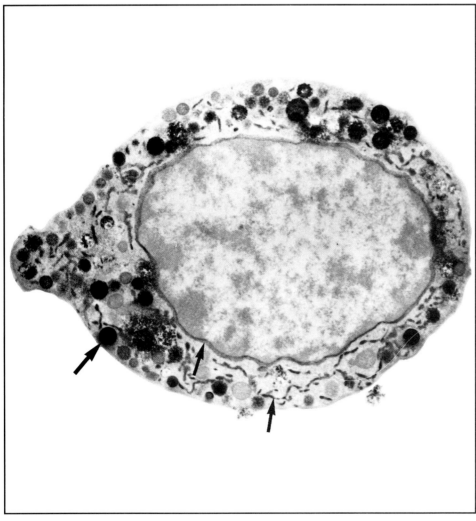

Fig. A6 Myeloblast: from a patient with acute myeloblastic leukaemia. This cell has relatively abundant cytoplasmic granules (large arrow) and a positive myeloperoxidase reaction (black granules); the enzyme reaction is also seen in the short profiles of endoplasmic reticulum and nuclear membrane (small arrows). x 9800. Courtesy of Dr. E. Matutes and Dr. D. Catovsky.

INDEX